THIRD EDITION

CASE FILES®
Obstetrics and Gynecology

Eugene C. Toy, MD
The John S. Dunn, Senior Academic Chair and Program Director
The Methodist Hospital Ob/Gyn Residency Program
Houston, Texas

Vice Chair of Academic Affairs
Department of Obstetrics and Gynecology
The Methodist Hospital
Houston, Texas

Associate Clinical Professor and Clerkship Director
Department of Obstetrics and Gynecology
University of Texas Medical School at Houston
Houston, Texas

Associate Clinical Professor
Weill Cornell College of Medicine

Benton Baker III, MD
Professor of Obstetrics and Gynecology
University of Texas Medical School at Houston
Houston, Texas

Patti Jayne Ross, MD
Professor and Clerkship Director
Department of Obstetrics and Gynecology
Holder of the Patti Jayne Ross Professorship
University of Texas Medical School at Houston
Houston, Texas

John C. Jennings, MD
Regional Dean, School of Medicine/
Roden Professor of Obstetrics and Gynecology
Texas Tech University Health Sciences Center
Odessa, Texas

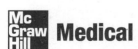 **Medical**

New York   Chicago   San Francisco   Lisbon   London   Madrid   Mexico City   Milan
New Delhi   San Juan   Seoul   Singapore   Sydney   Toronto

The McGraw·Hill Companies

Case Files®: Obstetrics and Gynecology, Third Edition

5 6 7 8 9 0   DOC/DOC   12 11

ISBN 978-0-07-160580-9
MHID 0-07-160580-0

Notice

Medicine is an ever-changing science. As new research and clinical experience broaden our knowledge, changes in treatment and drug therapy are required. The authors and the publisher of this work have checked with sources believed to be reliable in their efforts to provide information that is complete and generally in accord with the standards accepted at the time of publication. However, in view of the possibility of human error or changes in medical sciences, neither the authors nor the publisher nor any other party who has been involved in the preparation or publication of this work warrants that the information contained herein is in every respect accurate or complete, and they disclaim all responsibility for any errors or omissions or for the results obtained from use of the information contained in this work. Readers are encouraged to confirm the information contained herein with other sources. For example and in particular, readers are advised to check the product information sheet included in the package of each drug they plan to administer to be certain that the information contained in this work is accurate and that changes have not been made in the recommended dose or in the contraindications for administration. This recommendation is of particular importance in connection with new or infrequently used drugs.

This book was set in Goudy by International Typesetting and Composition.
The editors were Catherine A. Johnson and Cindy Yoo.
The production supervisor was Catherine H. Saggese.
Project management was provided by Gita Raman, International Typesetting and Composition.
The designer was Janice Bielawa; the cover designer was Aimee Nordin.
RR Donnelley was printer and binder.

This book is printed on acid-free paper.

Library of Congress Cataloging-in-Publication Data

Case files. Obstetrics and gynecology / Eugene C. Toy ... [et al.]. — 3rd ed.
    p. ; cm.
    Rev. ed. of: Case files. Obstetrics & gynecology / Eugene C. Toy ... [et al.]. 2nd ed. c2007.
    Includes bibliographical references and index.
    ISBN-13: 978-0-07-160580-9 (pbk. : alk. paper)
    ISBN-10: 0-07-160580-0 (pbk. : alk. paper)
    1. Gynecology—Examinations, questions, etc.   2. Obstetrics—Examinations, questions, etc.   3. Gynecology—Case studies.   4. Obstetrics—Examination Questions.
    I. Toy, Eugene C.   II. Case files.
    Obstetrics & gynecology. III. Title: Obstetrics and gynecology.
    [DNLM: 1. Gynecology—Case Reports.   2. Gynecology—Examination Questions.
3. Obstetrics—Case Reports.   4. Obstetrics—Examination Questions.   WQ 18.2 C337 2009]
RG111.C37 2009
618.0076—dc22   2009005749

To my loving and supportive wife, Terri, and my four delightful children, Andy, Michael, Allison, and Christina, who provide me with daily inspiration.

—ECT

With love and gratitude, to Mom, Joy, Ben, Anne, Jessica, Jim, John, and Col. Alvin Sholk.

—BB III

To the residents, faculty, and staff at Christus—St. Joseph Hospital and The Methodist Hospital—Houston Ob/Gyn Residency.

—ECT AND BB III

To Dr. James Knight, and Tulane Medical School, for giving me the opportunity to fulfill my dreams. To my parents, Mary and Jimmy Ross, for their love, inspiration, and devotion.

—PJR

To my wife, Sue Ellen, my three daughters, Beth, Allison, and Amy, their husbands, and my five grandchildren.

—JCJ

Finally, to the wonderful medical students from the University of Texas—Houston Medical School, who graciously gave constructive feedback and enthusiastically received this curriculum.

—THE AUTHORS

CONTENTS

Barrett R. Blaue, MD
Resident
Department of Obstetrics and Gynecology
The Methodist Hospital—Houston
Houston, Texas
Normal labor
Pulmonary embolism in pregnancy

Katie Bolt, MD
Resident
Department of Obstetrics and Gynecology
The Methodist Hospital—Houston
Houston, Texas
Thyroid storm in pregnancy

Kelli V. Burroughs, MD
Resident
Department of Obstetrics and Gynecology
The Methodist Hospital—Houston
Houston, Texas
Gonococcal cervicitis
Herpes simplex virus infection in labor

Kristin B. Chapman, MD
Resident
Department of Obstetrics and Gynecology
The Methodist Hospital—Houston
Houston, Texas
Pyelonephritis, unresponsive

Tina Barbaro Dieber, MD
Medical Genetics Fellow
Division of Medical Genetics
Department of Pediatrics
The University of Texas Medical School at Houston
Houston, Texas
Abdominal pain in pregnancy

Tri A. Dinh, MD
Assistant Professor
Department of Obstetrics and Gynecology
Weill Cornell Medical College
The Methodist Hospital—Houston
Houston, Texas
Fascial disruption
Hirsutism, Sertoli Leydig cell tumor

Juan Franco, MD
Faculty
Department of Obstetrics and Gynecology
The Methodist Hospital—Houston
Houston, Texas
Pruritus (cholestasis) of pregnancy
Galactorrhea due to hypothyroidism

Alfredo Gei, MD, FACOG
Director
Division of Maternal Fetal Medicine
The Methodist Hospital—Houston
Houston, Texas
Preterm labor
Serum screening in pregnancy

Lauren Giacobbe, MD
Resident
Department of Obstetrics and Gynecology
The Methodist Hospital—Houston
Houston, Texas
Placental abruption
Placenta previa

Zuleika Goss, MD
Resident
Department of Obstetrics and Gynecology
The Methodist Hospital—Houston
Houston, Texas
Postpartum endomyometritis

Konrad Harms, MD, FACOG
Assistant Professor
Department of Obstetrics and Gynecology
Weill Cornell Medical College
Associate Program Director
Department of Obstetrics and Gynecology
The Methodist Hospital—Houston
Houston, Texas
Polycystic ovarian syndrome
Preeclampsia and hepatic rupture

Eric Haufrect, MD
Clinical Professor
Department of Obstetrics and Gynecology
Weill Cornell Medical College
Vice Chair
Department of Obstetrics and Gynecology
The Methodist Hospital—Houston
Houston, Texas
Uterine inversion
Perimenopause

Christopher Hobday, MD
Faculty
Department of Obstetrics and Gynecology
The Methodist Hospital—Houston
Houston, Texas
Ectopic pregnancy

Lisa M. Hollier, MD, MPH
Associate Professor
Department of Obstetrics, Gynecology, and Reproductive Sciences
University of Texas Medical School at Houston
Houston, Texas
Syphilitic chancre

Jeané Simmons Holmes, MD, FACOG
Assistant Professor
Weill Cornell Medical College
Faculty
The Methodist Obstetrics and Gynecology Residency
Houston, Texas
Chlamydial cervicitis and HIV in pregnancy
Ureteral injury after hysterectomy

Gene E. Huebner, MD
Director
Perinatal Services
The Methodist Hospital—SugarLand
Faculty and Site Coordinator
Obstetrics and Gynecology Residency Program
The Methodist Hospital—Houston
Houston, Texas
Approach to the patient

Jennifer Huebner, MD
Resident
Department of Obstetrics and Gynecology
The Methodist Hospital—Houston
Houston, Texas
Placenta accreta
Shoulder dystocia

Alan L. Kaplan, MD
Chairman
Department of Obstetrics and Gynecology
The Methodist Hospital—Houston
Professor
Department of Obstetrics and Gynecology
Weill Cornell Medical College
Houston, Texas
Cervical cancer
Ovarian tumor (struma ovarii)

Amr Khalil, MD
Resident
Department of Obstetrics and Gynecology
The Methodist Hospital—Houston
Houston, TX
Deep venous thrombosis in pregnancy

Kathryn A. Karges, MD
Resident
Department of Obstetrics and Gynecology
The Methodist Hospital—Houston
Houston, Texas
Pubertal delay, gonadal dysgenesis

Charlie C. Kilpatrick, MD
Assistant Professor
Department of Obstetrics and Gynecology
University of Texas Medical School at Houston
LBJ Hospital
Houston, Texas
Urinary tract infection (cystitis)
Lichen sclerosis of vulva

G. T. Kuhn, MD, FACOG

Assistant Professor
Department of Obstetrics and Gynecology
Weill Cornell Medical College
The Methodist Hospital—Houston
Houston, Texas
Fibroadenoma of the breast
Dominant breast mass
Breast, abnormal mammogram

Sam Law II, MD

Clinical Associate Professor
Department of Obstetrics and Gynecology
Weill Cornell Medical College
The Methodist Hospital—Houston
Clinical Associate Professor
Department of Obstetrics and Gynecology
Baylor College of Medicine
Houston, Texas
Fetal bradycardia (cord prolapse)
Uterine leiomyomata

Carl E. Lee II, MD

Faculty
Obstetrics and Gynecology Residency Program
The Methodist Hospital—Houston
Houston, Texas
Salpingitis, acute
Herpes simplex infection in labor
Abortion, septic

Jodi M. Little, MS

Resident
Memorial Health University Medical Center
Savannah, Georgia
Parvovirus infection in pregnancy

Nancy Aguilar Magsino, MD

Resident
Department of Obstetrics and Gynecology
The Methodist Hospital—Houston
Houston, Texas
Amenorrhea (Sheehan syndrome)

John C. McBride, MD
Faculty
Obstetrics and Gynecology Residency Program
The Methodist Hospital—Houston
Houston, Texas
Anemia in pregnancy (thalassemia)
Postpartum hemorrhage
Salpingitis, acute

Jessica Coté Miller, MD
Resident
Department of Obstetrics and Gynecology
The Methodist Hospital—Houston
Houston, Texas
Amenorrhea (primary), Müllerian agenesis

Tiffany Montegut, DO
Resident
The Methodist Obstetrics and Gynecology Residency
Houston, Texas
Intra-amniotic infection

Stacy L. Norton, MD
Private Practice
Northwest Women's Center
Chairman
Department of Obstetrics and Gynecology
The Methodist Hospital—Willowbrook
Houston, Texas
Approach to clinical problem solving

Cristo Papasakelariou, MD
Clinical Professor
Department of Obstetrics and Gynecology
University of Texas Medical Branch
Galveston, Texas
Clinical Director
Department of Gynecologic Surgery
St. Joseph Medical Center
Houston, Texas
Infertility, peritoneal factor

Waverly F. Peakes, MD
Obstetrician, Private Practice
The Methodist Hospital—Houston
Houston, Texas
Approach to reading

Ana Lisa Ramirez-Chapman
Medical Student
University of Texas Medical School at Houston
Primay Student Reviewer
Anemia in Pregnancy

Keith O. Reeves, MD
Clinical Professor
Department of Obstetrics and Gynecology
Weill Cornell Medical College
Medical Director
Methodist Center for Restorative Pelvic Medicine
Houston, Texas
Urinary incontinence
Pelvic organ prolapse

Brandon Sass
Medical Student
University of Texas Medical School at Houston
Houston, Texas
Threatened abortion

Priti P. Schachel, MD, FACOG
Assistant Professor
Department of Obstetrics and Gynecology
Weill Cornell Medical College
Faculty
Obstetrics and Gynecology Residency Program
The Methodist Hospital—Houston
Houston, Texas
Health maintenance, age 66 years
Contraception

Tamika Sea, MD
Resident
The Methodist Obstetrics and Gynecology Residency
Houston, Texas
Bacterial vaginosis

Steven V. Whipp, MD
Resident
The Methodist Obstetrics and Gynecology Residency
Houston, Texas
Completed spontaneous abortion
Amenorrhea (Sheehan syndrome)

Stanley Wright, MD
Resident
The Methodist Obstetrics and Gynecology Residency
Houston, Texas
Breast abscess and mastitis

I have been deeply amazed and grateful to see how the Case Files books have been so well received, and have helped students to learn more effectively. In the 7 short years since *Case Files: Obstetrics and Gynecology* has first made it in print, the series has now multiplied to span the most of the clinical and the basic science disciplines, and been translated into over a dozen foreign languages. Numerous students have sent encouraging remarks, suggestions, and recommendations, many of which have been incorporated in this third edition. Questions have been improved to better reflect the USMLE format, and explanations have been expanded to help the student understand the mechanisms and the reason that the other choices are incorrect. Five completely new cases have been written. Updated or new sections include health maintenance, cervical cytology with human papilloma virus subtyping, contraception, polycystic ovarian syndrome, osteoporosis, neonatal complications, and human immunodeficiency virus. This third edition has been a collaborative work with my wonderful co-authors and contributors, and with the suggestions from three generations of students. Truly, the enthusiastic encouragement from students throughout not just the United States but worldwide provides me the inspiration and energy to continue to write. It is thus with humility that I offer my sincere thanks to students everywhere ... for without students, how can a teacher teach?

Eugene C. Toy

ACKNOWLEDGMENTS

The curriculum that evolved into the ideas for this series was inspired by two talented and forthright students, Philbert Yao and Chuck Rosipal, who have since graduated from medical school. It has been a tremendous joy to work with my friend, colleague, and program director, Dr. Bentor Baker III. It is also a privilege to work with Dr. Ross, who has been a steady hand in administrating the medical student clerkship for so many years. Unfortunately Dr. Larry Gilstrap could no longer collaborate on this book due to his many other duties; I owe him so much in being the motivation and "fire" behind this series. It is with fondness that I recall the many hours in his office as he scratched red through my manuscript to bring it up to his exacting standards, and it is those standards that I still strive for with each book. It is a personal honor and with extreme gratitude that I am able to work with Dr. John Jennings, a visionary, brilliant obstetrician gynecologist, leader, and friend. Also, I am awed by the many excellent contributors who continue to work under the deadlines and pleas of perfectionists. I am greatly indebted to my editor, Catherine Johnson, whose exuberance, experience, and vision helped to shape this series. I appreciate McGraw-Hill's believing in the concept of teaching through clinical cases. I am also grateful to Catherine Saggese for her excellent production expertise, and Cindy Yoo for her wonderful editing. I cherish the ever-organized and precise Gita Raman, senior project manager, whose friendship and talent I greatly value; she keeps me focused, and nurtures each of my books from manuscript to print. At Methodist Hospital, I appreciate the great support from Drs. Marc Boom, Dirk Sostman, Alan Kaplan, and Karin Larsen-Pollock. Likewise, without Ayse McCracken, Reggie Abraham, and Marla Buffington for their advice and support, this book may never have been completed. Without my dear colleagues, Drs. Konrad Harms, Jeané Holmes, Priti Schachel, and Christopher Hobday, this book could not have been written. I appreciate Yaki Bryant, who has faithfully and energetically served as the extraordinary student coordinator for literally thousands and thousands of students at the University of Texas Medical School at Houston. Most of all, I appreciate my loving wife, Terri, and my four wonderful children, Andy, Michael, Allison, and Christina, for their patience and understanding.

Eugene C. Toy

Mastering the cognitive knowledge within a field such as obstetrics and gynecology is a formidable task. It is even more difficult to draw on that knowledge, to procure and filter through the clinical and laboratory data, to develop a differential diagnosis, and finally to make a rational treatment plan. To gain these skills, the student often learns best at the bedside, guided and instructed by experienced teachers, and inspired toward self-directed, diligent reading. Clearly, there is no replacement for education at the bedside. Unfortunately, clinical situations usually do not encompass the breadth of the specialty. Perhaps the best alternative is a carefully crafted patient case designed to stimulate the clinical approach and decision making. In an attempt to achieve that goal, we have constructed a collection of clinical vignettes to teach diagnostic or therapeutic approaches relevant to obstetrics and gynecology. Most importantly, the explanations for the cases emphasize the mechanisms and underlying principles, rather than merely rote questions and answers.

This book is organized for versatility: It allows the student "in a rush" to go quickly through the scenarios and check the corresponding answers, and it provides more detailed information for the student who wants thought-provoking explanations. The answers are arranged from simple to complex: a summary of the pertinent points, the bare answers, an analysis of the case, an approach to the topic, a comprehension test at the end for reinforcement and emphasis, and a list of resources for further reading. The clinical vignettes are purposely placed in random order to simulate the way that real patients present to the practitioner. A listing of cases is included in Section III to aid the students who desire to test their knowledge of a specific area, or who want to review a topic including basic definitions. Finally, we intentionally did not use a multiple-choice question (MCQ) format in our clinical case scenarios, since clues (or distractions) are not available in the real world. Nevertheless, several MCQs are included at the end of each case discussion (comprehension questions) to reinforce concepts or introduce related topics.

HOW TO GET THE MOST OUT OF THIS BOOK

Each case is designed to simulate a patient encounter with open-ended questions. At times, the patient's complaint is different from the most concerning issue, and sometimes extraneous information is given. The answers are organized into four different parts:

PART I

1. **Summary:** The salient aspects of the case are identified, filtering out the extraneous information. Students should formulate their summary from the case before looking at the answers. A comparison to the summation in the answer will help to improve their ability to focus on the important data, while appropriately discarding the irrelevant information—a fundamental skill in clinical problem solving.
2. **A Straightforward Answer** is given to each open-ended question.
3. The **Analysis of the Case** is comprised of two parts:

    a) **Objectives of the Case:** A listing of the two or three main principles that are crucial for a practitioner to manage the patient. Again, the students are challenged to make educated "guesses" about the objectives of the case upon initial review of the case scenario, which helps to sharpen their clinical and analytical skills.

    b) **Considerations:** A discussion of the relevant points and brief approach to the specific patient.

PART II

Approach to the Disease Process: It consists of two distinct parts:

    a) **Definitions:** Terminology pertinent to the disease process.

    b) **Clinical Approach:** A discussion of the approach to the clinical problem in general, including tables, figures, and algorithms.

PART III

Comprehension Questions: Each case contains several multiple-choice questions, which reinforce the material, or which introduce new and related concepts. Questions about material not found in the text will have explanations in the answers.

PART IV

Clinical Pearls: Several clinically important points are reiterated as a summation of the text. This allows for easy review, such as before an examination.

How to Approach Clinical Problems

Part 1. Approach to the Patient

The transition from textbook and/or journal article learning to the application of the information in a specific clinical situation is one of the most challenging tasks in medicine. It requires retention of information, organization of the facts, and recall of a myriad of data in precise application to the patient. The purpose of this book is to facilitate this process. The first step is gathering information, also known as establishing the database. This includes taking the history; performing the physical examination; and obtaining selective laboratory examinations or special evaluations, such as urodynamic testing and/or imaging tests. Of these, the historical examination is the most important and useful. Sensitivity and respect should always be exercised during the interview of patients.

Clinical Pearl

> ➤ The history is usually the single most important tool in obtaining a diagnosis. The art of seeking the information in a nonjudgmental, sensitive, and thorough manner cannot be overemphasized.

HISTORY

1. Basic information:
   a. Age: Age must be recorded because some conditions are more common at certain ages; for instance, pregnant women younger than 17 years or older than 35 years are at greater risk for preterm labor, preeclampsia, or miscarriage.
   b. Gravidity: Number of pregnancies including current pregnancy (includes miscarriages, ectopic pregnancies, and stillbirths).
   c. Parity: Number of pregnancies that have ended at gestational age(s) greater than 20 weeks.
   d. Abortuses: Number of pregnancies that have ended at gestational age(s) less than 20 weeks (includes ectopic pregnancies, induced abortions, and spontaneous abortions).

Clinical Pearl

> ➤ Some practitioners use a four-digit parity system to designate the number of term deliveries, number of preterm deliveries, number of abortuses, and number of live births (TPAL system). For example, G2 P1001 indicates gravidity 2 (two pregnancies including the current one), parity 1001; 1 prior term delivery, no preterm deliveries, no abortuses, and 1 living.

2. Last menstrual period (LMP): The first day of the last menstrual period. In obstetric patients, the certainty of the LMP is important in determining the gestational age. The estimated gestational age (EGA) is calculated from the LMP or by ultrasound. A simple rule for calculating the expected due date (EDD) is to subtract 3 months from the LMP and add 7 days to the first day of the LMP (eg, an LMP of 1 November would equal an EDD of 8 August). Because of delay in ovulation in some cycles, this is not always accurate.

3. Chief complaint: What is it that brought the patient into the hospital or office? Is it a scheduled appointment, or an unexpected symptom, such as abdominal pain or vaginal bleeding in pregnancy? The duration and character of the complaint, associated symptoms, and exacerbating and relieving factors should be recorded. The chief complaint engenders a differential diagnosis, and the possible etiologies should be explored by further inquiry. For example, if the chief complaint is postmenopausal bleeding, the concern is endometrial cancer. Thus, some of the questions should be related to the risk factors for endometrial cancer, such as hypertension, diabetes, anovulation, early age of menarche, late age of menopause, obesity, infertility, nulliparity, and so forth.

Clinical Pearl

> The first line of any obstetric presentation should include age, gravidity, parity, LMP, estimated gestational age, and chief complaint.
> Example: A 32-year-old G3 P1011 woman, whose LMP was April 2 and who has a pregnancy with an estimated gestational age of 32 4/7 weeks' gestation, complains of lower abdominal cramping.

4. Past gynecologic history:
   a. Menstrual history
      i. Age of menarche (should normally be older than 9 years and younger than 16 years).
      ii. Character of menstrual cycles: Interval from the first day of one menses to the first day of the next menses (normal is 28 ± 7 days, or between 21 and 35 days).
      iii. Quantity of menses: Menstrual flow should last less than 7 days (or be <80 mL in total volume). If menstrual flow is excessive, then it is called menorrhagia.
      iv. Irregular *and* heavy menses is called menometrorrhagia.
   b. Contraceptive history: Duration, type, and last use of contraception, and any side effects.
   c. Sexually transmitted diseases: A positive or negative history of herpes simplex virus, syphilis, gonorrhea, Chlamydia, human immunodeficiency

   virus (HIV), pelvic inflammatory disease, or human papillomavirus.
   Number of sexual partners, whether a recent change in partners, and use
   of barrier contraception.

5. Obstetric history: Date and gestational age of each pregnancy at termination, and outcome; if induced abortion, then gestational age and method. If delivered, then whether the delivery was vaginal or cesarean; if applicable, vacuum or forceps delivery, or type of cesarean (low-transverse vs classical). All complications of pregnancies should be listed.

6. Past medical history: Any illnesses, such as hypertension, hepatitis, diabetes mellitus, cancer, heart disease, pulmonary disease, and thyroid disease should be elicited. Duration, severity, and therapies should be included. Any hospitalizations should be listed with reason for admission, intervention, and location of hospital.

7. Past surgical history: Year and type of surgery should be elucidated and any complications documented. Type of incision (laparoscopy vs laparotomy) should be recorded.

8. Allergies: Reactions to medications should be recorded, including severity and temporal relationship to medication. Nonmedicine allergies, such as to latex or iodine, are also important to note. Immediate hypersensitivity should be distinguished from an adverse reaction.

9. Medications: A list of medications, dosage, route of administration and frequency, and duration of use should be obtained. Prescription, over-the-counter, and herbal remedies are all relevant. Use or abuse of illicit drugs, tobacco, or alcohol should also be recorded.

10. Review of systems: A systematic review should be performed but focused on the more common diseases. For example, in pregnant women, the presence of symptoms referable to preeclampsia, such as headache, visual disturbances, epigastric pain, or facial swelling, should be queried. In an elderly woman, symptoms suggestive of cardiac disease, such as chest pain, shortness of breath, fatigue, weakness, or palpitations, should be elicited.

Clinical Pearl

➤ In every pregnancy greater than 20 weeks' gestation, the patient should be questioned about symptoms of preeclampsia (headaches, visual disturbances, dyspnea, epigastric pain, and face/hand swelling).

PHYSICAL EXAMINATION

1. General appearance: Cachectic versus well-nourished, anxious versus calm, alert versus obtunded.

2. Vital signs: Temperature, blood pressure, heart rate, and respiratory rate. Height and weight are often placed here.

3. Head and neck examination: Evidence of trauma, tumors, facial edema, goiter, and carotid bruits should be sought. Cervical and supraclavicular nodes should be palpated.

4. Breast examination: Inspection for symmetry, skin or nipple retraction with the patient's hands on her hips (to accentuate the pectoral muscles), and with arms raised. With the patient supine, the breasts should then be palpated systematically to assess for masses. The nipple should be assessed for discharge, and the axillary and supraclavicular regions should be examined for adenopathy.

5. Cardiac examination: The point of maximal impulse (PMI) should be ascertained, and the heart auscultated at the apex of the heart as well as base. Heart sounds, murmurs, and clicks should be characterized. Systolic flow murmurs are fairly common in pregnant women due to the increased cardiac output, but significant diastolic murmurs are unusual.

6. Pulmonary examination: The lung fields should be examined systematically and thoroughly. Wheezes, rales, rhonchi, and bronchial breath sounds should be recorded.

7. Abdominal examination: The abdomen should be inspected for scars, distension, masses or organomegaly (ie, spleen or liver), and discoloration. For instance, the Grey Turner sign of discoloration at the flank areas may indicate intra-abdominal or retroperitoneal hemorrhage. Auscultation of bowel sounds should be accomplished to identify normal versus high-pitched, and hyperactive versus hypoactive sounds. The abdomen should be percussed for the presence of shifting dullness (indicating ascites). Careful palpation should begin initially away from the area of pain, involving one hand on top of the other, to assess for masses, tenderness, and peritoneal signs. Tenderness should be recorded on a scale (eg, 1 to 4, where 4 is the most severe pain). Guarding, whether it is voluntary or involuntary, should be noted.

8. Back and spine examination: The back should be assessed for symmetry, tenderness, or masses. In particular, the flank regions are important to assess for pain on percussion since that may indicate renal disease.

9. Pelvic examination (adequate preparation of the patient is crucial, including counseling about what to expect, adequate lubrication, and sensitivity to pain and discomfort):

    a. The external genitalia should be observed for masses or lesions, discoloration, redness, or tenderness. Ulcers in this area may indicate herpes simplex virus, vulvar carcinoma, or syphilis; a vulvar mass at the 5:00 or 7:00 o'clock positions can suggest a Bartholin gland cyst or abscess. Pigmented lesions may require biopsy since malignant melanoma is not uncommon in the vulvar region.

    b. Speculum examination: The vagina should be inspected for lesions, discharge, estrogen effect (well-ruggated vs atrophic), and presence of a cystocele or a rectocele. The appearance of the cervix should be described, and masses, vesicles, or other lesions should be noted.

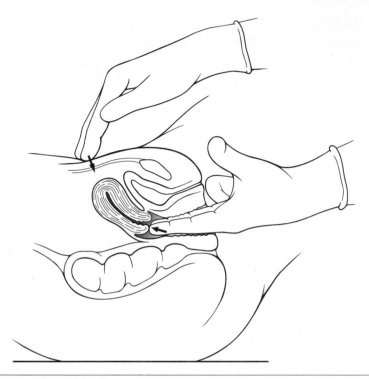

Figure I–1.   Bimanual pelvic examination. The examiner evaluates the patient's uterus by palpating her cervix vaginally while simultaneously assessing her uterine fundus abdominally.

    c. Bimanual examination: Initially, the index and middle finger of the one gloved hand should be inserted into the patient's vagina underneath the cervix, while the clinician's other hand is placed on the abdomen at the uterine fundus. With the uterus trapped between the two hands, the examiner should identify whether there is cervical motion tenderness, and evaluate the size, shape, and directional axis of the uterus. The adnexa should then be assessed with the vaginal hand in the lateral vaginal fornices. The normal ovary is approximately the size of a walnut (Figure I–1).

    d. Rectal examination: A rectal examination will reveal masses in the posterior pelvis, and may identify occult blood in the stool. Nodularity and tenderness in the uterosacral ligament can be signs of endometriosis. The posterior uterus and palpable masses in the cul-de-sac can be identified by rectal examination.

10. Extremities and skin: The presence of joint effusions, tenderness, skin edema, and cyanosis should be recorded.

11. Neurologic examination: Patients who present with neurologic complaints usually require a thorough assessment including evaluation of the cranial nerves, strength, sensation, and reflexes.

> Clinical Pearl

> ➤ The vaginal examination assesses the anterior pelvis, whereas the rectal examination is directed at the posterior pelvis.

12. Laboratory assessment for obstetric patients:
   a. Prenatal laboratory tests usually include the following:
      i. CBC, or complete blood count, to assess for anemia and thrombocytopenia.
      ii. Blood type, Rh, and antibody screen is of paramount importance for all pregnant women; for those women who are Rh negative, Rhogam is administered at 28 weeks' gestation and at delivery (if the baby proves Rh positive) to prevent isoimmunization.
      iii. Hepatitis B surface antigen (HBsAg): Indicates that the patient is infectious. At birth, the newborn should be given hepatitis B immune globulin (HBIG) and hepatitis B vaccine in an attempt to prevent neonatal hepatitis.
      iv. Rubella titer: If the patient is not immune to rubella, she should be vaccinated immediately postpartum; because it is a live-attenuated vaccine, this immunization is not given during pregnancy.
      v. Syphilis nontreponemal test (RPR [rapid plasma reagin] or VDRL [venereal disease research laboratory]): A positive test necessitates confirmation with a treponemal test, such as MHATP (micro-hemagglutination assay for antibodies to treponema pallidum) or FTA-ABS (fluorescent treponema antibody absorbed). Treatment during pregnancy is crucial to prevent congenital syphilis; penicillin is the agent of choice. Pregnant women who are allergic to penicillin usually undergo desensitization and receive penicillin.
      vi. Human immunodeficiency virus test: The screening test is usually the ELISA and, when positive, will necessitate the Western blot or other confirmatory test.
      vii. Urine culture or urinalysis: To assess for asymptomatic bacteriuria, which complicates 6% to 8% of pregnancies.
      viii. Pap smear: To assess for cervical dysplasia or cervical cancer; involves both ectocervical component and endocervical sampling (Figure I–2). Many clinicians prefer the liquid-based media because it may provide better cellular sampling and allows for HPV subtyping.
      ix. Endocervical assays for gonorrhea and/or *Chlamydia trachomatis* for high-risk patients.
   b. Timed prenatal tests:
      i. Serum screening for neural tube defects or Down syndrome offered; usually performed between 16 to 20 weeks' gestation. First-trimester screening for trisomies with serum pregnancy-associated plasma

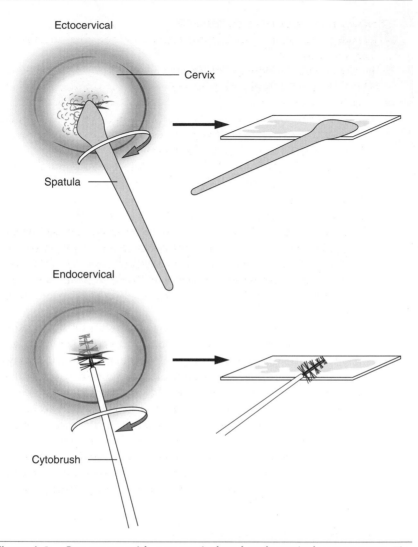

Figure I–2. Pap smear with ectocervical and endocervical components. The spatula is used to sample the exocervix. The endobrush is used to retrieve cells from the endocervix, and the cells are applied to the slide and fixative added.

protein-A (PAPP-A), beta human chorionic free gonadotropin (βhCG) and nuchal translucency (NT) has gained popularity as well.

ii. Screening for gestational diabetes at 26 to 28 weeks; generally consists of a 50-g oral glucose load and assessment of the serum glucose level after 1 hour.

iii. Some practitioners choose to repeat the complete blood count, cervical cultures, or syphilis serology in the third trimester.

iv. If the culture strategy for group B streptococcus is adopted, then introital cultures are obtained at 35 to 37 weeks' gestation.

13. Laboratory tests for gynecologic patients:
    a. Dependent on age, presence of coexisting disease, and chief complaint.
    b. Common scenarios:
        i. Threatened abortion: Quantitative hCG and/or progesterone levels may help to establish the viability of a pregnancy and risk of ectopic pregnancy.
        ii. Menorrhagia due to uterine fibroids: CBC, endometrial biopsy, and Pap smear. The endometrial biopsy is performed to assess for endometrial cancer and the Pap smear for cervical dysplasia or cancer.
        iii. A woman 55 years or older with an adnexal mass: CA-125 and CEA tumor markers for epithelial ovarian tumors.
14. Imaging procedures:
    a. Ultrasound examination:
        i. Obstetric patients: Ultrasound is the most commonly used imaging procedure in pregnant women. It can be used to establish the viability of the pregnancy, number of fetuses, location of the placenta, or establish the gestational age of the pregnancy. Targeted examinations can help to examine for structural abnormalities of the fetus.
        ii. Gynecologic patients: Adnexal masses evaluated by sonography are assessed for size and echogenic texture; simple (fluid filled) versus complex (fluid and solid components) versus solid. The uterus can be characterized for presence of masses, such as uterine fibroids, and the endometrial stripe can be measured. In postmenopausal women, a thickened endometrial stripe may indicate malignancy. Fluid in the cul-de-sac may indicate ascites. The gynecologic ultrasound examination usually also includes investigation of the kidneys, because hydronephrosis may suggest a pelvic process (ureteral obstruction). Saline infusion into the uterine cavity via a transcervical catheter can enhance the ultrasound examination of intrauterine growths such as polyps.

> ## Clinical Pearl
>
> ➤ Sonohysterography is a special ultrasound examination of the uterus that involves injecting a small amount of saline into the endometrial cavity to better define the intrauterine cavity. It can help to identify endometrial polyps or submucous myomata.

    b. Computed tomography (CT) scan:
        i. Because of the radiation concerns, this procedure is usually not performed on pregnant women unless sonography is not helpful, and it is deemed necessary.

   ii. The CT scan is useful in women with possible abdominal and/or
       pelvic masses, and may help to delineate the lymph nodes and
       retroperitoneal disorders.
   c. Magnetic resonance imaging (MRI):
      i. Identifies soft tissue planes very well and may assist in defining
         müllerian defects, such as vaginal agenesis or uterine didelphys
         (condition of double uterus and double cervix), and in selected
         circumstances may also aid in the evaluation of uterine anomalies.
     ii. May be helpful in establishing the location of a pregnancy, such as
         in differentiating a normal pregnancy from a cervical pregnancy.
   d. Intravenous pyelogram (IVP):
      i. Intravenous dye is used to assess the concentrating ability of the kid-
         neys, the patency of the ureters, and the integrity of the bladder.
     ii. It is also useful in detecting hydronephrosis, ureteral stone, or
         ureteral obstruction.
   e. Hysterosalpingogram (HSG):
      i. A small amount of radiopaque dye is introduced through a tran-
         scervical cannula and radiographs are taken.
     ii. It is useful for the detection of intrauterine abnormalities (submu-
         cous fibroids or intrauterine adhesions) and patency of the fallop-
         ian tubes (tubal obstruction or hydrosalpinx).

Part 2. Approach to Clinical Problem Solving

There are typically four distinct steps that a clinician undertakes to solve most
clinical problems systematically:
1. Making the diagnosis.
2. Assessing the severity and/or stage of the disease.
3. Rendering a treatment based on the stage of the disease.
4. Following the patient's response to the treatment.

MAKING THE DIAGNOSIS

The diagnosis is made by careful evaluation of the database, analysis of the
information, assessment of the risk factors, and development of the list of
possibilities (the differential diagnosis). The process includes knowing which
pieces of information are meaningful and which may be thrown out. Experience
and knowledge help to guide the physician to "key in" on the most important
possibilities. A good clinician also knows how to ask the same question in
several different ways, and use different terminology. For example, patients at
times may deny having been treated for "pelvic inflammatory disease," but
will answer affirmatively to being hospitalized for "a tubal infection."
Reaching a diagnosis may be achieved by systematically reading about each

possible cause and disease. The patient's presentation is then matched up against each of these possibilities, and each is either placed high up on the list as a potential etiology, or moved lower down because of disease prevalence, the patient's presentation, or other clues. A patient's risk factors may influence the probability of a diagnosis.

Usually, a long list of possible diagnoses can be pared down to two to three most likely ones, based on selective laboratory or imaging tests. For example, a woman who complains of lower abdominal pain *and* has a history of a prior sexually transmitted disease may have salpingitis; another patient who has abdominal pain, amenorrhea, *and* a history of prior tubal surgery may have an ectopic pregnancy. Furthermore, yet another woman with a one-day history of periumbilical pain localizing to the right lower quadrant may have acute appendicitis.

Clinical Pearl

> ➤ The first step in clinical problem-solving is making the diagnosis.

ASSESSING THE SEVERITY OF THE DISEASE

After ascertaining the diagnosis, the next step is to characterize the severity of the disease process; in other words, describe "how bad" a disease is. With malignancy, this is done formally by staging the cancer. Most cancers are categorized from stage I (least severe) to stage IV (most severe). Some diseases, such as preeclampsia, may be designated as mild or severe. With other ailments, there is a moderate category. With some infections, such as syphilis, the staging depends on the duration and extent of the infection, and follows along the natural history of the infection (ie, primary syphilis, secondary, latent period, and tertiary/neurosyphilis).

Clinical Pearl

> ➤ The second step in clinical problem-solving is to establish the severity or stage of disease. There is usually prognostic or treatment significance based on the stage.

TREATMENT BASED ON STAGE

Many illnesses are stratified according to severity because prognosis and treatment often vary based on the severity. If neither the prognosis nor the treatment was influenced by the stage of the disease process, there would not be a reason to subcategorize a disease as mild or severe. As an example, a pregnant woman at 32 weeks' gestation with mild preeclampsia is at less risk from the disease than if she developed severe preeclampsia (particularly if the severe preeclampsia were pulmonary edema or eclampsia). Accordingly, with mild preeclampsia, the management may be expectant, letting the pregnancy continue while watching for any danger signs (severe disease). In contrast, if severe preeclampsia complicated this same 32-week pregnancy, the treatment would be magnesium sulfate to prevent seizures (eclampsia) and, most importantly, delivery. It is primarily delivery that "cures" the preeclampsia. In this disease, severe preeclampsia means both maternal and fetal risks are increased. As another example, urinary tract infections may be subdivided into lower tract infections (cystitis) that are treated by oral antibiotics on an outpatient basis, versus upper tract infections (pyelonephritis) that generally require hospitalization and intravenous antibiotics.

Bacterial vaginosis (BV), which has been associated with preterm delivery, endometritis, and vaginal cuff cellulitis (following hysterectomy), does not have a severe or mild substaging. The presence of BV may slightly increase the risk of problems, but neither the prognosis nor the treatment is affected by "more" BV or "less" BV. Hence, the student should approach a new disease by learning the mechanism, clinical presentation, staging, and the treatment based on stage.

Clinical Pearl

> ➤ The third step in clinical problem-solving is that, for most conditions, the treatment is tailored to the extent or "stage" of the disease.

FOLLOWING THE RESPONSE TO TREATMENT

The final step in the approach to disease is to follow the patient's response to the therapy. The "measure" of response should be recorded and monitored. Some responses are clinical, such as improvement (or lack of improvement) in a patient's abdominal pain, temperature, or pulmonary examination. Obviously, the student must work on being more skilled in eliciting the data in an unbiased and standardized manner. Other responses may be followed by imaging tests, such as a CT scan to establish retroperitoneal node size in a patient receiving chemotherapy, or a tumor marker, such as the CA-125 level in a woman receiving chemotherapy for ovarian cancer. For syphilis, it may be the results of the nonspecific treponemal antibody test RPR titer over time. The student must be prepared to know what to do if the measured marker does not respond according to what is expected. Is the next step to retreat, or to reconsider the diagnosis, or to repeat the metastatic work-up, or to follow up with another more specific test?

Clinical Pearl

> The fourth step in clinical problem-solving is to monitor treatment response or efficacy, which may be measured in different ways. It may be symptomatic (patient feels better), or based on physical examination (fever), a laboratory test (CA-125 level), or an imaging test (ultrasound size of ovarian cyst).

Part 3. Approach to Reading

The clinical problem-oriented approach to reading is different from the classic "systematic" research of a disease. Patients rarely present with a clear diagnosis; hence, the student must become skilled in applying the textbook information to the clinical setting. Furthermore, a reader retains more information when reading with a purpose. In other words, the student should read with the goal of answering specific questions. Likewise, the student should have a plan for the acquisition and use of the information; the process is similar to having a mental "flow chart" and each step sifting through diagnostic possibilities, therapy, complications, and risk factors. There are several fundamental questions that facilitate clinical thinking. These are:

1. What is the most likely diagnosis?
2. What should be your next step?
3. What is the most likely mechanism for this process?
4. What are the risk factors for this condition?
5. What are the complications associated with the disease process?
6. What is the best therapy?
7. How would you confirm the diagnosis?

Clinical Pearl

> Reading with the purpose of answering the seven fundamental clinical questions improves retention of information and facilitates the application of "book knowledge" to "clinical knowledge."

WHAT IS THE MOST LIKELY DIAGNOSIS?

The method of establishing the diagnosis has been covered in the previous section. One way of attacking this problem is to develop standard "approaches" to common clinical situations. It is helpful to understand the most common causes of various presentations, such as "the most common cause of postpartum hemorrhage is uterine atony." (Clinical Pearls appear at the end of each case.)

The clinical scenario would be something such as:

An 18-year-old G1 P0 adolescent female undergoes an uncomplicated vaginal delivery at term. After the placenta is delivered, she has 1500 cc of vaginal bleeding. What is the most likely diagnosis?

With no other information to go on, the student would note that this patient has postpartum hemorrhage (blood loss of >500 mL with a vaginal delivery). Using the "most common cause" information, the student would make an educated guess that the patient has uterine atony.

However, what if the scenario also included the following phrase?

The uterus is noted to be firm.

Now the most likely diagnosis is a genital tract laceration, usually involving the cervix. With a firm well contracted uterus, atony is not likely.

Clinical Pearls

▶ The most common cause of postpartum hemorrhage is uterine atony. Thus, the first step in patient assessment and management is uterine massage to check if the uterus is boggy.

▶ If the uterus is firm, and the woman is still bleeding, then the clinician should consider a genital tract laceration.

▶ Now, the student would use the clinical pearl: "The most common cause of postpartum hemorrhage with a firm uterus is a genital tract laceration."

WHAT SHOULD BE YOUR NEXT STEP?

This question is difficult because the next step has many possibilities; the answer may be to obtain more diagnostic information, stage the illness, or introduce therapy. It is often a more challenging question than "What is the most likely diagnosis?" because there may be insufficient information to make a diagnosis and the next step may be to pursue more diagnostic information. Another possibility is that there is enough information for a probable diagnosis, and the next step is to stage the disease. Finally, the most appropriate answer may be to treat. Hence, from clinical data, a judgment needs to be rendered regarding how far along one is on the road of:

Make a diagnosis → Stage the disease →
Treat based on stage → Follow response

Frequently, the student is taught to "regurgitate" the information that someone has written about a particular disease, but is not skilled at giving the next step. This talent is learned optimally at the bedside, in a supportive environment, with freedom to make educated guesses, and with constructive feedback. A sample scenario describes a student's thought process as follows.

1. Make the diagnosis: "Based on the information I have, I believe that this patient has a pelvic inflammatory disease because she is not pregnant and has lower abdominal tenderness, cervical motion tenderness, and adnexal tenderness."
2. Stage the disease: "I don't believe that this is severe disease, since she does not have high fever, evidence of sepsis, or peritoneal signs. An ultrasound has already been done showing no abscess (tubo-ovarian abscess would put her in a severe category)."
3. Treat based on stage: "Therefore, my next step is to treat her with intramuscular ceftriaxone and oral doxycycline."
4. Follow response: "I want to follow the treatment by assessing her pain (I will ask her to rate the pain on a scale of 1 to 10 every day), her temperature, and abdominal examination, and reassess her in 48 hours."

In a similar patient, when the clinical presentation is unclear, perhaps the best "next step" may be diagnostic in nature, such as laparoscopy to visualize the tubes. This information is sometimes tested by the dictum, "the gold standard for the diagnosis of acute salpingitis is laparoscopy to visualize the tubes, and particularly seeing purulent material drain from the tubes."

Clinical Pearl

➤ Usually, the vague query, "What is your next step?" is the most difficult question, because the answer may be diagnostic, staging, or therapeutic.

WHAT IS THE LIKELY MECHANISM FOR THIS PROCESS?

This question goes further than making the diagnosis, but also requires the student to understand the underlying mechanism for the process. For example, a clinical scenario may describe an 18-year-old adolescent female at 24 weeks' gestation who develops dyspnea 2 days after being treated for pyelonephritis. The student must first diagnose the acute respiratory distress syndrome, which often occurs 1 to 2 days after antibiotics are instituted. Then, the student must understand that the endotoxins that arise from gram-negative organisms cause pulmonary injury, leading to capillary leakage of fluid into the pulmonary interstitial space. The mechanism is, therefore, endotoxin-induced "capillary leakage." Answers that a student may also entertain, but would be less likely to be causative, include pneumonia, pulmonary embolism, or pleural effusion.

The student is advised to learn the mechanisms for each disease process, and not merely memorize a constellation of symptoms. In other words, rather than solely committing to memorizing the classic presentation of pyelonephritis (fever, flank tenderness, and pyuria), the student should understand that gram-negative rods, such as *Escherichia coli*, would ascend from the external genitalia to the urethra to the bladder. From the bladder, the bacteria would ascend further to the kidneys and cause an infection in the renal parenchyma. The involvement of the kidney now causes fever (vs an infection of only the bladder, which usually does not induce a fever) and flank tenderness—a systemic response not seen with lower urinary tract infection (ie, bacteriuria or cystitis). Furthermore, the body's reaction to the bacteria brings about leukocytes in the urine (pyuria).

WHAT ARE THE RISK FACTORS FOR THIS PROCESS?

Understanding the risk factors helps the practitioner to establish a diagnosis and to determine how to interpret tests. For example, understanding the risk factor analysis may help to manage a 55-year-old woman with postmenopausal bleeding after an endometrial biopsy shows no pathologic changes. If the woman does not have any risk factors for endometrial cancer, the patient may be observed because the likelihood for uterine malignancy is not so great. On the other hand, if the same 55-year-old woman were diabetic, had a long history of anovulation (irregular menses), was nulliparous, and was hypertensive, a practitioner should pursue the postmenopausal bleeding further, even after a normal endometrial biopsy. The physician may want to perform a hysteroscopy to visualize the endometrial cavity directly and biopsy the abnormal-appearing areas. Thus, the presence of risk factors helps to categorize the likelihood of a disease process.

Clinical Pearl

➤ When patients are at high risk for a disease, based on risk factors, more testing may be indicated.

WHAT ARE THE COMPLICATIONS OF THIS PROCESS?

Clinicians must be cognizant of the complications of a disease, so that they will understand how to follow and monitor the patient. Sometimes, the student will have to make the diagnosis from clinical clues, and then apply his or her knowledge of the consequences of the pathologic process. For example, a woman who presents with lower abdominal pain, vaginal discharge, and dyspareunia is first diagnosed as having pelvic inflammatory disease or salpingitis (infection of the fallopian tubes). Long-term complications of this process would include ectopic pregnancy or infertility from tubal damage. Understanding the types of consequences also helps the clinician to be aware of the dangers to a patient. One life-threatening complication of a tubo-ovarian abscess (which is the end-stage of a tubal infection leading to a collection of pus in the region of the tubes and ovary) is rupture of the abscess. The clinical presentation is shock with hypotension, and the appropriate therapy is immediate surgery. In fact, not recognizing the rupture is commonly associated with patient mortality. The student applies this information when she or he sees a woman with a tubo-ovarian abscess on daily rounds, and monitors for hypotension, confusion, apprehension, and tachycardia. The clinician advises the team to be vigilant for any signs of abscess rupture, and to be prepared to undertake immediate surgery should the need arise.

WHAT IS THE BEST THERAPY?

To answer this question, the clinician needs to reach the correct diagnosis, and assess the severity of the condition, and then he or she must weigh the situation to reach the appropriate intervention. For the student, knowing exact dosages is not as important as understanding the best medication, the route of delivery, mechanism of action, and possible complications. It is important for the student to be able to verbalize the diagnosis and the rationale for the therapy. A common error is for the student to "jump to a treatment," like a random guess, and, therefore, he or she is given "right or wrong" feedback. In fact, the student's guess may be correct, but for the wrong reason; conversely, the answer may be a very reasonable one, with only one small error in thinking. Instead, the student should verbalize the steps so that feedback may be given at every reasoning point.

For example, if the question is, "What is the best therapy for a 19-year-old woman with a nontender ulcer of the vulva and painless adenopathy who is pregnant at 12 weeks' gestation?" the incorrect manner of response for the student to is to blurt out "azithromycin." Rather, the student should reason it in a way such as the following: "The most common cause of a nontender infectious ulcer of the vulva is syphilis. Painless adenopathy is usually associated. In pregnancy, penicillin is the only effective therapy to prevent congenital syphilis. Therefore, the best treatment for this woman with probable syphilis is intramuscular penicillin (after confirming the diagnosis)."

A related question is, "What would have best prevented this condition?" For instance, if the scenario presented is a 23-year-old woman with tubal factor infertility, then the most likely etiology is *Chlamydia trachomatis* cervicitis which had ascended to the tubes causing damage. The best preventive measure would be a barrier contraception such as condom use.

Clinical Pearl

➤ Therapy should be logical based on the severity of disease. Antibiotic therapy should be tailored for specific organism(s).

HOW WOULD YOU CONFIRM THE DIAGNOSIS?

In the previous scenario, the woman with a nontender vulvar ulcer is likely to have syphilis. Confirmation can be achieved by serology (RPR or VDRL test) and specific treponemal test; however, there is a significant possibility that patients with primary syphilis may not have developed an antibody response yet, and have negative serology. Thus, confirmation of the diagnosis would be attained with darkfield microscopy. The student should strive to know the limitations of various diagnostic tests, and the manifestations of disease.

Summary

1. There is no replacement for a meticulous history and physical examination.
2. There are four steps to the clinical approach to the patient: making the diagnosis, assessing severity, treating based on severity, and following response.
3. There are seven questions that help to bridge the gap between the textbook and the clinical arena.

REFERENCES

Cunningham FG, Leveno KJ, Bloom SL, Gilstrap LC III, Hauth JC, Wenstrom KD. Prenatal care. In: *Williams Obstetrics.* 22nd ed. New York, NY: McGraw-Hill; 2005:221-247.

Lentz GM. History, physical examination, and preventive health care. In: Katz VL, Lentz GM, Lobo RA, Gersenson DM, eds. *Comprehensive Gynecology.* 5th ed. St. Louis, MO: Mosby-Year Book; 2007:137-150.

Moore GJ. Obstetric and gynecologic evaluation. In: Hacker NF, Moore JG, eds. *Essentials of Obstetrics and Gynecology.* 4th ed. Philadelphia, PA: Saunders; 2005:12-26.

Clinical Cases

Case 1

A 48-year-old G3 P3 woman complains of a 2-year history of loss of urine four to five times each day, typically occurring with coughing, sneezing, or lifting; she denies dysuria or the urge to void during these episodes. These events cause her embarrassment and interfere with her daily activities. The patient is otherwise in good health. A urine culture performed 1 month previously was negative. On examination, she is slightly obese. Her blood pressure is 130/80 mm Hg, her heart rate is 80 beats per minute, and her temperature 99°F (37.2°C). The breast examination is normal without masses. Her heart has a regular rate and rhythm without murmurs. The abdominal examination reveals no masses or tenderness. A midstream voided urinalysis is unremarkable.

➤ What is the most likely diagnosis?

➤ What physical examination finding is most likely to be present?

➤ What is the best initial treatment?

ANSWERS TO CASE 1:
Urinary Incontinence

Summary: A 48-year-old multiparous woman complains of urinary incontinence, which is related to stress activities. There is no urge component, and no delay from the Valsalva maneuver to the loss of urine.

➤ **Most likely diagnosis:** Genuine stress incontinence.

➤ **Physical examination finding:** Hypermobile urethra, cystocele, or loss of urethrovesical angle.

➤ **Best initial treatment:** Kegel exercises and timed voiding.

ANALYSIS

Objectives

1. Discern between the typical history of genuine stress urinary incontinence (GSUI) versus urge urinary incontinence (UUI).
2. Know that the cystometric examination can be used to distinguish between the two etiologies.
3. Know the treatments for both entities (GSUI and UUI).

Considerations

This patient's history is very typical for genuine stress incontinence. She has loss of urine concurrent with coughing, sneezing, or lifting. There is no urge component or a delay from cough as these findings would be consistent with urge incontinence. There is no evidence of diabetes or a neuropathy, making overflow incontinence unlikely. The pelvic examination likely reveals a cystocele (bladder bulging into the anterior vagina) or a loss of the normal bladder-urethral angle (hypermobile urethra); both of these findings of pelvic relaxation may be associated with the anatomic problem of GSUI, the bladder neck being below the abdominal cavity. In patients with urge incontinence, or mixed symptoms (loss of urine with Valsalva, and urge to void), cystometric examination can be helpful to differentiate between genuine stress and urge incontinence. An accurate diagnosis is important, since the therapies for these two conditions are very different, and surgical therapy may actually worsen urge incontinence.

With genuine stress urinary incontinence, initial treatment usually entails pelvic floor strengthening exercises, called Kegel exercises. If this is unsuccessful, then options for treatment include urethropexy (surgical fixation of the proximal urethra above the pelvic diaphragm, suburethral sling, or transobturator) or transvaginal fixation.

APPROACH TO
Urinary Incontinence

DEFINITIONS

URINARY INCONTINENCE: The involuntary loss of urine that is objectively demonstrable and creates social or hygienic concern.

GENUINE STRESS INCONTINENCE: Incontinence through the urethra due to sudden increases in intra-abdominal pressure, in the absence of bladder muscle spasm.

URGE INCONTINENCE: Loss of urine due to an uninhibited and sudden bladder detrusor muscle contraction.

OVERFLOW INCONTINENCE: Loss of urine associated with an overdistended, hypotonic bladder in the absence of detrusor contractions. This is often associated with diabetes mellitus, spinal cord injuries, or lower motor neuropathies. It may also be caused by urethral edema after pelvic surgery.

CYSTOMETRIC EVALUATION: Investigation of pressure and volume changes in the bladder with the filling of known volumes. It is often used to discern between GSUI and UUI.

MIDURETHRAL SLING PROCEDURES: Supporting the midurethra with a hammock-like effect, with procedures such as tensionless transvaginal tape (TVT), or transobturator tape (TOT).

TRANSVAGINAL TAPE PROCEDURE: A minimally invasive procedure used to fix the proximal urethra retropubic via a blind technique using a special hook-like instrument to place a synthehic tape under the urethra.

TRANSOBTURATOR TAPE PROCEDURE: A minimally invasive procedure similar to the TVT but originating laterally to try to avoid the bladder or bowel injuries that have been reported with the TVT procedures.

CLINICAL APPROACH

Normal Physiology

Urinary continence is maintained when the urethral pressure exceeds the intravesicular (bladder) pressure. The bladder and proximal urethra are normally intra-abdominal in position, that is, above the pelvic diaphragm. In this situation, a Valsalva maneuver transmits pressure to both the bladder and proximal urethra so that continence is maintained. In the normal anatomic situation, the urethral pressure exceeds the bladder pressure, and also the pelvic diaphragm supports the bladder and urethra.

Mechanisms of Incontinence

Genuine Stress Incontinence: Following trauma and/or other causes of weakness of the pelvic diaphragm (such as childbearing), the proximal urethra may fall below the pelvic diaphragm. When the patient coughs, intra-abdominal pressure is exerted to the bladder, but not to the proximal urethra. When the bladder pressure equals or exceeds the maximal urethral pressure, urinary flow occurs. Because this is a mechanical problem, the patient feels no urge to void, and the loss of urine occurs simultaneously with coughing. There is no delay from cough to incontinence. Urethropexy replaces the proximal urethra back to its intra-abdominal position (Figure 1–1). More recently, narrow strips of polypropylene mesh have been used to suspend the mid-urethra due to the theory that urinary incontinence occurs due to pubourethral ligament insufficiency. These procedures act as a hammock to support the urethra, and also act to compress the urethra somewhat. These include various tension-free vaginal tape procedures, and outcomes are favorable as compared to urethropexy. Because of the minimally invasive nature of these procedures, they have gained popularity. Nevertheless, there is concern about erosion of the synthetic material into the bladder or urethra prompting an FDA warning in 2008. A large NIH-funded study is being conducted to try to ascertain which procedure is best to treat GSUI.

Urge Incontinence: With uninhibited spasms of the detrusor muscle, the bladder pressure overcomes the urethral pressure. Dysuria and/or the urge to void are prominent symptoms, reflecting the bladder spasms. Sometimes, coughing or sneezing can provoke a bladder spasm, so that a delay of several seconds is noted before urine loss.

Overflow Incontinence: With an overdistended bladder, coughing will increase the bladder pressure and eventually lead to dribbling or small loss of urine.

Work-up

The history, physical examination, urinalysis, and postvoid residual are part of the initial evaluation of urinary incontinence (Table 1–1).

Behavior therapy, including timed voiding, and pelvic musculature strengthening, seem to have a role and generally should be the first line of treatment.

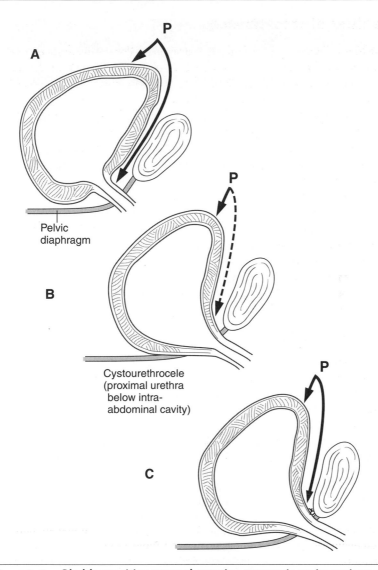

Pelvic diaphragm

Cystourethrocele
(proximal urethra
below intra-
abdominal cavity)

Figure 1–1.   Bladder position: normal, genuine stress urinary incontinence, and after urethropexy. Normally, a Valsalva maneuver causes the increased intra-abdominal pressure *(P)* to be transmitted equally to the bladder and urethra (**A**). With genuine stress urinary incontinence, the proximal urethra has fallen outside the abdominal cavity (**B**) so that the intraabdominal pressure no longer is transferred to the proximal urethra, leading to incontinence. After urethropexy (**C**), pressure is again transmitted to the urethra.

Table 1–1 DIFFERENTIAL DIAGNOSIS OF URINARY INCONTINENCE

	MECHANISM	HISTORY	DIAGNOSTIC TEST	TREATMENT
Genuine stress urinary incontinence	Bladder neck has fallen out of its normal intra-abdominal position	Painless loss of urine concurrent with Valsalva; no urge to void.	Physical examination: loss of bladder angle; cystometric examination	Urethropexy (Burch procedure or urethral sling) to return proximal urethra back to intra-abdominal position
Urge incontinence	Detrusor muscle is overactive and contracts unpredictably	Urge component, "I have to go to the bathroom and can't make it there in time".	Cystometric examination shows uninhibited contractions	Anticholinergic medication to relax detrusor muscle (surgery may worsen)
Overflow incontinence	Overdistended bladder due to hypotonic bladder	Loss of urine with Valsalva; dribbling; diabetes or spinal cord injury.	Postvoid residual (catheterization) shows large amount of urine	Intermittent self-catheterization
Fistula	Communication between bladder or ureter and vagina	Constant leakage after surgery or prolonged labor.	Dye into bladder shows vaginal discoloration	Surgical repair of fistulous tract

Comprehension Questions

1.1 A 55-year-old woman notes constant wetness from her vagina following a total vaginal hysterectomy procedure, which she had undergone 2 months previously. She denies dysuria or urgency to void. The urinanalysis is normal. Which of the following is the best method to diagnose the etiology of urinary incontinence?

    A. Cystometric examination
    B. Dye instillation into bladder
    C. Postvoid catheterization of the bladder
    D. Neurological profile of the sacral nerves

Match the following *single* best therapy (A-G) that will most likely help in the clinical situation described (1.2-1.4):

    A. Burch urethropexy
    B. Oxybutynin (Ditropan, an anticholinergic medication)
    C. Placement of ureteral stents
    D. Surgical repair of the fistulous tract
    E. Propranolol (inderal)
    F. Placement of an artificial urethral sphincter
    G. Intermittent self-catheterization

1.2 A 42-year-old woman with long-standing diabetes mellitus complains of small amounts of constant dribbling of urine loss with coughing or lifting.

1.3 A 39-year-old woman wets her underpants two to three times each day. She feels as though she needs to void, but cannot make it to the restroom in time.

1.4 A 35-year-old woman has undergone four vaginal deliveries. She notes urinary loss six to seven times a day concurrently with coughing or sneezing. She denies dysuria or an urge to void. Her urine culture is negative.

ANSWERS

1.1 **B.** This patient likely has a vesicovaginal (between bladder and vagina) fistula from the surgery. A dye instilled into the bladder would be seen leaking into the vagina. If the leakage is slow, sometimes a tampon is placed into the vagina and removed after 30 to 60 minutes. Constant wetness after a pelvic operation suggests a fistula, such as vesicovaginal fistula, which is best treated with surgical repair. This situation is best treated with surgical repair since it is an anatomic problem. Medications would not be helpful in this situation. The operation would include excision of the fistulous tract which usually may be infected or weakened, and then closure of the opening. Other common fistulae that may occur after pelvic surgery include ureterovaginal (between ureter and vagina) and rectovaginal fistulas (between rectum and vagina).

1.2   **G.** This patient has long-standing diabetes mellitus, which is a risk factor for a neurogenic bladder, leading to overflow incontinence. Other causes include spinal cord injury or multiple sclerosis. These patients generally do not feel the urge to void and accumulate large amounts of urine in their bladders. The best therapy for overflow incontinence (neurogenic bladder) is intermittent self-catheterization. Neither surgery (indicated for fistula repair), nor Burch urethropexy (indicated for genuine stress incontinence) would be appropriate for this scenario because it is not an anatomic problem. The medications listed would also not be indicated for neurogenic bladder, however, Bethanechol is a commonly prescribed drug to help stimulate bladder contractions by selectively acting on muscarinic receptors in the bladder muscles in individuals with overflow incontinence.

1.3   **B.** This woman's prominent urge component makes urge incontinence the most likely diagnosis, best treated with anticholinergic medications. Anticholinergics relax the overactive detrusor muscle. Surgery would not be indicated in this situation, and in fact, may worsen the situation by further damaging nerves and muscles of the bladder. An artificial urethral sphincter would not improve the patient's symptoms because the problem has to do with the detrusor muscle, and not the urethral sphincter. The patient is not having a problem with overflow, so self-catheterization would not be helpful either.

1.4   **A.** This clinical presentation is consistent with GSUI and is best treated by urethropexy. There is some evidence that vaginal deliveries may increase the incidence of GSUI due to trauma to the pelvic diaphragm. The medications listed would not be indicated for this patient because her symptoms are due to a weakening of the pelvic diaphragm versus a problem with the bladder itself, or muscles of the bladder, as with urge incontinence. Unlike urge incontinence, the patient feels no urge to void, and there is no delay noted before urine loss after a cough or sneeze. A cytometric or urodynamic evaluation helps to differentiate between urge and genuine stress incontinence.

Clinical Pearls

➤ The primary treatment of genuine stress incontinence is surgical, whereas the best treatment of urge incontinence is medical.

➤ Although midurethral sling procedures have emerged as the most commonly performed procedures to treat GSUI, it is unclear that they are the best procedures.

➤ Cystometric or urodynamic evaluation helps to differentiate genuine from urge incontinence.

➤ A postvoid catheterization showing a large residual volume suggests overflow incontinence.

➤ Loss of urine occurs when the intravesicular pressure equals (or exceeds) the sphincter pressure.

REFERENCES

American College of Obstetricians and Gynecologists. Urinary incontinence in women. In: ACOG *Practice Bulletin 63*. Washington DC: 2005.

American College of Obstetricians and Gynecologists. Pelvic organ prolapse. ACOG *Practice Bulletin 85*. Washington, DC: 2007.

Lentz GM. Urogynecology. In: Katz VL, Lentz GM, Lobo RA, Gersenson DM, eds. *Comprehensive Gynecology*. 5th ed. St. Louis, MO: Mosby-Year Book; 2007:537-568.

Tarnay CM, Bhatia NN. Genitourinary dysfunction, pelvic organ prolapse, urinary incontinence, and infections. In: Hacker NF, Gambone JC, Hobel CJ, eds. *Essentials of Obstetrics and Gynecology*, 5th ed. Philadelphia, PA: Saunders; 2009:276-289.

Case 2

A 66-year-old woman comes in for a routine physical examination. Her menopause occurred at age 51 years, and she is currently taking an estrogen pill along with a progestin pill each day. The past medical history is unremarkable. Her family history includes one maternal cousin with ovarian cancer. On examination, she is found to have a blood pressure of 120/70 mm Hg, heart rate of 70 beats per minute, and temperature of 98°F (36.6°C). She weighs 140 lb and is 5 ft 4 in tall. The thyroid is normal to palpation. Examination of her breasts reveals no masses or discharge. The abdominal, cardiac, and lung evaluations are within normal limits. The pelvic examination shows a normal, multiparous cervix, a normal-sized uterus, and no adnexal masses. She had undergone mammography 3 months previously.

➤ What is your next step?

➤ What would be the most common cause of mortality for this patient?

ANSWERS TO CASE 2:

Health Maintenance, Age 66 Years

Summary: A 66-year-old woman presents for health maintenance. A mammogram has been performed 3 months previously.

➤ **Next step:** Each of the following should be performed: Stool for occult blood, colonoscopy or barium enema/flexible sigmoidoscopy, pneumococcal vaccine, influenza vaccine, tetanus vaccine (if not within 10 years), cholesterol screening, fasting blood sugar, thyroid function tests, bone mineral density screening, and urinalysis.

➤ **Most common cause of mortality:** Cardiovascular disease.

ANALYSIS

Objectives

1. Understand which health maintenance studies should be performed for a 66-year-old woman.
2. Know the most common cause of mortality for a woman in this age group.
3. Understand that preventive maintenance consists of cancer screening, immunizations, and screening for common diseases.

Considerations

The approach to health maintenance includes three parts: (1) cancer screening, (2) immunizations, and (3) addressing common diseases for the particular patient group. For a 66-year-old woman, this includes annual mammography for breast cancer screening, colon cancer screening (annual stool test for occult blood and either intermittent colonoscopy or barium enema/flexible sigmoidoscopy), tetanus booster every 10 years, the pneumococcal vaccine, and a yearly influenza immunization. Screening for hypercholesterolemia every 5 years up to age 75 years, thyroid function testing every 5 years, and fasting blood sugar levels every 3 years are also recommended. Because urosepsis is common in geriatric patients, a urinalysis is also usually performed. Osteoporosis screening is indicated for women over the age of 65. Finally, the most common cause of mortality in a woman in this age group is cardiovascular disease.

/ **APPROACH TO**
Health Maintenance in Older Women

DEFINITIONS

SCREENING TEST: A device used to identify asymptomatic disease in the hope that early detection will lead to an improved outcome. An optimal screening test has high sensitivity and specificity, is inexpensive, and is easy to perform.

PRIMARY PREVENTION: Identifying and modifying risk factors in people who have never had the disease of concern.

SECONDARY PREVENTION: Actions taken to reduce morbidity or mortality once a disease has been diagnosed.

COST EFFECTIVENESS: A comparison of resources expended (dollars) in an intervention versus the benefit, which may be measured in life-years, or quality-adjusted life years.

CLINICAL APPROACH

In each age group, particular screening tests are recommended (Table 2–1).

Rationale

When the patient does not have any apparent disease or complaint, then the goal of medical intervention is disease prevention. One method of targeting diseases is by using the patient's age. For example, the most common cause of death for a 16-year-old person is a motor vehicle accident; hence the teenage patient would be well served by the physician encouraging him or her to wear seat belts and to avoid alcohol intoxication when driving. In contrast, a 56-year-old woman will most likely die of cardiovascular disease, so the physician should focus on exercise, weight loss, and screening for hyperlipidemia. In a woman beyond 65 years of age, if prior Pap smears have been normal cervical cancer screening is not cost-effective. Patients who have had a total hysterectomy (removal of uterine corpus and cervix) do not require vaginal cytology (Pap smears) as long as the patient had no history of cervical dysplasia.

Table 2-1 SCREENING BASED ON AGE

	13-18 YR	19-39 YR	40-64 YR	65+ YR
Cancer screening	Pap smear approximately 3 y after onset of sexual activity	Annual Pap smear after age 21 or approximately 3 y after onset of sexual activity; every 2-3 y after age 30 if three consecutive negative Pap smears	Pap smear, *age 50*: stool for occult blood, barium enema with flexible sigmoidoscopy q 5 y, or colonoscopy q 10 y, annual mammography*	Annual stool for occult blood Colonoscopy or barium enema with flexible sigmoidoscopy every 5 y annual mammography* Pap smears until age 65-70 y
Immunizations	Tetanus booster once between ages 11-16 y Hepatitis B vaccine Human papillomavirus vaccine ages 9-26	Tetanus every 10 y Human papillomavirus vaccine ages 9-26	Tetanus every 10 y *Age 50*: annual influenza vaccine *Age 60*: varicella zoster vaccine	Tetanus every 10 y Pneumococcal vaccine Annual influenza vaccine
Other diseases	Motor vehicle accidents Depression Firearms	Cardiovascular diseases	Cholesterol screening every 5 y at age 45 Fasting blood sugar level every 3 y at age 45 TSH every 5 y at age 50	Cholesterol screening every 5 y at age 45 Fasting blood sugar level every 3 y at 45 Bone mineral density study at 65
Most common causes of mortality	• Motor vehicle accidents • Malignant neoplams • Homicide	• Malignant neoplasms • Accidents • Cardiovascular disease	• Cancer • Cardiovascular disease	• Heart disease • Cancer. • Cerebrovascular disease

*Some experts recommend mammography beginning at age 40 yr whereas others question its efficacy in decreasing mortality.
Adapted from ACOG Committee Opinion No. 357, 2006. Washington, DC: American College of Obstetricians and Gynecologists; 2003.

Comprehension Questions

2.1   A 59-year-old woman is being seen for a health maintenance appoint-
        ment. She has not seen a doctor for over 10 years. She had undergone
        a total hysterectomy for uterine fibroids 12 years ago. The patient
        takes supplemental calcium. The physician orders a fasting glucose
        level, lipid panel, mammogram, colonoscopy, and a Pap smear of the
        vaginal cuff. Which of the following statements is most accurate
        regarding the screening for this patient?
        A. The Pap smear of the vaginal cuff is unnecessary.
        B. In general colon cancer screening should be initiated at age 60
           but this patient has very sporadic care, therefore colonoscopy is
           reasonable.
        C. Because the patient takes supplemental calcium, a DEXA scan is
           not needed.
        D. Pneumococcal vaccination should be recommended.

2.2   A 63-year-old woman has had annual health maintenance appoint-
        ments and has followed all the recommendations offered by her physi-
        cian. The physician counsels her about varicella zoster vaccine. Which
        of the following is the most accurate statement about this vaccine?
        A. This vaccine is recommended for patients who are aged 50 and older.
        B. This vaccine is not recommended if a patient has already devel-
           oped the shingles.
        C. This vaccine is a live attenuated immunization.
        D. This vaccine has some cross-reactivity with herpes simplex virus
           and offers some protection against HSV.

2.3   An 18-year-old adolescent female is being seen for a health mainte-
        nance appointment. She has not had a Pap smear previously. She cur-
        rently takes oral contraceptive pills. She began sexual intercourse 1 year
        previously. Which of the following statements is most accurate regard-
        ing health maintenance for this individual?
        A. A Pap smear should not be performed in this patient at this time.
        B. The HPV vaccine should be administered only if she has a history
           of genital warts.
        C. The most common cause of mortality for this patient would be
           suicide.
        D. Hepatitis C vaccination should be offered to this patient.

ANSWERS

2.1   **A.** Cervical cytology of the vaginal cuff is unnecessary when the hys-
        terectomy was for benign indications (not cervical dysplasia or cer-
        vical cancer), and when there is no history of abnormal Pap smears.

Colon cancer screening is generally started at age 50. DEXA scan for osteoporosis screening should be considered in any postmenopausal woman at risk, such as having an osteoporosis-related fracture, a family history, or being thin and Caucasian. Pneumococcal vaccine is generally given at age 65.

2.2   **C.** The varicella zoster vaccine is a live attenuated vaccine, recommended for individuals aged 60 and above, and has been shown to greatly reduce the incidence of herpes zoster (shingles), and the severity and likelihood of post-herpetic neuralgia. It has no efficacy in preventing HSV.

2.3   **A.** Cervical cytology should be deferred until age 21 or 3 years after initiation of sexual intercourse. This is due to the fact that adolescents many times will clear the HPV infection, and cause an abnormal Pap smear to normalized. The HPV vaccine should be recommended to all females between the age of 9 and 26, regardless of exposures. The most common cause of mortality for adolescent females is motor vehicle accidents. The hepatitis C vaccine is currently not available, but hopefully in several years, it may be developed.

Clinical Pearls

➤ The basic approach to health maintenance is threefold: (1) cancer screening, (2) age-appropriate immunizations, and (3) screening for common diseases.

➤ The most common cause of mortality in a woman younger than 20 years is motor vehicle accidents.

➤ The most common cause of mortality of a woman older than 39 years is cardiovascular disease.

➤ Major conditions in women aged 65 years and older include osteoporosis, heart disease, breast cancer, and depression.

➤ Cervical cytology screening does not appear to be cost-effective in women older than age 65 when prior Pap smears have been normal.

REFERENCES

American College of Obstetricians and Gynecologists. Primary and preventive care: periodic assessments. *ACOG Committee Opinion 357*. Washington, DC: 2006.

American College of Obstetricians and Gynecologists. Low bone mass (osteopenia) and fracture risk. *ACOG Committee Opinion 407*. Washington, DC: 2008.

Centers for Disease Control. Immunization schedule for adults, 2008. www.cdc.gov/mmwr/acip/rr5515a1.htm. Accessed Feb 6, 2009.

Case 3

After a 4-hour labor, a 31-year-old G4 P3 woman undergoes an uneventful vaginal delivery of a 7 lb 8 oz infant over an intact perineum. During her labor, she is noted to have mild variable decelerations and accelerations that increase 20 beats per minute (bpm) above the baseline heart rate. At delivery, the male baby has Apgar scores of 8 at 1 minute, and 9 at 5 minute. Slight lengthening of the cord occurs after 28 minute along with a small gush of blood per vagina. As the placenta is being delivered, a shaggy, reddish, bulging mass is noted at the introitus around the placenta.

➤ What is the most likely diagnosis?

➤ What is the most likely complication to occur in this patient?

ANSWERS TO CASE 3:
Uterine Inversion

Summary: A 31-year-old G4 P3 woman has a normal vaginal delivery of her baby, and after slight lengthening of the cord, a reddish mass is noted bulging in the introitus.

➤ **Most likely diagnosis:** Uterine inversion.

➤ **Most likely complication:** Postpartum hemorrhage.

ANALYSIS

Objectives

1. Know the signs of spontaneous placental separation.
2. Recognize the clinical presentation of uterine inversion.
3. Understand that the most common cause of uterine inversion is undue traction of the cord before placental separation.

Considerations

This patient's history reveals that the first and second stages of labor are normal. The third stage of labor (placental delivery) reaches close to the upper limits of normal. The evidence for placental separation is never definite. The four signs of placental separation are: (1) gush of blood, (2) lengthening of the cord, (3) globular and firm shape of the uterus, and (4) the uterus rises up to the anterior abdominal wall. In this case, although there is not good evidence for placental separation, traction on the cord is exerted, which results in an inverted uterus. The reddish bulging mass noted adjacent to the placenta is the endometrial surface; hence, the mass will have a shaggy appearance and be all around the placenta. Other masses and/or organs may at times prolapse, such as vaginal or cervical tissue, but these will have a smooth appearance.

APPROACH TO
Inverted Uterus

DEFINITIONS

THIRD STAGE OF LABOR: From delivery of infant to the delivery of the placenta (upper limit of normal is 30 minutes).

ABNORMALLY RETAINED PLACENTA: Third stage of labor that has exceeded 30 minutes.

UTERINE INVERSION: A "turning inside out" of the uterus; whereupon the fundus of the uterus moves through the cervix, into the vagina (Figure 3–1).

SIGNS OF PLACENTAL SEPARATION: Cord lengthening, gush of blood, globular uterine shape, and uterus lifting up to the anterior abdominal wall.

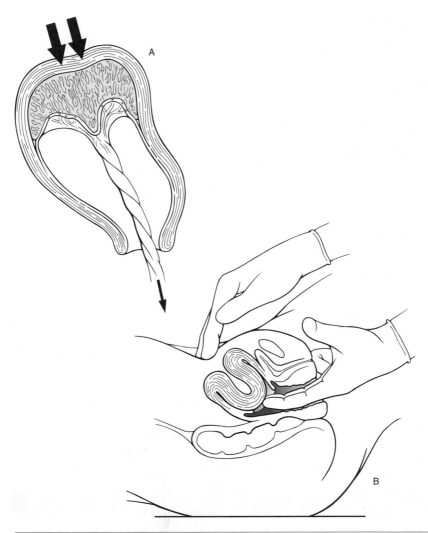

Figure 3–1.   Inverted uterus. Uterine inversion can occur when excessive umbilical cord traction is exerted on a fundally implanted, unseparated placenta (**A**). Upon recognition, the operator attempts to reposition the inverted uterus using cupped fingers (**B**).

CLINICAL APPROACH

After a vaginal delivery, 95% of women experience spontaneous placenta separation within 30 minutes. Because the uterus and placenta are no longer joined, the placenta is usually in the lower segment of the uterus, just inside the cervix, and the uterus is often contracted. The umbilical cord lengthens due to the placenta having dropped into the lower portion of the uterus. The gush of blood represents bleeding from the placental bed, usually coinciding with placental separation. If the placenta has not separated, excessive force on the cord may lead to uterine inversion. Massive hemorrhage usually results; thus, in this situation, the practitioner must be prepared for rapid volume replacement. Although it was classically taught by some that the shock was out of proportion to the actual amount of blood loss, this is not the case. In other words, shock is due to massive hemorrhage.

The best method of averting a uterine inversion is to await spontaneous separation from the placenta from the uterus before placing traction on the umbilical cord. Even after one or two of the signs of placental separation are present, the operator should be cautious not to put undue tension on the cord. At times, part of the placenta may separate, revealing the gush of blood, but the remaining attached placenta may induce a uterine inversion or traumatic severing of the cord. The grand-multiparous patient with the placenta implanted in the fundus (top of uterus) is at particular risk for uterine inversion. A placenta accreta, an abnormally adherent placenta, is also a risk factor.

Treatment

With the diagnosis of an inverted uterus, immediate assistance—including that of an anesthesiologist—is essential because a uterine relaxation anesthetic agent, such as halothane (for uterine replacement), and/or emergency surgery may be necessary. If the placenta has already separated, the recently inverted uterus may sometimes be replaced by using the gloved palm and cupped fingers. Two intravenous lines should be started as soon as possible and preferably prior to placental separation, since profuse hemorrhage may follow placental removal. Terbutaline or magnesium sulfate can also be utilized to relax the uterus if necessary prior to uterine replacement. Upon replacing the uterine fundus to the normal location, the relaxation agents are stopped, and then uterotonic agents, such as oxytocin, are given. Placement of the clinician's fist inside the uterus to maintain the normal structure of the uterus is important.

Note: Even with optimal treatment of uterine inversion, hemorrhage is almost a certainty.

Comprehension Questions

3.1 A 23-year-old G1 P0 woman at 38 weeks' gestation delivered a 7 lb 4 oz baby boy vaginally. Upon delivery of the placenta, there was noted to be an inverted uterus, which was successfully managed including replacement of the uterus. Which of the following placental implantation sites would most likely predispose to an inverted uterus?

A. Fundal
B. Anterior
C. Posterior
D. Lateral
E. Lower segment

3.2 A 24-year-old woman underwent a normal vaginal delivery of a term infant female. After the delivery, the placenta does not deliver even after 30 minutes. Which of the following would be the next step for this patient?

A. Initiate oxytocin.
B. Wait for an additional 30 minutes.
C. Hysterectomy.
D. Attempt a manual extraction of the placenta.
E. Misoprostol estrogen intravaginally.

3.3 A 32-year-old G1 P0 woman at 40 weeks' gestation undergoes a normal vaginal delivery. Delivery of the placenta is complicated by an inverted uterus, with subsequent hemorrhage leading to 1500 mL of blood loss. She is managed with a transfusion of erythrocytes. Which of the following is the best explanation of the mechanism of hemorrhage?

A. Inverted uterus stretches the uterus, causing trauma to blood vessels leading to bleeding.
B. Inverted uterus leads to inability for an adequate myometrial contraction effect.
C. Inverted uterus causes a local coagulopathic reaction to the uterus and endometrium.
D. Inverted uterus causes muscular abrasions and lacerations leading to bleeding.

3.4 A 33-year-old G5 P5 woman, who is being induced for preeclampsia delivers a 9 lb baby. Upon delivery of the placenta, uterine inversion is noted. The physician attempts to replace the uterus, but the cervix is tightly contracted, preventing the fundus of the uterus from being repositioned. Which of the following is the best therapy for this patient?

A. Vaginal hysterectomy.
B. Dührssen incisions of the cervix.
C. Halothane anesthesia.
D. Discontinue the magnesium sulfate.
E. Infuse oxytocin intravenously.

ANSWERS

3.1 **A.** A fundally implanted placenta predisposes to uterine inversion. A placenta implanted in either the anterior, posterior, lateral, or lower segment of the uterus does not have the direct angle that a fundally implanted placenta has through the cervix and out the vagina. The best method for preventing inversion is to await spontaneous separation of the placenta from the uterus before placing traction on the umbilical cord.

3.2 **D.** After 30 minutes, the placenta is abnormally retained, and a manual extraction is generally attempted. Waiting for another 30 minutes may lead to maternal hemorrhage, which may then lead to an indication for a hysterectomy. However, a hysterectomy would not be the initial step after 30 minutes have passed during the third stage of labor. Oxytocin should not be given until the uterine fundus is placed back to its normal location. Oxytocin is a uterotonic agent that aids in allowing the uterus to contract down on itself in an effort to stop bleeding after the placenta has been removed. Intravaginal estrogen is not indicated for this scenario and is typically prescribed to patient with vaginal atrophy.

3.3 **B.** An inverted uterus makes it impossible for the uterus to establish its normal tone, and to contract. Thus, the myometrial fibers do not exert their normal tourniquet effect on the spiral arteries. The endometrial placental bed pours out blood, which previously had been perfusing the intervillous space. Thus, uterine atony is the most common reason for hemorrhage in inverted uterus. The muscle of the uterus and the vasculature is seldom damaged. Replacing the uterus to its normal position and assisting tonicity of the uterus will alleviate the bleeding.

3.4 **C.** A uterine relaxing agent (such as halothane anesthesia) is the best initial therapy for a nonreducible uterus. Terbutaline and magnesium sulfate can also be used to relax the uterus if necessary. Oxytocin is a uterotonic agent and may be used following replacement of the uterine fundus to its normal location. Dührssen incisions are used to treat the entrapped fetal head of a breech vaginal delivery and would not be indicated for uterine inversion. A vaginal hysterectomy would not be the best treatment option for this patient either.

Clinical Pearls

➤ Although it can occur spontaneously, one of the most common causes of inverted uterus is undue traction on the cord when the placenta has not yet separated.

➤ The signs of placental separation are (1) gush of blood, (2) lengthening of the cord, (3) globular-shaped uterus, and (4) the uterus rising to the anterior abdominal wall.

➤ Hemorrhage is a common complication of an inverted uterus.

➤ The upper limit of normal for the third stage of labor (time between delivery of the infant to delivery of the placenta) is 30 minutes.

➤ When the placenta does not deliver spontaneously after 30 minutes, then a manual extraction of the placenta should be attempted.

REFERENCES

American College of Obstetricians and Gynecologists. Postpartum hemorrhage. ACOG *Practice Bulletin 76*. Washington, DC: American College of Obstetricians and Gynecologists; 2006.

Cunningham FG, Leveno KJ, Bloom SL, Gilstrap LC III, Hauth JC, Wenstrom KD. Obstetrical hemorrhage. In: *Williams Obstetrics*. 22nd ed. New York, NY: McGraw-Hill; 2005:809-854.

Kim M, Hyashi RH, Gambone JC. Obstetrical hemorrhage and puerperal sepsis. In: Hacker NF, Gambone JC, Hobel CJ, eds. *Essentials of Obstetrics and Gynecology*, 5th ed. Philadelphia, PA: Saunders; 2009:128-138.

Case 4

A 49-year-old woman complains of irregular menses over the past 6 months, feelings of inadequacy, vaginal dryness, difficulty sleeping, and episodes of warmth and sweating at night. On examination, her blood pressure is 120/68 mm Hg, heart rate is 90 beats per minute, and temperature is 99°F (37.2°C). Her thyroid gland is normal to palpation. The cardiac and lung examinations are unremarkable. The breasts are symmetric, without masses or discharge. Examination of the external genitalia does not reveal any masses.

➤ What is the most likely diagnosis?

➤ What is your next diagnostic step?

ANSWERS TO CASE 4:
Perimenopause

Summary: A 49-year-old woman complains of irregular menses, feelings of inadequacy, sleeplessness, and episodes of warmth and sweating.

➤ **Most likely diagnosis:** Climacteric (perimenopausal state).

➤ **Next diagnostic step:** Serum follicle-stimulating hormone (FSH) and luteinizing hormone (LH).

ANALYSIS

Objectives

1. Understand the normal clinical presentation of women in the perimenopausal state.
2. Understand that elevated serum FSH and LH levels help to confirm the diagnosis.
3. Know that estrogen replacement therapy is usually effective in treating the hot flushes.
4. Know the risks of continuous estrogen-progestin therapy.

Considerations

This 49-year-old woman complains of irregular menses, feelings of inadequacy, and intermittent sensations of warmth and sweating. This constellation of symptoms is consistent with the perimenopause, or climacteric state. Between the age of 40 and 51 years, the majority of women begin to experience symptoms of hypoestrogenemia, primarily hot flushes. Hot flushes, which are the typical vasomotor change due to decreased estrogen levels, are associated with skin temperature elevation and sweating lasting for 2 to 4 minutes. The low estrogen concentration also has an effect on the vagina by decreasing the epithelial thickness, leading to atrophy and dryness. Elevated serum FSH and LH levels are helpful in confirming the diagnosis of the perimenopause. Treatment for hot flushes includes estrogen replacement therapy with progestin. When a woman still has her uterus, the addition of progestin to estrogen replacement is important in preventing endometrial cancer.

Note: The selective estrogen receptor modulator (SERM), raloxifene, does not treat hot flushes.

APPROACH TO
Menopause

DEFINITIONS

MENOPAUSE: The point in time in a woman's life when there is cessation of menses due to follicular atresia occurring after age 40 years (mean age 51 years).

PERIMENOPAUSE (CLIMACTERIC): The transitional 2 to 4 years spanning from immediately before to immediately after the menopause.

HOT FLUSHES: Irregular unpredictable episodes of increased skin temperature and sweating lasting about 3 to 4 minutes caused by vasomotor changes.

PREMATURE OVARIAN FAILURE: The cessation of ovarian function due to atresia of follicles prior to age 40 years. At ages younger than 30 years, autoimmune diseases or karyotypic abnormalities should be considered.

CLINICAL APPROACH

At about 47 years of age, most women experience perimenopausal symptoms due to the ovaries' impending failure. Symptoms include irregular menses due to anovulatory cycles; vasomotor symptoms, such as hot flushes; and decreased estrogen and androgen levels. Because ovarian inhibin levels are decreased, FSH and LH levels rise even before estradiol levels fall. The decreased estradiol concentrations lead to vaginal atrophy, bone loss, and vasomotor symptoms. While most clinicians agree that estrogen replacement therapy is currently the best treatment for the vasomotor symptoms and to prevent osteoporosis, scientific data raises concerns about the risks of this therapy. The Women's Health Initiative Study of continuous estrogen-progestin treatment reported a small but significant increased risk of breast cancer, heart disease, pulmonary embolism, and stroke. Women on hormone replacement therapy had fewer fractures and a lower incidence of colon cancer.

It should be noted that there is no evidence of adverse effects from short-term (<6 months) estrogen therapy for the acute relief of menopausal symptoms. Currently, hormone replacement therapy is indicated for vasomotor symptoms, and should be used for as short a duration as possible in the smallest dose. For women who cannot or choose not to take estrogen, the antihypertensive agent clonidine may help with the vasomotor symptoms. A selective estrogen receptor modulator (SERM), such as raloxifene, is helpful in preventing bone loss, but does not alter the hot flushes. Weight-bearing exercise, calcium and vitamin D supplementation, and estrogen replacement are important cornerstones in maintaining bone mass. Because the FSH responds to the inhibin and not to estrogen, the FSH level cannot be used to titrate the estrogen replacement dose. In other words, the FSH concentration is still elevated even though the estrogen replacement may be sufficient.

Other diseases that are important to consider in the perimenopausal woman include hypothyroidism, diabetes mellitus, hypertension, and breast cancer. Women in this stage of life may also experience depression, whether spontaneous in its onset or situational due to grief or midlife adjustments. The practitioner should advocate aerobic exercise at least three times a week, again, with weight-bearing exercise being advantageous for the prevention of osteoporosis. Bone mineral density (BMD) testing, such as by dual-energy x-ray absorptiometry (DEXA), is useful in the early identification of osteoporosis and osteopenia. BMD testing is indicated for all postmenopausal women aged 65 years or older and postmenopausal women at risk for osteoporosis and presenting with a bone fracture. Alcohol abuse may be seen in up to 10% of postmenopausal women, and requires clinical suspicion to establish the diagnosis.

Comprehension Questions

Which of the following single best mechanisms (A-H) best matches the clinical situations described (4.1-4.6)?

    A. Gonadotropin receptor insensitivity
    B. Pituitary dysfunction
    C. Ovarian failure
    D. Ovarian cortical atrophy syndrome
    E. Peritoneal interference with ovulation
    F. Hypothalamic dysfunction
    G. Estrogen excess
    H. Immune down-regulation of ovary

4.1   A 51-year-old woman with oligomenorrhea and hot flushes.

4.2   A 22-year-old nonpregnant woman with galactorrhea and hyperprolactinemia.

4.3   A 25-year-old woman slightly obese, slightly hirsute, and with a long history of irregular menses.

4.4   An 18-year-old adolescent female with infantile breast development has not started her menses. She has some webbing of the neck region.

4.5   A 19-year-old nonpregnant woman marathon runner with amenorrhea.

4.6   A 33-year-old woman who has not started her menses since a vaginal delivery 1 year previously complicated by postpartum hemorrhage. She was unable to breastfeed her baby.

4.7   A 25-year-old woman has a history of 1 year of amenorrhea due to hyper-prolactinemia. She has bilateral galactorrhea due to a prolactin-secreting adenoma. Which of the following tests is also likely to reveal an abnormal finding?

A. DEXA scan of the spine
B. Endometrial biopsy
C. Mammography of the breasts
D. Thyroid-stimulating hormone (TSH) level

ANSWERS

4.1   **C.** Ovarian failure due to follicular atresia is the reason for oligo-ovulation in the perimenopausal years. During perimenopause (or climacteric), follicular atresia occurs from *hypo*estrogenemia, as do the vasomotor changes that lead to hot flushes. There is nothing dysfunctional occurring in this scenario, as it is a common occurrence in a perimenopausal patient.

4.2   **F.** Both hypothyroidism and hyperprolactinemia may cause hypothalamic dysfunction, which inhibits gonadotropin-releasing hormone pulsations, which in turn inhibit pituitary FSH and LH release. The lack of gonadotropins, FSH and LH, leads to hypoestrogenic amenorrhea. A common cause of hyperprolactinemia in a girl *hypot.* of this age is a prolactinoma. This is not a pituitary problem, nor a receptor insensitivity issue. There is no pathology related to the ovaries, however this patient will most likely be amenorrheic due to the lack of stimulation to the ovaries by the gonadotropins.

4.3   **G.** This patient most likely has polycystic ovarian syndrome (PCOS). *estrogen + androgen↑* Women with PCOS often are obese and hirsute, have anovulation and insulin resistance, but an estrogen excess. Because of this, they are often prescribed progesterone alone or combination oral contraceptive pills to induce vaginal bleeding and to prevent endometrial hyperplasia.

4.4   **C.** Ovarian failure is the most likely etiology in this woman with probable Turner syndrome (45,X). It would be reflected by elevated gonadotropin levels and streaked ovaries. She most likely has decreased estrogen levels as well, which predisposes her to complications such as osteoporosis later in life. This patient's symptoms result from a chromosomal abnormality and not a hypothalamic or pituitary dysfunction.

4.5   **F.** Excessive exercise may lead to hypothalamic dysfunction, but many times simple weight gain will lead to its restoration of function. This patient has amenorrhea, and therefore is in a hypoestrogenic state. This puts this patient at an increased risk of bone fractures. Many times these individuals are placed on OCPs in order to maintain normal hypothalamic function. There is no pathology related to the ovaries or pituitary in this scenario.

4.6   **B.** Sheehan syndrome is when the anterior pituitary suffers from hemorrhagic necrosis associated with postpartum hemorrhage. She is unable to breastfeed due to her inability to release prolactin from the anterior pituitary. This patient's symptoms are unrelated to the ovaries and hypothalamus. This patient would be in a hypoestrogenic state due to the lack of gonadotropin stimulation. Treatment for this would be supplemental hormonal replacement.

4.7   **A.** Amenorrhea due to hyperprolactinemia causes a hypoestrogenic state due to decreased GnRH release, and decreased FSH and LH secretion. Ovarian estrogen levels are decreased, leading to decreased bone mineral density. Hence the DEXA scan is most likely to be abnormal. The endometrial biopsy is likely to be normal, or perhaps show atrophic changes due to the hypoestrogenic state, and certainly not likely to show hyperplasia or cancer. The mammogram would not be affected. The thyroid gland is not affected by hyperprolactinemia; rather, hypothyroidism can lead to hyperprolactinemia, not vice versa.

Clinical Pearls

➤ Hot flushes and irregular menses after the age of 45 years are most likely due to the climacteric, and the symptoms usually respond to estrogen replacement therapy.

➤ The current indication for hormone replacement therapy in the menopausal woman is significant vasomotor symptoms, and the lowest dose should be used for the shortest duration feasible.

➤ The most common location of an osteoporosis-associated fracture is the thoracic spine as a compression fracture.

➤ Weight-bearing exercise, calcium and vitamin D supplementation, and estrogen replacement therapy are the important cornerstones in the prevention of osteoporosis.

➤ Progestin should be added to estrogen replacement therapy when a woman has her uterus, to prevent endometrial cancer.

➤ Continuous estrogen-progestin therapy may be associated with a small but significant risk of cardiovascular disease and breast cancer.

REFERENCES

American College of Obstetricians and Gynecologists. Hormone therapy and heart disease. ACOG *Committee Opinion 420*. Washington, DC: 2008.

American College of Obstetricians and Gynecologists. Low bone mass (osteopenia) and fracture risk. ACOG *Committee Opinion 407*. Washington, DC: 2008.

Laufer LR, Gambone JC. Climacteric: menopause and peri- and post-menopause. In: Hacker NF, Gambone JC, Hobel CJ, eds. *Essentials of Obstetrics and Gynecology*, 5th ed. Philadelphia, PA: Saunders; 2009:379-385.

Lobo RA. Menopause. In: Katz VL, Lentz GM, Lobo RA, Gersenson DM, eds. *Comprehensive Gynecology*. 5th ed. St. Louis, MO: Mosby-Year Book; 2007:1039-1072.

Writing Group for the Women's Health Initiative Investigators. Risks and benefits of estrogen plus progestin in healthy postmenopausal women. *JAMA*. 2002;288(3):321-333.

Case 5

A 28-year-old woman who underwent a cesarean delivery 1 week ago is brought into the emergency room with a blood pressure of 60/40 mm Hg. The patient's husband states that she had 2 days of nausea and vomiting, fever to 102°F (38.8°C), and myalgias. The reason for the cesarean was arrest of active phase, with cervical dilation at 5 cm for 3 hours despite strong uterine contractions. She was discharged home on postoperative day 3 in good condition. On examination, the patient appears lethargic and has mental confusion. Auscultation of her heart reveals tachycardia. The lung examination demonstrates slight crackles at the lung bases. The abdomen is tender throughout, and the fundus of the uterus is slightly tender. The skin incision is tender, red, and indurated. Upon opening the incision, purulent material is expressed. The underlying tissue is palpated and has a brawny texture with crepitance noted. The laboratory evaluation reveals a hemoglobin level of 15 g/dL and a serum creatinine of 2.1 mg/dL.

➤ What is the most likely diagnosis?

➤ What is the next step in therapy?

ANSWERS TO CASE 5:
Necrotizing Fasciitis

Summary: A 28-year-old woman has fever to 102°F (38.8°C), myalgias, vomiting, hypotension, confusion, and a skin incision that is infected with underlying tissue revealing brawny and crepitance. She has evidence of hemoconcentration and renal insufficiency.

> ➤ **Most likely diagnosis:** Necrotizing fasciitis.

> ➤ **Next step in therapy:** Isotonic intravenous fluids, broad-spectrum antibiotics, and immediate surgical debridement.

ANALYSIS

Objectives

1. Recognize the manifestations of shock.
2. Understand that necrotizing fasciitis is a rare but potentially fatal infection that can affect patients.
3. Understand that aggressive fluid resuscitation, broad-spectrum antibiotics, and immediate surgical debridement are fundamental in the treatment of necrotizing fasciitis.

Considerations

This patient presents with multiple life-threatening issues. First the hypotension must be recognized, since her blood pressure is 60/40 mm Hg. Her mean arterial pressure is 47 mm Hg, which is insufficient to maintain cerebral perfusion. Regardless of the etiology, the blood pressure needs to be supported immediately. Because the patient has a fever of 102°F (38.8°C) with hypotension, and no history of hemorrhage or postpartum bleeding, septic shock is the most likely diagnosis. The first step in resuscitation should therefore be addressed at supporting the blood pressure, with aggressive use of intravenous isotonic fluids. A Foley catheter measuring urine output can help to assess urine output and indirectly kidney perfusion, particularly since the patient has an elevated serum creatinine level. The goal is to keep the mean arterial blood pressure at least 65 mm Hg to perfuse her vital organs. Ideally, this patient would have a urine output of at least 25 to 30 mL/h (depending on the degree of renal insufficiency). Furthermore, this woman most likely has necrotizing fasciitis since she has the wound infection complicated by the underlying tissue having an abnormal consistency upon palpation. The crepitance is due to gas in the soft tissue. This is likely due to anaerobic bacteria. Her myalgias, fever, nausea, and vomiting indicate the systemic nature of the infection.

APPROACH TO
Necrotizing Fasciitis

DEFINITIONS

NECROTIZING FASCIITIS: A serious infection of the muscle and fascia usually caused by multiple organisms or anaerobes. It can involve surgical infections, traumatic injury, or rarely Group A Streptococci (flesh-eating bacteria).

GROUP A STREPTOCOCCAL TOXIC SHOCK SYNDROME: Rapidly progressing infection of the episiotomy or cesarean delivery incision ("flesh-eating bacteria" syndrome).

SHOCK: Condition of circulatory insufficiency where tissue perfusion needs are not met.

SEPTIC SHOCK: Circulatory insufficiency due to infection or the body's response to infection, commonly caused by gram-negative endotoxins.

$$\text{Mean arterial pressure (MAP)} = [(2 \times \text{Diastolic blood pressure}) + (1 \times \text{Systolic blood pressure})]/3$$

CLINICAL APPROACH

The management of septic shock includes copious intravenous fluids with close monitoring of urine output and blood pressure. At times, invasive hemodynamic monitoring with a central venous catheter or Swan-Ganz line is needed. Intravenous antibiotics should be broad spectrum to include penicillin, gentamicin, and metronidazole or other anaerobic agent, and dopamine or dobutamine are sometimes required when fluids alone are insufficient to maintain the blood pressure. Addressing the underlying etiology of the septic shock is important. When dealing with an aggressive wound infection, immediate surgical debridement, sometimes very radical or wide excisional procedures, is warranted. Necrotic and infected tissue must be removed, and sometimes requires multiple surgeries. Monitoring of blood pressure, heart ratio, oxygen saturation, urine output, and neutral status is important. Once the patient is stabilized, treating the underlying cause typically leads to resolution. Septic shock initially presents as decreased urine output and if untreated, proceeds to ischemia of vital organs and death.

Comprehension Questions

5.1   A 35-year-old woman is noted to have a blood pressure of 80/40 mm Hg, fever, and abdominal pain. Which of the following is the likely mechanism of the patient's hypotension?
        A. Cardiac contractility dysfunction
        B. Cardiac bradycardia
        C. Third spacing of fluid
        D. Vasodilation

5.2   A 45-year-old woman is noted to have a surgical incision site that is suspicious for necrotizing fasciitis. Which of the following is most consistent with necrotizing fasciitis?
        A. Redness of the surgical incision
        B. Induration and edema of the surgical incision
        C. Gas in the surgical tissue
        D. Gram-negative rods growing from blood culture

5.3   A 30-year-old woman is brought into the emergency department with fever and a blood pressure of 70/40 mm Hg. She is presumed to be in septic shock. Which of the following is a fundamental principle for the treatment?
        A. Intravenous normal saline
        B. Plasmapheresis
        C. Oral fluid resuscitation
        D. Await blood culture results prior to initiation of antibiotic therapy

ANSWERS

5.1   **D.** The pathophysiology of septic shock is vasodilation usually due to endotoxins, although at times, such as with *Staphylococcus aureus* (toxic shock syndrome), exotoxins can be causative. The vasodilation leads to hypotension, and is treated with IV fluids. If the IV fluids are insufficient to produce a correction in hypotension, then vasoconstrictors are indicated, such as dopamine. Late in the course of septic shock, cardiac dysfunction can occur; however, at this stage, the patient is typically in a near terminal condition.

5.2   **C.** Gas in the muscle or fascia is indicative of necrotizing fasciitis, likely due to a clostridial species. Induration and redness of the surgical wound is suggestive of a superficial wound infection, in which the skin and subcutaneous tissue is infected. This is a superficial surgical site infection, and needs to be opened. The superficial wound infection is not as life-threatening as when a deep surgical site infection occurs.

5.3   **A.** Intravenous isotonic fluids are the initial treatment of choice for septic shock. The cornerstones of therapy include removing the nidus of infection, antibiotic therapy, and support of the blood pressure. Plasmapheresis is not a major part of the treatment of septic shock.

Clinical Pearls

➤ The cornerstones of treatment of septic shock include aggressive intravenous fluids, source control, antibiotic therapy, and monitoring perfusion and organ function.

➤ Source control in septic shock means removing the etiology of the infection.

➤ The sunburn-like rash and/or desquamation is typical for *S aureus* infections.

➤ The initial antibiotic therapy for serious *S aureus* infections is generally intravenous nafcillin or methicillin unless methicillin resistance is suspected, in which case vancomycin is used.

➤ Hypotension that persists despite intravenous isotonic fluid replacement generally requires pressor support such as with intravenous infusion of dopamine.

REFERENCES

Cunningham FG, Leveno KJ, Bloom SL, Hauth JC, Gilstrap LC III, Wenstrom KD. Puerperal infection. In: *Williams Obstetrics*. 22nd ed. New York, NY: McGraw-Hill; 2005:671-688.

Katz VL. Postoperative counseling and management. In: Katz VL, Lentz GM, Lobo RA, Gersenson DM, eds. *Comprehensive Gynecology*. 5th ed. St. Louis, MO: Mosby-Year Book; 2007:661-710.

Gambone JC. Gynecologic procedures. In: Hacker NF, Gambone JC, Hobel CJ, eds. *Essentials of Obstetrics and Gynecology*, 5th ed. Philadelphia, PA: Saunders; 2009: 332-344.

Case 6

A 26-year-old G1 P0 woman at 39 weeks' gestation is admitted to the hospital in labor. She is noted to have uterine contractions every 7 to 10 minutes. Her antepartum history is significant for a nonimmune rubella status. On examination, her blood pressure (BP) is 110/70 mm Hg, and heart rate (HR) is 80 beats per minute (bpm). The estimated fetal weight is 7 lb. On pelvic examination, she has been noted to have a change in cervical examinations from 4-cm dilation to 7 cm over the last 2 hours. The pelvis is assessed to be adequate on digital examination.

➤ What is your next step in the management of this patient?

ANSWER TO CASE 6:
Labor (Normal Active Phase)

Summary: A 26-year-old G1 P0 woman at term with an adequate pelvis on clinical pelvimetry, nonimmune rubella status, is in labor. Her cervix has changed from 4-cm to 7-cm dilation over 2 hours with uterine contractions noted every 7 to 10 minutes.

➤ **Next step in management:** Continue to observe the labor.

ANALYSIS

Objectives

1. Know the normal labor parameters in the latent and active phase for nulliparous and multiparous patients.
2. Be familiar with the management of common labor abnormalities and know that normal labor does not require intervention.
3. Know that rubella vaccination, as a live-attenuated preparation, should not be administered during pregnancy.

Considerations

This 26-year-old G1 P0 woman is at term (defined as between 37 to 42 completed weeks from the last menstrual period). She is in the active phase of labor (generally about 4 cm of dilation) and her cervix has changed from 4 cm to 7 cm over 2 hours; her contractions are only every 7 to 10 minutes. Because she is nulliparous, the expectation is that her cervix will dilate at a rate of at least 1.2 cm/h during the active phase of labor. She has met these norms by a change of 1.5 cm/h (3 cm over 2 hours). The uterine contraction pattern appears suboptimal, but it is the change in the cervix per time and not the uterine contraction pattern that dictates normalcy in labor. Because she has had a normal labor, the appropriate management is to observe her course without intervention. The clinical pelvimetry is accomplished by digital palpation of the pelvic bones. This patient's pelvis was judged to be adequate. Unfortunately, this estimation is not very precise, and in clinical practice, the clinician would generally observe the labor of a nulliparous patient. Finally, the nonimmune rubella status should alert the practitioner to immunize for rubella during the postpartum time (since the rubella vaccine is live-attenuated and is contraindicated during pregnancy).

APPROACH TO
Labor Evaluation

DEFINITIONS

LABOR: Cervical change accompanied by regular uterine contractions.

LATENT PHASE: The initial part of labor where the cervix mainly effaces (thins) rather than dilates (usually cervical dilation >4 cm).

ACTIVE PHASE: The portion of labor where dilation occurs more rapidly, usually when the cervix is greater than 4-cm dilation.

PROTRACTION OF ACTIVE PHASE: Cervical dilation in the active phase that is less than expected (normal ≥1.2 cm/h for a nulliparous woman, and ≥ 1.5 cm/h for a woman who has had at least one vaginal delivery).

ARREST OF ACTIVE PHASE: No progress in the active phase of labor for 2 hours.

STAGES OF LABOR: First stage: onset of labor to complete dilation of cervix. Second stage: complete cervical dilation to delivery of infant. Third stage: delivery of infant to delivery of placenta.

FETAL HEART RATE BASELINE: Normally between 110 and 160 bpm. Fetal bradycardia is a baseline less than 110 bpm, and fetal tachycardia is exceeding 160 bpm.

DECELERATIONS: Fetal heart rate episodic changes below the baseline. There are three types of decelerations: early (mirror image of uterine contractions), variable (abrupt jagged dips below the baseline), and late which are offset following the uterine contraction.

ACCELERATIONS: Episodes of the fetal heart rate that increase above the baseline for at least 15 bpm and last for at least 15 seconds.

CLINICAL APPROACH TO LABOR

The assessment of labor is based on cervical change versus time (Table 6–1). Normal labor should be expectantly managed. When a labor abnormality is diagnosed, then the three Ps should be evaluated (powers, passenger, and pelvis). When inadequate "powers" are thought to be the etiology, then oxytocin may be initiated to augment the uterine contraction strength and/or frequency. When the latent phase exceeds the upper limits of normal, then it is called a prolonged latent phase. When the cervix has exceeded 4 to 5 cm, particularly with near-complete effacement, then the active phase has been reached. When there is cervical dilation but less than the minimum expected change, then this is called protraction of active phase. When the

Table 6–1 NORMAL LABOR PARAMETERS

	NULLIPARA (LOWER LIMITS OF NORMAL)	MULTIPARA (LOWER LIMITS OF NORMAL)
Latent phase (dilation <4 cm)	≤18-20 h	≤14 h
Active phase	≥1.2 cm/h	≤1.5 cm/h
Second stage of labor (complete dilation to expulsion of infant)	≤2h ≤3h if epidural	≤1 h ≤2h if epidural
Third stage of labor	≤30 min	≤30 min

Data from Friedman EA. *Labor: Evaluation and Management.* 2nd ed. East Norwalk, CT: Appleton-Century-Crofts; 1978.

cervix does not dilate for 2 hours in the active phase, then it is called arrest of active phase.

When there is cephalopelvic disproportion, where the pelvis is too small for the fetus (either due to an abnormal pelvis or an excessively large baby), then cesarean delivery must be considered. When the "powers" are thought to be the factor, then intravenous oxytocin may be initiated via a dilute titration. Clinically adequate uterine contractions are defined as contractions every 2 to 3 minutes, firm on palpation, and lasting for at least 40 to 60 seconds (Figure 6–1). Some clinicians choose to use internal uterine catheters to evaluate the adequacy of the powers. One common assessment tool is to examine a 10-minute window and add each contraction's rise above baseline (each mm Hg rise is called a Montevideo unit). A calculation that meets or exceeds 200 Montevideo units is commonly accepted as an adequate uterine contraction pattern (Figure 6–2).

Fetal heart rate assessment can help to assess the fetal status. A normal baseline between 110 and 160 bpm, with accelerations, and variability are indicative of a normal well-oxygenated fetus. Fetal tachycardia can occur due to a variety of disorders such as maternal fever. Fetal bradycardia, if profound and prolonged, necessitates intervention. The most common decelerations are variable, caused by cord compression. If these are intermittent with abrupt return to baseline, then they can be observed. Early decelerations, caused by fetal head compression, are benign. Late decelerations are "offset" from the uterine contraction with their onset after the onset of the contraction, the nadir following the contraction peak, and the return to baseline following the contraction resolution. Late decelerations suggest fetal hypoxia, and if persistent, can indicate fetal acidemia. (See Figure 6-3).

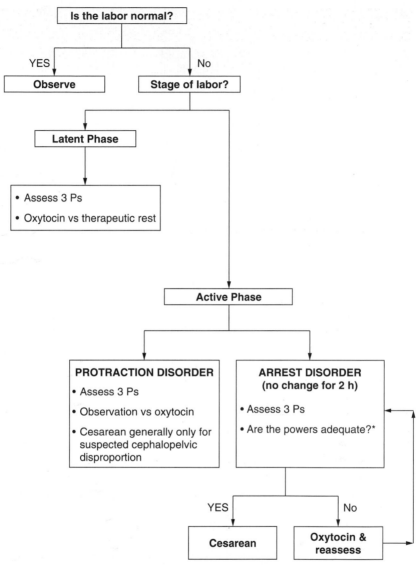

* Adequate contractions generally > 200 Montevideo units or clinically contractions q 2-3 min, firm, lasting 40-60 sec.

Figure 6–1.   Algorithm for management of labor.

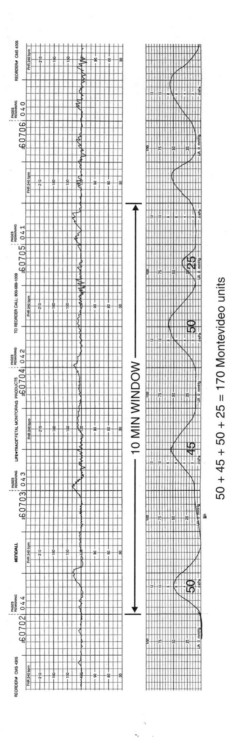

50 + 45 + 50 + 25 = 170 Montevideo units

Figure 6–2. Calculating Montevideo units. Montevideo units are calculated by the sum of the amplitudes (in mm Hg) above baseline of the uterine contractions within a 10-minute window.

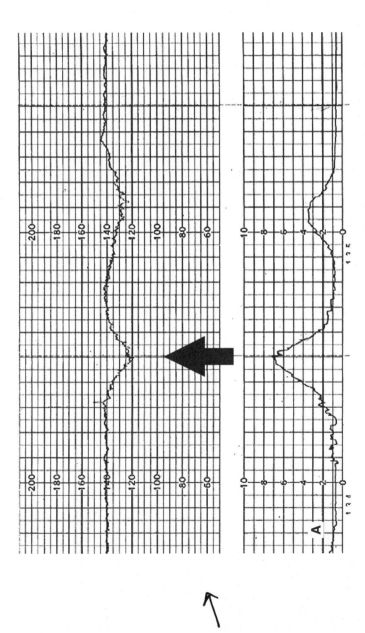

Figure 6–3. Fetal heart rate decelerations. A: Early Deceleration- note arrow shows deceleration is gradual and a mirror image to the uterine contraction; B. Late Deceleration- note arrow shows deceleration nadir is after the peak of the uterine contraction; C. Variable Deceleration- note arrow shows the deceleration is abrupt in its decline and resolution.

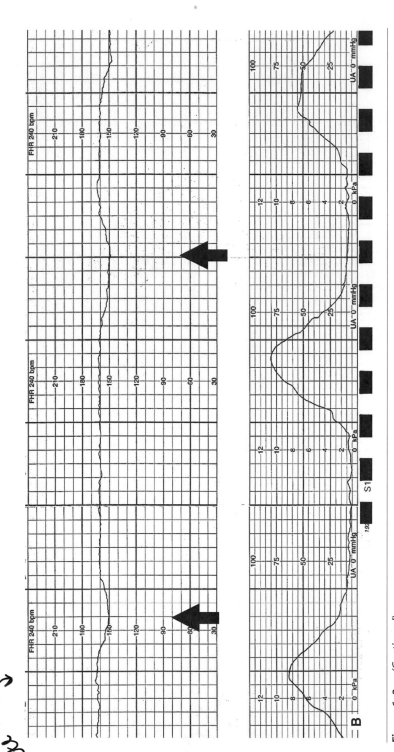

Figure 6-3. *(Continued)*

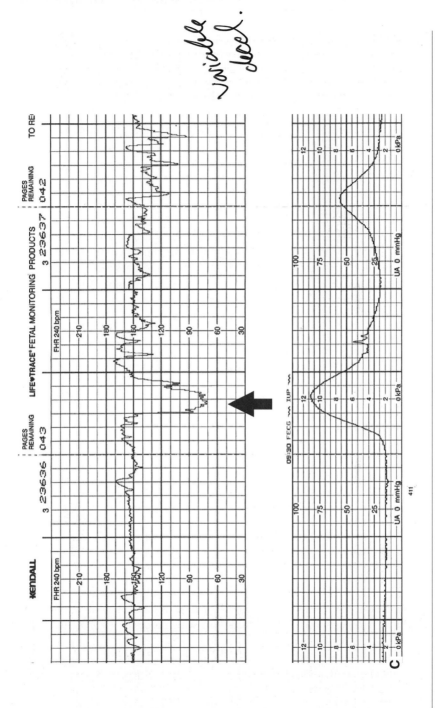

Figure 6-3. *(Continued)*

Comprehension Questions

6.1   A 31-year old G2 P1 woman at 39 weeks' gestation complains of painful
        uterine contractions that are occurring every 3 to 4 minutes. Her cervix
        has changed from 1-cm dilation to 2-cm dilation over 3 hours. Which
        one of the following management plans is most appropriate?
        A. Cesarean delivery
        B. Intravenous oxytocin
        C. Observation
        D. Fetal scalp pH monitoring
        E. Intranasal gonadotropin therapy

6.2   A 26-year-old G2 P1 woman at 41 weeks' gestation has been pushing for
        3 hours without progress. Throughout this time, her vaginal examina-
        tion has remained completely dilated, completely effaced, and 0 station,
        with the head persistently in the occiput posterior (OP) position.
        Which of the following statements accurately describes the situation?
        A. The occiput posterior position is frequently associated with a gynecoid
            pelvis.
        B. The labor progress is normal if the patient does not have an
            epidural catheter for analgesia, but is abnormal if epidural analge-
            sia is being used.
        C. The patient is best described as having an arrest of descent.
        D. The bony part of the fetal head is likely to be at the plane of the
            pelvic inlet.

6.3   A 31-year-old G2 P1 woman at 40 weeks' gestation has progressed in
        labor from 5-cm to 6-cm cervical dilation over 2 hours. Which of the
        following best describes the labor?
        A. Prolonged latent phase
        B. Prolonged active phase
        C. Arrest of active phase
        D. Protracted active phase
        E. Normal labor

6.4   A 24-year-old G2 P1 woman at 39 weeks' gestation presents with painful
        uterine contractions. She also complains of dark, vaginal blood mixed
        with some mucus. Which of the following describes the most likely eti-
        ology of her bleeding?
        A. Placenta previa
        B. Placenta abruption
        C. Bloody show
        D. Vasa previa
        E. Cervical laceration

ANSWERS

6.1   **C.** This patient is still in the (normal) latent phase; the upper limit
        is 14 hours. A fetal scalp pH monitor is a method for obtaining a
        small amount of capillary blood from the fetal scalp to assess for fetal
        academia, procedure that is very infrequently performed. It is not
        indicated in this scenario and does not aid in the progress of labor.
        Intravenous oxytocin enhances contraction strength and/or fre-
        quency, but does not affect cervical dilation. A cesarean delivery is
        considered if there is a disorder during the active phase of labor and
        not the latent phase. Intranasal gonadotropin therapy is not indi-
        cated during any phase of labor.

6.2   **C.** A 3-hour second stage of labor still is abnormal, even with epidural
        analgesia. An anthropoid pelvis, which predisposes to the persistent
        fetal occiput posterior position, is characterized by a pelvis with an
        anteroposterior diameter greater than the transverse diameter with
        prominent ischial spines and a narrow anterior segment. The baby is
        at "0" station, meaning the presenting part (in most cases, the bony
        part of the fetal head) is right at the plane of the ischial spines and
        not at the pelvic inlet. Station refers to the relationship of the pre-
        senting bony part of the fetal head in relation to the ischial spines,
        and not the pelvic inlet. Engagement refers to the relationship of the
        widest diameter of the presenting part and its location with reference
        to the pelvic inlet.

6.3   **D.** Protracted active phase means some progress but less than
        expected (1.5 cm/h) in the active phase of labor. This patient is
        >4 cm dilated, so she is in active phase and not latent phase of
        labor. This would have been an arrest of active phase if there had
        been no progress at all. The cervix has changed 1 cm over 2 hours
        when the expected change would be 3 cm, therefore this is not nor-
        mal labor.

6.4   **C.** Bloody show or loss of cervical mucus plug often is a sign of
        impending labor. The sticky mucus admixed with blood can differ-
        entiate bloody show from antepartum bleeding. Placenta previa, pla-
        centa abruption, and vasa previa are all associated with antepartum
        bleeding. A cervical laceration typically occurs during a vaginal
        delivery. They may be associated with postpartum hemorrhage.

Clinical Pearls

➤ The normalcy of labor is determined by assessing the cervical change versus time. Normal labor should be observed.

➤ Cesarean delivery (for labor abnormalities) in the absence of clear cephalopelvic disproportion is generally reserved for arrest of active phase with adequate uterine contractions.

➤ Adequate uterine contractions is not a precise definition, but is commonly judged as greater than 200 Montevideo units with an internal uterine pressure catheter, or by uterine contractions every 2 to 3 minutes, firm on palpation, and lasting at least 40 to 60 seconds.

➤ In general, latent labor occurs when the cervix is less than 4-cm dilated and active labor when the cervix is greater than 4-cm dilated.

➤ Early decelerations are mirror images of uterine contractions, caused by fetal head compressions.

➤ Variable decelerations are abrupt in decline and abrupt in resolution and are caused by cord compression.

➤ Late decelerations are gradual in shape and are offset from the uterine contractions, caused by uteroplacental insufficiency (hypoxia).

➤ The normal fetal heart rate baseline is between 110 and 160 bpm.

REFERENCES

American College of Obstetricians and Gynecologists. Intrapartum fetal heart rate monitoring. ACOG Practice Bulletin 70. Washington, DC: 2005.

Cunningham FG, Leveno KJ, Bloom SL, Hauth JC, Gilstrap LC III, Wenstrom KD. Dystocia: abnormal labor and fetopelvic disproportion. In: Williams Obstetrics. 22nd ed. New York, NY: McGraw-Hill; 2005:495-520.

Hobel CJ, Zakowski M. Normal labor, delivery, and postpartum care: anatomic considerations, obstetric and analgesia, and resuscitation of the newborn. In: Hacker NF, Gambone JC, Hobel CJ, eds. Essentials of Obstetrics and Gynecology, 5th ed. Philadelphia, PA: Saunders; 2009:91-118.

Case 7

An 18-year-old G1 P0 adolescent female, who is pregnant at 7 weeks' gestation by last menstrual period, complains of a 2-day history of vaginal spotting and lower abdominal pain. She denies a history of sexually transmitted diseases. On examination, her blood pressure (BP) is 130/60 mm Hg, heart rate (HR) is 70 beats per minute, and temperature is 99°F (37.2°C). Her neck is supple and the heart examination is normal. The lungs are clear bilaterally. The abdomen is nontender and no masses are palpated. On pelvic examination, the uterus is 4-week size and nontender. There are no adnexal masses on pelvic examination. The quantitative β-hCG level is 700 mIU/mL and a transvaginal ultrasound reveals an empty uterus and no adnexal masses.

➤ What is your next step in the management of this patient?

ANSWER TO CASE 7:
Threatened Abortion

Summary: An 18-year-old adolescent female at 7 weeks' gestation by LMP complains of a 2-day history of vaginal spotting and lower abdomen pain. The physical examination reveals a 4-week-sized uterus and unremarkable adnexa. The β-hCG level is 700 mIU/mL and no intrauterine gestational sac is noted on endovaginal sonography.

➤ **Next step in management:** Follow up β-hCG in 48 hours.

ANALYSIS

Objectives

1. Understand the concept of the hCG discriminatory zone or threshold, and its utility with transvaginal sonography.
2. Understand the principle of obtaining a follow-up hCG level when a patient is asymptomatic and has an hCG level that is below the discriminatory zone.
3. Know that a normal ultrasound examination does not rule out the presence of an ectopic pregnancy.

Considerations

This 18-year-old patient complains of lower abdominal pain and vaginal spotting, which in a woman of childbearing potential should be considered an ectopic pregnancy until otherwise proven. She does not have a history of sexually transmitted diseases, which if present would be a risk factor for an ectopic pregnancy. The physical examination is unremarkable and ultrasound does not show any adnexal masses. Significantly, the hCG level is below the threshold whereby transvaginal sonography should reveal an intrauterine pregnancy (hCG threshold of 1500 to 2000 mIU/mL). Thus, the goal is to establish whether this pregnancy is a normal intrauterine gestation or an abnormal pregnancy. This may be accomplished by following serial hCG levels. After 48 hours, if the follow-up hCG level rises by at least 66%, then the patient most likely has a normal intrauterine pregnancy. If the follow-up hCG does not rise by 66% (particularly if it rises by only 20%), then she most likely has an abnormal pregnancy. The subnormal rise in hCG does not indicate whether the abnormal pregnancy is in the uterus or the tube. Notably, the gestational age based on last menstrual period is not very reliable. Thus, the hCG levels and transvaginal ultrasound are generally the best tools for evaluating a possible ectopic pregnancy.

HCG rise 66% in 48 hr → NL
20% → ectopic↑

APPROACH TO
Threatened Abortion

DEFINITIONS

THREATENED ABORTION: Pregnancy with vaginal spotting during the first half of pregnancy. This does not delineate the viability of the pregnancy.

ECTOPIC PREGNANCY: Pregnancy outside of the normal uterine implantation site. Most of the time, this means a pregnancy in the fallopian tube.

HUMAN CHORIONIC GONADOTROPIN: "The pregnancy hormone," which is a glycoprotein that is secreted by the chorionic villi of a pregnancy. It is the hormone on which pregnancy tests are based. The normal pregnancy will have a logarithmic rise in early pregnancy. Usually the β-subunit is assayed to prevent cross-reactivity with LH.

HCG THRESHOLD: Level of serum hCG such that an intrauterine pregnancy should be seen on ultrasound. For endovaginal sonography, this level is 1500 to 2000 mIU/mL. When an intrauterine pregnancy is not seen on sonography and the hCG level exceeds the threshold, then it is highly probable that an ectopic pregnancy is present.

CLINICAL APPROACH

The possibility of ectopic pregnancy must be considered when assessing a pregnant woman with vaginal spotting and/or lower abdominal pain. It is of paramount importance to determine if the woman is hypotensive, volume depleted, or has severe abdominal or adnexal pain. These patients will most likely need laparoscopy or laparotomy since ectopic pregnancy is probable. For asymptomatic women, the quantitative human chorionic gonadotropin (hCG) level is useful. When the hCG level is below the threshold for sonographic visualization of an intrauterine gestational sac, then a repeat hCG level is generally performed in 48 hours to establish the viability of pregnancy. Another option would be a single progesterone level: levels greater than 25 ng/mL almost always indicate a normal intrauterine gestation, whereas values less than 5 ng/mL usually correlate with a nonviable gestation. When a nonviable pregnancy is diagnosed either by an abnormal hCG rise or single progesterone assay (< 5 ng/mL), it is still unclear whether the patient has a spontaneous abortion or an ectopic pregnancy. Many clinicians will perform a uterine curettage at this time to assess whether the patient has a miscarriage (histologic confirmation of chorionic villi) or an ectopic pregnancy (no villi from the curettage). Women with asymptomatic, small (< 3.5 cm) ectopic pregnancies are ideal candidates for intramuscular methotrexate. A nonviable intrauterine pregnancy may be managed expectantly, surgically via dilation and curettage, or medically with vaginal misoprostol. Vaginal misoprostol has been reported to be effective in evacuating the pregnancy in about 80% of cases.

When the hCG level is greater than the ultrasound threshold, then a transvaginal sonogram will dictate the next step. A patient in whom an intrauterine gestational sac is seen may be sent home with a diagnosis of threatened abortion and should have close follow-up. There is still a significant risk of miscarriage. When the hCG level is above the threshold, and there is no sonographic evidence of intrauterine pregnancy, the risk of ectopic pregnancy is high (about 85%), and thus laparoscopy is often undertaken to diagnose and treat the ectopic pregnancy. Because an intrauterine gestation is possible in this circumstance (about 15% of the time), methotrexate is usually not given; however, a high hCG level in the face of a sonographically empty uterus is almost always caused by an extrauterine gestation. (See Figure 7–1 for one

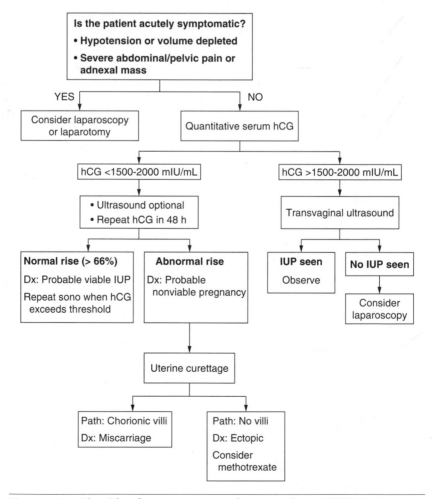

Figure 7–1.   Algorithm for management of suspected ectopic pregnancy.

example of a management scheme.) Finally, Rh-negative women with threat-ened abortion, spontaneous abortion, or ectopic pregnancy should receive Rhogam to prevent isoimmunization.

Comprehension Questions

7.1 Which of the following is the most significant risk factor for the devel-opment of an ectopic pregnancy?
A. Prior chlamydial cervical infection
B. History of a tubal ligation
C. Prior molar pregnancy
D. Prior miscarriage
E. Combination oral contraceptive pill use

7.2 A 32-year-old woman is diagnosed with an ectopic pregnancy based on hCG levels that have plateaued in the range of 1400 mIU/mL and no chorionic villi found on uterine curettage. She is given 50 mg/m² of methotrexate intramuscularly. Five days later, she complains of increased lower abdominal pain. Her blood pressure and heart rate are normal. Her abdomen shows some tenderness in the lower quadrants without guard-ing or rebound. Which of the following is the best course of action?
A. Immediate laparotomy
B. Repeat dose of methotrexate
C. Observation
D. Folic acid rescue
E. Epidural analgesia

7.3 An 18-year-old adolescent female who is brought to the emergency room complains of vaginal spotting and lower abdominal pain. Her abdominal and pelvic examinations are normal. The hCG level is 700 mIU/mL and transvaginal sonogram shows no intrauterine gestational sac and no adnexal masses. Which of the following statements is most accurate regarding this patient's situation?
A. She has an unruptured ectopic pregnancy.
B. She has a viable intrauterine pregnancy that is too early to assess on ultrasound.
C. She has a nonviable intrauterine pregnancy.
D. There is insufficient information to draw a conclusion about the viability of this pregnancy.
E. An MRI scan would be useful in further assessing the possibility of an ectopic pregnancy.

7.4   A 22-year-old woman, who is pregnant at 5 weeks' gestation, com-
       plains of severe lower abdominal pain. On examination, she is noted
       to have a blood pressure of 86/44 mm Hg and heart rate of 120 bpm.
       Her abdomen is tender. The pelvic examination is difficult to perform
       due to guarding. The hCG level is 500 mIU/mL and the transvaginal
       sonogram reveals no intrauterine gestational sac and no adnexal masses.
       There is some free fluid in the cul-de-sac. Which of the following is the
       best management for this patient?
       A. Repeat hCG level in 48 hours to assess for a rise of 66%.
       B. Check the serum progesterone level.
       C. Immediate surgery.
       D. Intramuscular methotrexate.
       E. Repeat sonography in 48 hours.

ANSWERS

7.1   **A.** Chlamydial infection increases the risk of ectopic pregnancy. The
       use of combination oral contraceptives tends to prevent all pregnan-
       cies, both ectopic and intrauterine, and is not a risk factor. A history
       of a tubal ligation by itself does not increase the risk of ectopic preg-
       nancy. However, if a woman has had a tubal ligation and then becomes
       pregnant, there is a significant risk of tubal pregnancy. Prior ectopic
       pregnancy greatly increases the risk of future ectopic pregnancy.

7.2   **C.** Many women treated with methotrexate will have mild abdomi-
       nal pain, which may be observed in the absence of severe peritoneal
       signs of hypotension, or overt signs of rupture. However, if these
       signs are present, a laparotomy would be indicated. Pain associated
       with resolution of tubal pregnancy is usually distinguishable from
       tubal rupture. The pain of resolution is typically much milder than
       the pain of tubal rupture and is not associated with acute abdomen
       or hemodynamic instability. An epidural is not indicated for this
       type of pain or scenario. Repeating the dose of methotrexate will not
       alleviate the patient's pain, and may just worsen the painful side
       effects of the drug. A folic acid rescue is sometimes used in cancer
       patients experiencing toxic side effects of methotrexate such as
       inflammation of the digestive tract.

7.3   **D.** There is insufficient information in this scenario to establish via-
       bility of the pregnancy. A repeat hCG in 48 hours may be able to
       assess the state of the pregnancy. Since no conclusion may be drawn,
       it would be difficult to say whether this patient has an unruptured
       ectopic pregnancy, an intrauterine pregnancy that is too early to
       assess by ultrasound, or a nonviable intrauterine pregnancy. An MRI

is not specific in evaluating for an ectopic versus viable intrauterine pregnancy, plus it is costly and time consuming.

7.4   C. Surgery is indicated because this patient is hypotensive and tachycardic due to a likely ruptured ectopic pregnancy. This patient is in shock, and immediate surgery is indicated to prevent end organ damage that may immediately lead to or eventually result in death. Delaying treatment or relying on intramuscular (IM) methotrexate is not indicated for a patient in hemodynamic instability. Considering the patient's symptoms, methotrexate would be an ineffective treatment anyway since the ectopic pregnancy has most likely ruptured. A progesterone level would not be of use because tubal rupture in itself would indicate a nonviable gestation was present.

Clinical Pearls

➤ When the hCG level is above the threshold and no intrauterine pregnancy is seen on transvaginal ultrasound, the patient most likely has an ectopic pregnancy.

➤ Early in the course of a normal intrauterine pregnancy, the β-hCG should rise by at least 66% over 48 hours.

➤ The presence of a true intrauterine gestational sac on ultrasound makes the risk of ectopic pregnancy very unlikely.

➤ Surgery is usually the best therapy in a patient with an early pregnancy who is hypotensive or has severe adnexal pain.

REFERENCES

American College of Obstetricians and Gynecologists. Medical management of ectopic pregnancy. *ACOG Practice Bulletin 94*. Washington, DC: 2008.

Lobo RA. Ectopic pregnancy. In: Katz VL, Lentz GM, Lobo RA, Gersenson DM, eds. *Comprehensive Gynecology*. 5th ed. St. Louis, MO: Mosby-Year Book; 2007:389-410.

Lu MC, Williams III, J, Hobel CJ. Antepartum care: preconception and prenatal care, genetic evaluation and teratology, and antenatal fetal assessment. In: Hacker NF, Gambone JC, Hobel CJ, eds. *Essentials of Obstetrics and Gynecology*, 5th ed. Philadelphia, PA: Saunders; 2009:71-90.

Shamonki M, Nelson AL, Gambone JC. Ectopic pregnancy. In: Hacker NF, Gambone JC, Hobel CJ, eds. *Essentials of Obstetrics and Gynecology*, 5th ed. Philadelphia, PA: Saunders; 2009:290-297.

Zhang J. A comparison of medical management with misoprostol and surgical management of early pregnancy failure. *N Eng J Med*. 2005;253(8):761-769.

Case 8

A 35-year-old G5 P4 woman at 39 weeks' gestation is undergoing a vaginal delivery. She has a history of a previous myomectomy and one prior low-transverse cesarean delivery. She was counseled about the risks, benefit, and alternatives of vaginal birth after cesarean, and elected a trial of labor. She proceeded through a normal labor. The delivery of the baby is uneventful. The placenta does not deliver after 30 minutes, and a manual extraction of the placenta is undertaken. The placenta seems to be firmly adherent to the uterus.

➤ What is the most likely diagnosis?

➤ What is your next step in management for this patient?

ANSWERS TO CASE 8:
Placenta Accreta

Summary: A 35-year-old G5 P4 woman at term with a prior history of a myomectomy and cesarean delivery is undergoing a vaginal delivery. The retained placenta is firmly adherent to the uterus when there is an attempt at manual extraction.

➤ **Most likely diagnosis:** Placenta accreta.

➤ **Next step in management for this patient:** Hysterectomy.

ANALYSIS

Objectives

1. Know the risk factors for and the clinical diagnosis of placenta accreta.
2. Understand that hysterectomy is usually the best treatment for placenta accreta.

Considerations

This patient has had two previous uterine incisions, which increases the risk of placenta accreta. The placenta is noted to be very adherent to the uterus, which is the clinical definition of placenta accreta, although the histologic diagnosis requires a defect of the decidua basalis layer. The usual management of true placental accreta is hysterectomy since attempts to remove a firmly attached placenta often lead to hemorrhage and/or maternal death. Conservative management of placenta accreta, such as removal of as much placenta as possible and packing the uterus, often leads to excess mortality as compared to immediate hysterectomy. Nevertheless in a younger patient who strongly desires more children, this option may rarely be entertained.

APPROACH TO
Placenta Accreta

DEFINITIONS

PLACENTA ACCRETA: Abnormal adherence of the placenta to the uterine wall due to an abnormality of the decidua basalis layer of the uterus. The placental villi are attached to the myometrium.

PLACENTA INCRETA: The abnormally implanted placenta penetrates into the myometrium.

PLACENTA PERCRETA: The abnormally implanted placenta penetrates entirely through the myometrium to the serosa. Often invasion into the bladder is noted.

CLINICAL APPROACH

Risk factors for placental adherence include low-lying placentation or placenta previa, prior cesarean delivery or uterine curettage, or prior myomectomy. Antepartum bleeding may occur. With complete placenta accreta, there may be no bleeding and only a retained placenta. Undue traction on the cord may lead to uterine inversion. With a retained placenta, clinicians will usually attempt a manual extraction of the placenta, in an effort to find a cleavage plane between the placenta and the uterus. With placenta accreta, no cleavage plane is found. Hysterectomy is usually the best choice in this circumstance. Because the placenta is so firmly adherent, attempts to conserve the uterus, such as curettage of the placenta or removing the placenta "piecemeal," are often unsuccessful, and may lead to hemorrhage and exsanguination.

Placenta accreta should be suspected in circumstances of placenta previa, particularly with a history of a prior cesarean delivery (Table 8–1). The greater the number of prior cesareans in the face of current placenta previa, the higher the risk of accreta. For example, a woman with three or more prior cesarean deliveries and a low-lying anterior placenta suggestive of partial previa or a known placenta previa has up to a 40% to 50% chance of having placenta accreta. Some practitioners advise performing ultrasound examinations to assess the placental location in those women who have had a prior cesarean delivery. Studies examining the accuracy of MRI to diagnose placenta accreta prior to delivery reveal a sensitivity of only 38%. When the placenta is anterior or low-lying in position, there is a greater risk of accreta. One caution is that a low-lying placenta or placenta previa diagnosed in the second trimester may resolve in the third trimester as the lower uterine segment grows more rapidly, a phenomenon known as "transmigration of the placenta."

Table 8–1 RISK FACTORS FOR PLACENTA ACCRETA

Placenta previa
Implantation over the lower uterine segment
Prior cesarean scar or other uterine scar
Uterine curettage
Fetal Down syndrome

Comprehension Questions

8.1   A 33-year-old woman G3 P2002 who had two prior cesareans is cur-
       rently at 38 weeks' gestation. She is noted to have a posterior placenta.
       On ultrasound, there is evidence of possible placenta accreta. The
       patient is counseled about the possible risk of need for hysterectomy.
       Which of the following is the most accurate statement?
       A. Having two prior cesareans is associated with a 50% risk for pla-
          centa accreta.
       B. Placenta accreta is associated with a defect in the myometrial layer
          of the uterus.
       C. If the patient had gestational diabetes, the risk for placenta accreta
          would be even higher.
       D. The posterior placenta is associated with less of a risk for accreta
          than an anterior placenta.

8.2   A 25-year-old woman at 34 weeks' gestation is noted to have a placenta
       previa, after she presented with vaginal bleeding and has undergone
       sonography. At 37 weeks, she has a scheduled cesarean. Upon cesarean
       section, bluish tissue densely adherent between the uterus and maternal
       bladder is noted. Which of the following is the most likely diagnosis?
       A. Placenta accreta
       B. Placenta melanoma
       C. Placenta percreta
       D. Placental polyp

8.3   A 29-year-old G1 P0 woman at 39 weeks' gestation delivered vaginally.
       Her placenta does not deliver easily. A manual extraction of the pla-
       centa is attempted and the placenta seems to be adherent to the uterus.
       A hysterectomy is contemplated, but the patient refuses due to strongly
       desiring more children. The cord is ligated with suture as high as possi-
       ble. The patient is given the option of methotrexate therapy. Which of
       the following is the most likely complication after this intervention?
       A. Coagulopathy
       B. Utero-vaginal fistula
       C. Infection
       D. Malignant degeneration

8.4   A 32-year-old woman undergoes myomectomy for symptomatic uter-
       ine fibroids, all of which are subserosal. The endometrial cavity was
       not entered during the procedure. Which of the following statements
       is most likely to be correct regarding the risk of placental accreta?
       A. Her risk of accreta is most likely to be increased due to the
          myomectomy.
       B. Her risk of accreta is most likely to be decreased due to the
          myomectomy.
       C. Her risk of accreta is most likely not affected by the myomectomy.
       D. If the myomectomy incisions are anterior, then she has an increased
          risk of a placental polyp.

ANSWERS

8.1   **D.** Placenta accreta is more common with increasing number of
       cesareans and placenta previa. Three prior cesareans *with* placenta
       previa are associated with up to a 50% risk for placenta accreta, in
       which the decidua basalis layer is defective. It is the endometrial
       layer that is defective and not the myometrial layer. Nevertheless,
       the placenta may grow into the myometrium or even through the
       entire uterus to the serosa.

8.2   **C.** The blue tissue densely adherent between the uterus and bladder
       is very characteristic of percreta, where the placenta penetrates
       entirely through the myometrium to the serosa and adheres to the
       bladder. These findings are not typically found with placenta accreta
       or polyps. Malignant melanoma can metastasize to the placenta, but
       this is much less common under these circumstances.

8.3   **A.** The best management of placenta accreta is hysterectomy due
       to the great risk of hemorrhage if the placenta is attempted to be
       removed. When the patient refuses hysterectomy, then ligation of
       the umbilical cord as high as possible and attempt at IV methotrex-
       ate therapy has been attempted with limited success. Other than
       hemorrhage, the other complication to be concerned about is
       infection. The necrosis of the placental tissue can be a nidus for
       infection.

8.4   **C.** In general, myomectomy incisions on the serosal (outside) surface
       of the uterus do not predispose to accreta because the endometrium
       is not disturbed. However, the risk of accreta is not decreased due to
       the myomectomy either. Placental polyps result from retained prod-
       ucts after either a term pregnancy or incomplete abortion, and occur
       inside the uterus. Therefore, the location of the incisions for a
       myomectomy will not influence whether or not a patient develops
       polyps.

Clinical Pearls

➤ The usual management of placenta accreta (abnormal adherence of the placenta to the uterus) is hysterectomy.

➤ Placenta accreta is associated with a defect in the decidua basalis.

➤ The risk of placenta accreta increases in a woman with a prior uterine incision and placenta previa. The greater the number of cesareans, the higher the risk of accreta.

➤ Low-lying or marginal placenta previa diagnosed in the second trimester will often resolve later in pregnancy, so repeat sonography is prudent.

REFERENCES

American College of Obstetricians and Gynecologists. Postpartum hemorrhage. *ACOG Practice Bulletin 76*. Washington, DC; 2006.

Cunningham FG, Leveno KJ, Bloom SL, Hauth JC, Gilstrap LC III, Wenstrom KD. Obstetrical hemorrhage. In: *Williams Obstetrics*. 22nd ed. New York, NY: McGraw-Hill; 2005;830-832.

Kim M, Hyashi RH, Gambone JC. Obstetrical hemorrhage and puerperal sepsis. In: Hacker NF, Gambone JC, Hobel CJ, eds. *Essentials of Obstetrics and Gynecology*, 5th ed. Philadelphia, PA: Saunders; 2009:128-138.

Case 9

A 22-year-old nulliparous woman complains of a 2-week history of vaginal discharge and vaginal spotting after intercourse. She denies a history of sexually transmitted diseases and currently does not use any contraceptive agents. Her past medical history is unremarkable. Her last menstrual period began 1 week ago and was normal. On examination, her blood pressure (BP) is 100/60 mm Hg, heart rate (HR) 80 beats per minute (bpm), and temperature is 99°F (37.2°C). The heart and lung examinations are normal. Her abdomen is nontender and without masses. Her pelvic examination shows purulent vaginal discharge, which on Gram stain shows intracellular gram-negative diplococci. Her pregnancy test is negative.

➤ What is the most likely diagnosis?

➤ What is the next step in therapy?

➤ What are the complications of this problem?

ANSWERS TO CASE 9:
Gonococcal Cervicitis

Summary: A 22-year-old nonpregnant nulliparous woman complains of a vaginal discharge and postcoital spotting. A purulent vaginal discharge on Gram stain shows intracellular gram-negative diplococci.

➤ **Most likely diagnosis:** Gonococcal cervicitis.

➤ **Next step in therapy:** Intramuscular ceftriaxone for gonorrhea, and oral azithromycin (or doxycycline) for chlamydial infection.

➤ **Complications of this problem:** Salpingitis, which may lead to infertility or increased risk of ectopic pregnancy. Disseminated gonorrhea is also possible.

ANALYSIS

Objectives

1. Know that gram-negative intracellular diplococci are highly suggestive of *Neisseria gonorrhoeae*.
2. Know the clinical presentation and treatment of gonococcal cervicitis.
3. Understand the complications of gonococcal cervicitis.

Considerations

This 22-year-old nulliparous woman complains of a vaginal discharge and postcoital spotting. The first disease that should be ruled out with abnormal vaginal bleeding is a pregnancy-related disorder, such as ectopic pregnancy or threatened abortion. In this case, the patient's pregnancy test is negative. The purulent vaginal discharge is found to be diagnostic of gonorrhea by Gram stain. Because of gonorrhea's propensity to invade the endocervix, this woman almost certainly has at least cervicitis. Thus, the endocervix should be sampled for culture or DNA probe. The next step is to assess the extent of the disease. This patient had no evidence of salpingitis (tubal infection) since she did not have adnexal tenderness. She did not complain of abdominal tenderness or heavy menses (uterine involvement), which would be more indicative of upper genital tract disease. Likewise, she has no joint complaints to indicate gonococcal arthritis, or painful skin lesions to suggest disseminated gonorrhea.

One common treatment for gonococcal cervicitis is ceftriaxone 125 to 250 mg intramuscularly. Because Chlamydia often coexists with gonorrhea, therapy with azithromycin 1 g orally or doxycycline 100 mg twice daily for 7 to 10 days is also indicated. The gonococcal organisms appear to be confined to the endocervix in this case, but complications can include ascension to the tubes causing infertility (tubal disease) or a development of ectopic pregnancy in the future.

APPROACH TO
Gonococcal Cervicitis

DEFINITIONS

MUCOPURULENT CERVICITIS: Yellow exudative discharge arising from the endocervix with 10 or more polymorphonucleocytes per high-power field on microscopy.

LOWER GENITAL TRACT: The vulva, vagina, and cervix.

UPPER GENITAL TRACT: The uterine corpus, fallopian tubes, and ovaries.

CLINICAL APPROACH

An infection of the cervix is analogous to an infection of the urethra in the male. Thus, sexually transmitted pathogens, such as *Chlamydia trachomatis*, *N gonorrhoeae*, or herpes simplex virus, may infect the cervix. Gonococcal and chlamydial organisms have a propensity for the columnar cells of the endocervix. Often, erythema of the endocervix is noted, leading to friability; these patients may complain of postcoital spotting. Mucopurulent cervical discharge is a common complaint, again analogous to the exudative urethral discharge of the male. The most common organism implicated in mucopurulent cervical discharge is *C trachomatis*, although gonorrhea may also be a pathogen.

When a patient presents with this type of cervical discharge, Gram stain may be done; if evidence of gonorrhea is present, that is, intracellular gram-negative diplococci, then treatment should be directed toward gonococcal disease (ceftriaxone 125 to 250 mg IM). Because of the frequency of coexisting chlamydial infection, azithromycin 1 g orally or doxycycline 100 mg orally bid for 7 to 10 days is also often given. If the Gram stain of the cervical discharge is negative, then antimicrobial therapy directed at *Chlamydia* is warranted. Nevertheless, cultures or tests for both organisms should be performed. If the symptoms resolve, no follow-up cultures need to be done (see Figure 9–1 for one suggested management scheme). Finally, the patient and partner should be counseled and offered testing for other sexually transmitted organisms such as HIV, syphilis, and hepatitis B and C.

Gonococcal cervicitis may lead to more serious complications. The organism may ascend and infect the fallopian tubes, causing salpingitis. The term pelvic inflammatory disease is usually synonymous with acute salpingitis. The tubal infection in turn predisposes the patient to infertility and ectopic pregnancies

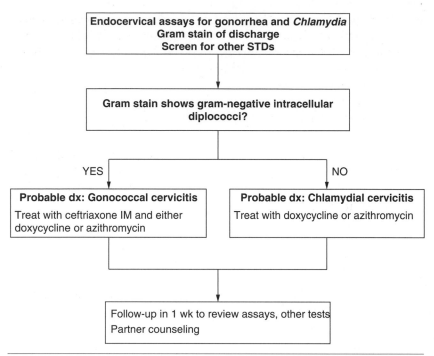

Figure 9–1. Algorithm for evaluation of mucopurulent cervical discharge.

due to tubal occlusion and/or adhesions. The gonococcal organism may lead to an infectious arthritis, usually involving the large joints, and classically is migratory. In fact, in the United States, gonorrhea is the most common cause of septic arthritis in young women. Disseminated gonorrhea can occur also; affected individuals will usually have eruptions of painful pustules with an erythematous base on the skin. The diagnosis is made by Gram stain and culture of the pustules.

Comprehension Questions

9.1 An 18-year-old adolescent female has a yellowish vaginal discharge. On examination, the cervix is erythematous and the discharge reveals numerous leukocytes. Which of the following is the most likely etiology?

A. *Neisseria gonorrhea*
B. *Chlamydia trachomatis*
C. Ureaplasma species
D. Bacterial vaginosis

9.2 A 22-year-old woman, who uses a barrier method for contraception, complains of lower abdominal tenderness and dyspareunia. On laparoscopy, hyperemic fallopian tubes are noted. Which of the following is most likely to be an isolated pathogen in this process?
A. *Pseudomonas aerugenosa*
B. *Chlamydia trachomatis*
C. *Treponema pallidum*
D. Actinomyces species

9.3 A 34-year-old woman is diagnosed as having a vaginitis based on a "fishy odor" to her vaginal discharge and vaginal pruritus. The cervix is normal in appearance. Which of the following most likely corresponds to the etiology?
A. *Neisseria gonorrhea*
B. *Chlamydia trachomatis*
C. Bacterial vaginosis
D. *Candida vaginitis*

9.4 A 21-year-old college student has a sexually transmitted pharyngitis. Which of the following most likely corresponds to the etiology?
A. *Neisseria gonorrhea*
B. *Chlamydia trachomatis*
C. Human papillomavirus
D. HIV pharyngitis

9.5 A 28-year-old woman has multiple painful pustules erupting throughout the skin of her body. Which of the following most likely corresponds to the etiology?
A. *Neisseria gonorrhea*
B. *Chlamydia trachomatis*
C. Meningococcus
D. Tuberculosis

9.6 A 19-year-old patient with a history of multiple sexually transmitted diseases presents to the labor and delivery area of a local hospital in active labor. She has not had prenatal care. The pediatrician is concerned about maternal infections which may cause blindness in the newborn. Due to the concern, a DNA assay should be performed for which of the following?
A. Human papillomavirus
B. *Chlamydia trachomatis*
C. Group B *Streptococcus*
D. *Treponema pallidum*

ANSWERS

9.1   **B.** Chlamydial cervicitis is the most common cause of mucopurulent cervical discharge. Although gonorrhea is also associated with a mucopurulent discharge, it is less common than *Chlamydia*. The mucus in the mucopurulent discharge is due to involvement of the columnar (mucin-containing) glandular cells of the endocervix.

9.2   **B.** This patient has salpingitis; common organisms include *Gonorrhea*, *Chlamydia*, gram-negative rods, and anaerobes. Risk factors for salpingitis include: use of an IUD, previous infection with either *Gonorrhea* or *Chlamydia*, surgery, or anything that breaks the cervical barrier and enhances transfer of organisms from the endocervix to the upper reproductive tract. *Pseudomonas aeruginosa* is a gram-negative nonfermenting bacillus that is commonly known to cause infections associated with hot tubs, contaminated contact lens solution, patients on ventilators (typically in the ICU), and immunocompromised patients (ie, burn patients). It is not associated with infecting the upper genital tract. *Treponema pallidum* is a spirochete bacterium that causes syphilis. There are multiple stages that this chronic disease may progress to if left untreated. The presenting symptom in the first stage of disease is a painless chancre typically located at the site of inoculation and not lower abdominal tenderness with dyspareunia. Treatment of choice is penicillin. *Actinomyces* is an organism considered part of the normal vaginal flora and is associated with intrauterine device use, but is not commonly encountered.

9.3   **C.** Neither gonorrhea nor chlamydial infection typically cause vaginitis. This patient likely has bacterial vaginosis, based on the fishy odor. *Candida* infection does not usually cause a fishy odor, and induces a heterogenous (cottage-cheese) discharge.

9.4   **A.** The diagnosis of gonococcal pharyngitis is made by swabbing the throat. The infection is typically located on the tonsils and back of the throat. Patients who engage in oral sex are at increased risk of acquiring gonococcal pharyngitis. Typically no symptoms are noted by the patient unless the disease disseminates. *Chlamydia* is not a common cause of pharyngitis most likely because, unlike *Neisseria gonorrhea*, it lacks the pili that allow the gonococcal bacteria to adhere to the surface of the columnar epithelium at the back of the throat.

9.5   **A.** Disseminated gonococcal disease leads to multiple, often painful, pustules on the skin. These pustules can be cultured and Gram stained for diagnostic purposes. Other signs of disseminated gonococcal disease include fever, malaise, chills, and joint pain or swelling. *Chlamydia* is not a common cause of a disseminated process; however, reinfection or persistent infections are common.

9.6   **B.** Both chlamydial infection and gonorrhea may cause conjunctivitis and blindness in a newborn. Gonococcal infections usually present between the second and fifth days of life, whereas chlamydial infections present between the fifth and fourteenth day of life. *Neisseria gonorrhea* was once the most common cause of blindness in the newborn. *Chlamydia trachomatis* may also cause infantile pneumonia, generally between 1 and 3 months of age.

Clinical Pearls

> ➤ The two most common etiologies of mucopurulent cervical discharge are chlamydial infection and gonorrhea (of which chlamydial infection is more common).
> ➤ Gram-negative intracellular diplococci are highly suggestive of *N gonorrhoeae*.
> ➤ *Chlamydia* often coexists with gonococcal cervicitis.
> ➤ Ceftriaxone treats gonorrhea, whereas doxycycline or azithromycin treat chlamydial infections.

REFERENCES

Eckert LO, Lentz GM. Infections of the lower genital tract. In: Katz VL, Lentz GM, Lobo RA, Gersenson DM, eds. *Comprehensive Gynecology*. 5th ed. St. Louis, MO: Mosby-Year Book; 2007:569-606.

McGregor JA, Lench JB. Vulvovaginitis, sexually transmitted infections, and pelvic inflammatory disease. In: Hacker NF, Gambone JC, Hobel CJ, eds. *Essentials of Obstetrics and Gynecology*, 5th ed. Philadelphia, PA: Saunders; 2009:265-275

Case 10

A 35-year-old woman at 8 weeks' gestation complains of crampy lower abdominal pain and vaginal bleeding. She states that the pain was intense last night, and that something that looked like liver passed per vagina. After that, the pain subsided tremendously as did the vaginal bleeding. On examination, her blood pressure (BP) is 130/80 mm Hg, heart rate (HR) 90 beats per minute, and temperature is 98°F (36.6°C). Her abdominal examination is unremarkable. The pelvic examination reveals normal external female genitalia. The cervix is closed and non-tender and no adnexal masses are appreciated.

➤ What is the most likely diagnosis?

➤ What is your next step in management?

ANSWERS TO CASE 10:
Completed Spontaneous Abortion

Summary: A 35-year-old woman at 8 weeks' gestational age had intense crampy lower abdominal pain and vaginal bleeding last night; after passing what looked like "liver," her pain and bleeding subsided tremendously. On examination, her cervix is closed.

➤ **Most likely diagnosis:** Completed abortion.

➤ **Next step in management:** Follow hCG levels to zero.

ANALYSIS

Objectives

1. Know the typical characteristics of the different types of spontaneous abortions.
2. Understand the clinical presentations of and the treatments for the different types of abortions.

Considerations

This woman is pregnant at 8 weeks' gestation, which is in the first trimester. She noted intense cramping pain the night before and passed something that looked like liver to her. This may be tissue, although the gross appearance of presumed tissue can be misleading. The patient's pain and bleeding have subsided since the passage of the "liver." This fits with the complete expulsion of the pregnancy tissue. The clinical picture of passage of tissue, resolution of cramping and bleeding, and a closed cervical os are consistent with a completed abortion. To confirm that all of the pregnancy (trophoblastic) tissue has been expelled from the uterus, the clinician should follow serum quantitative hCG levels. It is expected that the hCG levels should halve every 48 to 72 hours. If the hCG levels plateau instead of falling, then the patient has residual pregnancy tissue (which may be either an incomplete abortion or an ectopic pregnancy). Notably, this patient is of advanced maternal age, and spontaneous abortions are more common in older patients. The most common cause identified with spontaneous abortion is a chromosomal abnormality of the embryo.

APPROACH TO
Spontaneous Abortion

DEFINITIONS

THREATENED ABORTION: A pregnancy less than 20 weeks' gestation associated with vaginal bleeding, generally without cervical dilation.

INEVITABLE ABORTION: A pregnancy less than 20 weeks' gestation associated with cramping, bleeding, and cervical dilation; there is no passage of tissue.

INCOMPLETE ABORTION: A pregnancy less than 20 weeks' gestation associated with cramping, vaginal bleeding, an open cervical os, and some passage of tissue per vagina, but also some retained tissue in utero. The cervix remains open due to the continued uterine contractions; the uterus continues to contract in an effort to expel the retained tissue.

COMPLETED ABORTION: A pregnancy less than 20 weeks' gestation in which all the products of conception have passed; the cervix is generally closed. Because all the tissue has passed, the uterus no longer contracts, and the cervix closes.

MISSED ABORTION: A pregnancy less than 20 weeks' gestation with embryonic or fetal demise but no symptoms such as bleeding or cramping.

CLINICAL APPROACH

The history, physical examination, and/or sonography usually point to the category of spontaneous abortion (Table 10–1). Women with threatened abortion should be instructed to bring in any passed tissue for histologic analysis.

Note: An inevitable abortion must be differentiated from an incompetent cervix. With an inevitable abortion, the uterine contractions (cramping) lead to the cervical dilation. With an incompetent cervix, the cervix opens spontaneously without uterine contractions and, therefore, affected women present with painless cervical dilation. This disorder is treated with a surgical ligature at the level of the internal cervical os (cerclage). Hence, one of the main features used to distinguish between an incompetent cervix and an inevitable abortion is the presence or absence of uterine contractions.

The treatment of an **incomplete abortion**, characterized by the **passage of tissue and an open cervical os**, is dilatation and curettage of the uterus. The primary complications of persistently retained tissue are bleeding and infection. A completed abortion is suspected by the history of having passed tissue and experiencing cramping abdominal pain, now resolved. The cervix is closed.

Table 10–1 CLASSIFICATION OF SPONTANEOUS ABORTIONS

TERMINOLOGY	HISTORY	PASSAGE OF TISSUE?	CERVICAL OS	VIABILITY OF PREGNANCY?	TREATMENT
Threatened abortion	Vaginal bleeding	No	Closed	Uncertain; up to 50% will miscarry	Transvaginal ultrasound and hCG levels
Inevitable abortion	Cramping, bleeding	No	Open	Abortion is inevitable	D&C vs expectant management
Incomplete abortion	Cramping, bleeding (still continuing)	Some but not all tissues passed	Open	Nonviable	D&C
Complete abortion	Cramping, bleeding previously but now subsided	All tissues passed	Closed	Nonviable	Follow hCG levels to negative
Missed abortion	No symptoms	No	Closed	Nonviable (diagnosed on ultrasound)	D&C vs expectant management

Serum hCG levels are still followed to confirm that no further chorionic villi are contained in the uterus.

An unusual type of abnormal pregnancy is a **molar pregnancy**, which is trophoblastic tissue, or placenta-like tissue, usually without a fetus. The clinical presentation of molar pregnancy is vaginal spotting, absence of fetal heart tones, size greater than dates, and markedly elevated HCG levels. The diagnosis is by **ultrasound**, revealing a "snow storm" like pattern in the uterus. Uterine suction curettage is the treatment. After curettage, patients are followed with weekly hCG levels because sometimes gestational trophoblastic disease persists after evacuation of the molar pregnancy. In these instances, chemotherapy is used.

Comprehension Questions

Match the single best treatment (A-F) with the clinical scenario (10.1-10.4).

    A. Laparoscopy
    B. Follow up hCG level in 48 hours
    C. Cervical cerclage
    D. Dilation and curettage of uterus
    E. Expectant management

10.1   A 19-year-old G1 P0 woman at 18 weeks' gestation, who had a prior cervical conization procedure, states that she had felt no abdominal cramping. She has a cervical dilation of 2 cm and effacement of 70%.

10.2   A 33-year-old woman at 10 weeks' gestation complains of vaginal bleeding and passage of a whitish substance along with something "meat-like." She continues to have cramping, and her cervix is 2 cm dilated.

10.3   A 20-year-old G2 P1 woman at 12 weeks' gestation has had no problems with this pregnancy prior to today. She complains of some slight vaginal spotting. No fetal heart tones are heard on Doppler, and a transvaginal ultrasound reveals no uterine gestational sac and no adnexal masses. The hCG level is 700 mIU/mL.

10.4   A 28-year-old G3 P2 woman at 22 weeks' gestation is noted to have vaginal spotting, and fetal heart tones are in the 140 to 145 bpm range.

ANSWERS

10.1   **C.** The hallmark of cervical incompetence is painless dilation of the cervix. Cervical conization is a risk factor for incompetent cervix. Other risk factors for incompetent cervix include: congenital manifestations (ie, short cervix or collagen disorder), trauma to the cervix, prolonged second stage of labor, and uterine overdistention as with a multiple gestation pregnancy. No contractions were felt by the patient in this scenario, so the diagnosis is less likely to be inevitable abortion. Cervical incompetence may be treated with a surgical ligature known as a cerclage.

10.2   **D.** An open cervical os, a history of passing tissue, and continued cramping are all findings consistent with an incomplete abortion. If the cramping had stopped and the cervix closed, this would have been a complete abortion. The treatment of an incomplete abortion is dilation and curettage (D&C) of the uterus to prevent complications of retained tissue such as hemorrhage and infection. The products of conception obtained from the curettage are sent for pathology to confirm the diagnosis and to look for rare complications such as molar pregnancy.

10.3   **B.** This patient has a threatened abortion. Her hCG level is below the threshold when a gestational sac should be seen on transvaginal sonography (1500-2000 mIU/mL). Thus, it is unclear with the information at this time to discern whether she has a normal early intrauterine pregnancy, or an abnormal pregnancy (miscarriage or ectopic). Follow-up hCG level in 48 hours would be judicious; an appropriate rise in hCG of at least 66% is consistent with a normal intrauterine pregnancy, whereas a rise less than 66% is highly suggestive of an abnormal pregnancy.

10.4   **E.** This patient does not have an abortive process since she is at 22 weeks' gestation; she has antepartum bleeding. Abortions are described as less than 20 weeks' gestation. The two most common causes of antepartum bleeding are placenta previa and placental abruption. In abruption, the patient typically presents to triage with severe abdominal pain. The evaluation of this patient would include ultrasound to assess for placenta previa, and if this is ruled out, then speculum examination and assessment for abruption.

Clinical Pearls

➤ When a pregnant woman has an open cervical os with uterine cramping and history of passage of tissue, she usually has an incomplete abortion, best treated by uterine curettage.

➤ The typical history of a completed abortion is resolution of cramping and vaginal bleeding following passage of tissue, and the finding of a small firm uterus and a closed cervical os.

➤ The most common cause of a first-trimester miscarriage is a fetal karyotypic abnormality.

➤ Incompetent cervix, which is suspected with painless cervical dilation, is best treated with a cervical cerclage (stitch).

➤ A molar pregnancy is an unusual type of pregnancy characterized by vaginal spotting, absence of fetal heart tones, and size greater than dates. The diagnosis is made by sonography.

REFERENCES

American College of Obstetricians and Gynecologists. Medical management of abortion. ACOG *Practice Bulletin 67*. Washington, DC: 2005

American College of Obstetricians and Gynecologists. Diagnosis and treatment of gestational trophoblastic disease. ACOG *Practice Bulletin 53*. Washington, DC: 2004.

Katz VL. Recurrent and spontaneous abortion. In: Katz VL, Lentz GM, Lobo RA, Gersenson DM, eds. *Comprehensive Gynecology*. 5th ed. St. Louis, MO: Mosby-Year Book; 2007:359-388.

Lu MC, Williams III, J, Hobel CJ. Antepartum care: preconception and prenatal care, genetic evaluation and teratology, and antenatal fetal assessment. In: Hacker NF, Gambone JC, Hobel CJ, eds. *Essentials of Obstetrics and Gynecology*, 5th ed. Philadelphia, PA: Saunders; 2009:71-90.

Case 11

A 25-year-old G2 P1 woman is delivering at 42 weeks' gestation. She is moderately obese, but the fetus appears clinically to be of about 3700 g weight. After a 4-hour first stage of labor, and a 2-hour second stage of labor, the fetal head delivers but is noted to be retracted back toward the patient's introitus. The fetal shoulders do not deliver, even with maternal pushing.

➤ What is your next step in management?

➤ What is a likely complication that can occur because of this situation?

➤ What maternal condition would most likely put the patient at risk for this condition?

ANSWERS TO CASE 11:
Shoulder Dystocia

Summary: A 25-year-old obese G2 P1 woman is delivering at 42 weeks' gestation; the fetus appears clinically to be 3700 g (average weight). After a 4-hour first stage of labor, and a 2-hour second stage of labor, the head delivers but the shoulders do not easily deliver.

➤ **Next step in management:** McRoberts maneuver (hyperflexion of the maternal hips onto the maternal abdomen and/or suprapubic pressure).

➤ **Likely complication:** A likely maternal complication is postpartum hemorrhage; a common neonatal complication is a brachial plexus injury such as an Erb palsy.

➤ **Maternal condition:** Gestational diabetes, which increases the fetal weight on the shoulders and abdomen.

ANALYSIS

Objectives

1. Understand the risk factors for shoulder dystocia.
2. Understand that shoulder dystocia is an obstetric emergency, and be familiar with the initial maneuvers used to manage this condition.
3. Know the neonatal complications that can occur with shoulder dystocia.

Considerations

The patient is multiparous and obese, both of which are risk factors for shoulder dystocia. There is no indication of gestational diabetes, which would also be a significant risk factor. The patient is post-term at 42 weeks, which increases the likelihood of fetal macrosomia. The patient's prolonged second stage of labor (upper limits for a multiparous patient is 1 hour without and 2 hours with epidural analgesia) may be a nonspecific indicator of impending shoulder dystocia. Nevertheless, the diagnosis is straightforward in that the fetal shoulders are described as not easily delivering. The fetal head is retracted back toward the maternal introitus, the "turtle sign." Because most shoulder dystocia events are unpredictable, as in this case, the clinician must be proficient in the management of this entity, particularly because of the potential for fetal injury.

APPROACH TO
Shoulder Dystocia

DEFINITIONS

SHOULDER DYSTOCIA: Inability of the fetal shoulders to deliver spontaneously, usually due to the impaction of the anterior shoulder behind the maternal symphysis pubis.

MCROBERTS MANEUVER: The maternal thighs are sharply flexed against the maternal abdomen to straighten the sacrum relative to the lumbar spine and rotate the symphysis pubis anteriorly toward the maternal head (Figure 11–1).

SUPRAPUBIC PRESSURE: The operator's hand is used to push on the suprapubic region in a downward or lateral direction in an effort to push the fetal shoulder into an oblique plane and from behind the symphysis pubis.

ERB PALSY: A brachial plexus injury involving the C5-C6 nerve roots, which may result from the downward traction of the anterior shoulder; the baby usually has weakness of the deltoid and infraspinatus muscles as well as the flexor muscles of the forearm. The arm often hangs limply by the side and is internally rotated.

CLINICAL APPROACH

Because of the unpredictability and urgency of shoulder dystocia, the clinician should rehearse its management and be ready when the situation is encountered. Shoulder dystocia should be suspected with fetal macrosomia, maternal obesity, prolonged second stage of labor, and gestational diabetes. However, it must be noted that almost one-half of all cases occur in babies weighing less than 4000 g, and shoulder dystocia is frequently unsuspected. Significant fetal hypoxia may occur with undue delay from the delivery of the head to the body. Moreover, excessive traction on the fetal head may lead to a brachial plexus injury to the baby. It should be recognized that brachial plexus injury can occur with vaginal delivery not associated with shoulder dystocia, or even with cesarean delivery. Shoulder dystocia is not resolved with more traction, but by maneuvers to relieve the impaction of the anterior shoulder (Table 11–1).

The diagnosis is made when external rotation of the fetal head is difficult, and the fetal head may retract back toward the maternal introitus, the "turtle sign." The first actions are nonmanipulative of the fetus, such as the McRoberts maneuver and suprapubic pressure. Fundal pressure should be avoided when shoulder dystocia is diagnosed because of the increased associated neonatal injury. Other maneuvers include the Wood's corkscrew (progressively rotating the posterior shoulder in 180° in a corkscrew fashion), delivery of the posterior arm, and the Zavanelli maneuver (cephalic replacement with immediate cesarean section).

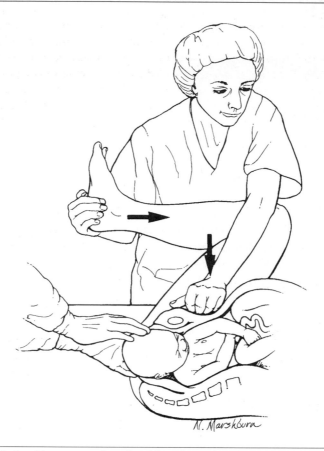

Figure 11–1. Maneuvers for shoulder dystocia. The McRoberts maneuver involves flexing the maternal thighs against the abdomen. Suprapubic pressure attempts to push the fetal shoulders into an oblique plane. *Reproduced with permission from Cunningham FG, et al.* Williams Obstetrics, *22nd ed. New York, NY: McGraw-Hill; 2005:515.*

Table 11–1 COMMON MANEUVERS FOR TREATMENT OF SHOULDER DYSTOCIA

Common McRoberts maneuver
Suprapubic pressure
Wood's corkscrew maneuver
Delivery of the posterior arm
Zavanelli maneuver

One area of controversy is the practice of cesarean delivery in certain circumstances in an attempt to avoid shoulder dystocia; indications include macrosomia diagnosed on ultrasound, particularly with maternal gestational diabetes. Because of the imprecision of estimated fetal weights and prediction of shoulder dystocia, there is no uniform agreement regarding this practice. Operative vaginal delivery, such as vacuum or forceps-assisted deliveries in the face of possible fetal macrosomia, may possibly increase the risk of shoulder dystocia.

Comprehension Questions

11.1   Which of the following is a risk factor for shoulder dystocia?
        A. Maternal gestational diabetes
        B. Fetal hydrocephalus
        C. Fetal prematurity
        D. Precipitous (fast) labor

11.2   A 30-year-old woman is noted to be in active labor at 40 weeks' gestation. Delivery of the fetal head occurs, but the fetal shoulders do not deliver with the normal traction. The fetal head is retracted toward the maternal introitus. Which of the following is a useful maneuver for this situation?
        A. Internal podalic version
        B. Suprapubic pressure
        C. Fundal pressure
        D. Intentional fracture of the fetal humerus
        E. Delivery of the anterior arm

Match the following mechanisms (A-E) to the stated maneuver (11.3-11.5):
        A. Anterior rotation of the symphysis pubis
        B. Decreases the fetal bony diameter from shoulder to axilla
        C. Fracture of the humerus
        D. Displaces the fetal shoulder axis from anterior-posterior to oblique
        E. Separates the maternal symphysis pubis

11.3   The clinician performs a delivery of the posterior fetal arm.

11.4   The McRoberts maneuver is utilized.

11.5   The nurse is instructed to apply the suprapubic pressure maneuver.

ANSWERS

11.1   **A.** Gestational diabetes is a risk factor because the fetal shoulders and abdomen are disproportionately bigger than the head, therefore the head may pass through with no problems, yet it is quite difficult to deliver the anterior shoulder since it is lodged behind the maternal symphysis pubis. The McRoberts maneuver and application of suprapubic pressure are two techniques that attempt to relieve the impaction of the anterior shoulder. Unlike gestational diabetes, the complication with hydrocephalus is that the fetal head is greater than the body. The head itself may have a difficult time passing through the pelvis, but if it does pass, the shoulders would have no problem passing through since their width would be smaller than the width of the fetal head. The premature fetus typically has a well-proportioned body, but is overall smaller in size than the average-sized baby. No part of a premature fetus' body should typically get impacted anywhere along the birth canal. With precipitous labor, there is a decreased chance that a shoulder dystocia will occur, whereas a prolonged second stage of labor should raise suspicion that a dystocia is present.

11.2   **B.** The patient in this question has shoulder dystocia. The McRoberts maneuver or suprapubic pressure is generally the first maneuver used. The McRoberts maneuver involves sharply flexing the maternal thighs against the maternal abdomen to straighten the sacrum relative to the lumbar spine and rotate the symphysis pubis anteriorly toward the maternal head. Applying suprapubic pressure, or pushing on the suprapubic region, relieves the fetal shoulder from being impacted behind the symphysis pubis. The internal podalic version is an obstetric procedure in which the fetus, typically in a transverse position, is rotated inside the womb to where the feet or a foot is the presenting part during labor and delivery. This method would not be applicable in this situation because the fetus is presenting in the proper cephalic position. Fracturing of the fetal humerus is a complication that can occur with shoulder dystocia if one of the fetal arms is pulled or tugged on too forcefully. Attempting to deliver the anterior shoulder in the setting of shoulder dystocia can result in a brachial plexus injury involving the C5-C6 nerve roots. As a result, the baby could have weakness of the deltoid and infraspinatus muscles as well as the flexor muscles of the forearm (Erb palsy/"Waiter's tip").

11.3   **B.** With delivery of the posterior arm, the shoulder girdle diameter is reduced from shoulder-to-shoulder to shoulder-to-axilla, which usually allows the fetus to deliver.

11.4 **A.** The McRoberts maneuver causes anterior rotation of the symphysis pubis and flattening of the lumbar spine. This relieves the anterior shoulder from impaction and allows for delivery of the fetus. Separating the symphysis pubis is not associated with any kind of mechanism or maneuver for relieving shoulder dystocia. Fracturing the humerus is never indicated either, and may also lead to brachial plexus injury.

11.5 **D.** The rationale of suprapubic pressure is to move the fetal shoulders from the anteroposterior to an oblique plane, allowing the shoulder to slip out from under the symphysis pubis. Applying fundal pressure would only supply a greater force of the fetal shoulder against the symphysis pubis and possibly cause a more complex and serious situation such as brachial plexus injury to the fetus.

Clinical Pearls

➤ Shoulder dystocia cannot be predicted nor prevented in the majority of cases.
➤ The biggest risk factor for shoulder dystocia is fetal macrosomia, particularly in a woman who has gestational diabetes.
➤ The estimation of fetal weight is most often inaccurate, as is the diagnosis of macrosomia.
➤ The most common injury to the neonate in a shoulder dystocia is brachial plexus injury, such as Erb palsy.
➤ The first actions for shoulder dystocia are generally the McRoberts maneuver or suprapubic pressure.
➤ Fundal pressure should not be used once shoulder dystocia is encountered.

REFERENCES

American College of Obstetricians and Gynecologists. Shoulder dystocia. ACOG *Practice Bulletin 40.* Washington, DC: 2002.

Bashore RA, Ogunyemi D Hayashi RH. Uterine contractility and dystocia. In: Hacker NF, Gambone JC, Hobel CJ, eds. *Essentials of Obstetrics and Gynecology,* 5th ed. Philadelphia, PA: Saunders; 2009:139-145.

Cunningham FG, Leveno KJ, Bloom SL, Hauth JC, Gilstrap LC III, Wenstrom KD. Dystocia: abnormal presentation, position, and development of the fetus. In: *Williams Obstetrics.* 22nd ed. New York, NY: McGraw-Hill; 2005:513-517.

Case 12

A 45-year-old woman underwent a total abdominal hysterectomy for symptomatic endometriosis 2 days previously. She complains of right flank tenderness. On examination, her temperature is 102°F (38.8°C), heart rate (HR) is 100 beats per minute, and blood pressure (BP) is 130/90 mm Hg. Her heart and lung examinations are normal. The abdomen is slightly tender diffusely with normal bowel sounds. The incision appears within normal limits. Exquisite right costovertebral angle tenderness is noted.

➤ What would be your next diagnostic step?

➤ What is the most likely diagnosis?

ANSWERS TO CASE 12:
Ureteral Injury after Hysterectomy

Summary: A 45-year-old woman who underwent a total abdominal hysterectomy for symptomatic endometriosis 2 days previously has right flank tenderness, fever of 102°F (38.8°C), and exquisite costovertebral angle tenderness. The incision appears normal.

> ➤ **Next step:** Intravenous pyelogram (IVP), or CT scan of the abdomen with intravenous contrast.

> ➤ **Most likely diagnosis:** Right ureteral obstruction or injury.

ANALYSIS

Objectives

1. Understand that the urinary tract is sometimes injured in pelvic surgery.
2. Know the common presentations of ureteral and bladder injuries after gynecologic surgery.
3. Know some of the conditions that predispose patients to urinary tract injury.

Considerations

This patient has a clinical picture identical to pyelonephritis; however, because she has recently undergone a hysterectomy, injury to or obstruction of the ureter is of paramount concern. Endometriosis tends to obliterate tissue planes, making ureteral injury more likely. The intravenous pyelogram (IVP) is the best initial test to evaluate this disorder, although a CT scan of the abdomen and pelvis with intravenous contrast would also be diagnostic. If the same clinical picture were present without the recent surgery, then the most likely diagnosis would be pyelonephritis and the next step would be intravenous antibiotics and urine culture. Finally, the wound is normal, which argues against a wound infection causing the postoperative fever.

APPROACH TO
Ureteral Injuries

DEFINITIONS

CARDINAL LIGAMENT: The attachments of the uterine cervix to the pelvic side walls through which the uterine arteries traverse.

INTRAVENOUS PYELOGRAM: Radiologic study in which intravenous dye is injected and radiographs are taken of the kidneys, ureters, and bladder.

HYDRONEPHROSIS: Dilation of the renal collecting system, which gives evidence of urinary obstruction.

CYSTOSCOPY: Procedure whereby a scope is placed into the bladder via the urethra. Various procedures, such as placement of stents into the ureters, can be performed.

PERCUTANEOUS NEPHROSTOMY: Placement of a stent into the renal pelvis through the skin under radiologic guidance to relieve a urinary obstruction.

CLINICAL APPROACH

Up to 1% of abdominal hysterectomies can be complicated by ureteral injury. Cancer, extensive adhesions, endometriosis, tubo-ovarian abscess, residual ovaries, and interligamentous leiomyomata are risk factors. Any gynecologic procedure, including laparoscopy or vaginal hysterectomy, may result in ureteral injury; however, the majority of the injuries are associated with abdominal hysterectomy. The most common location for ureteral injury is at the cardinal ligament, where the ureter is only 2- to 3-cm lateral to the cervix. The ureter is just under the uterine artery, "water under the bridge" (Figure 12–1). Other locations of ureteral injuries include the pelvic brim, which occur during the ligation of the ovarian vessels (infundibular pelvic ligament), and at the point at which the ureter enters the bladder (anterior to the vagina, when the vaginal cuff is ligated at the end of the hysterectomy). Ureteral injuries include suture ligation, transsection, crushing with clamps, ischemia-induced damage from stripping the blood supply, and laparoscopic injury.

If the IVP shows possible obstruction with hydronephrosis and/or hydroureter (Figure 12–2), the next steps include antibiotic administration and cystoscopy to attempt retrograde stent passage. This procedure is performed in the hope that the ureter is kinked but not occluded. Relief of the obstruction is paramount in preventing renal damage. The decision for immediate ureteral repair versus initial percutaneous nephrostomy with later ureteral repair should be individualized.

In general, bladder lacerations on the dome (top) of the bladder can be sutured at the time of surgery; however, injury in the trigone area (lower) may need ureteral stent placement to prevent ureteral stricture.

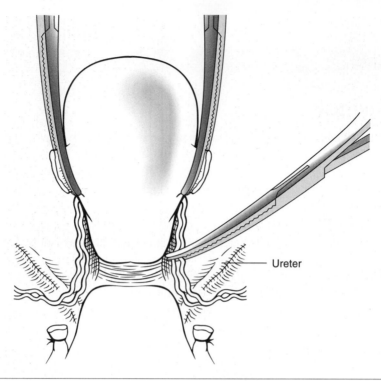

Figure 12–1.   Location of ureters during hysterectomy. The ureters are within 2 to 3 cm lateral to the internal cervical os and can be injured upon clamping of the uterine arteries.

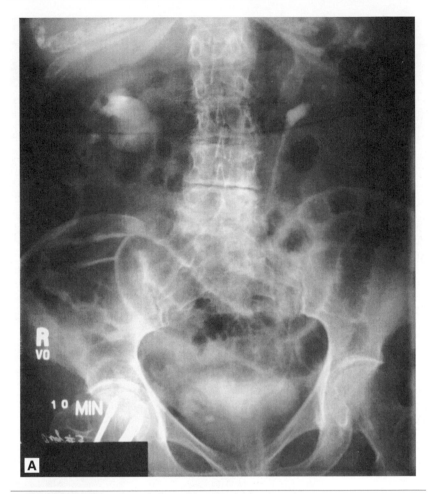

Figure 12–2.   Intravenous pyelogram. Right hydronephrosis is reflected by dilation of the renal collecting system and hydroureter, whereas the left collecting system is normal (A).

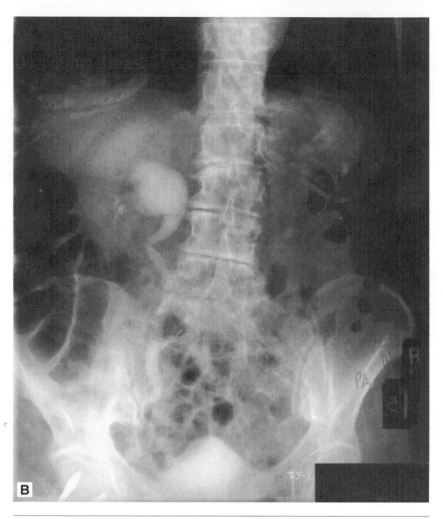

Figure 12–2.   Delayed film of the same patient shows the right hydroureter more prominently. *Images courtesy of Dr. John E. Bertini.*

Comprehension Questions

Match the following processes (A-E) to the most likely clinical situations (12.1-12.4).

    A. Vesicovaginal fistula

    B. Ureteral ligation

    C. Ureteral ischemia leading to injury

    D. Ureteral thermal injury

    E. Bladder perforation injury

12.1   A 55-year-old woman undergoes a total abdominal hysterectomy and develops fever and flank tenderness.

12.2   A 33-year-old woman undergoes pelvic lymphadenectomy for cervical cancer. During the procedure, the right ureter is meticulously and cleanly dissected free and a Penrose drain is placed around it to ensure its safety. She is asymptomatic until postoperative day 9, when she develops profuse nausea and vomiting, and is noted to have ascites on ultrasound.

12.3   A 55-year-old woman, who underwent a vaginal hysterectomy for third-degree vaginal prolapse 1 month ago, complains of constant leakage of fluid per vagina of 7 days duration.

12.4   A 44-year-old woman undergoes a right salpingo-ophorectomy laparoscopically. Bipolar cautery is used to ligate the infundibular pelvic ligament. The next day, she complains of fever and flank tenderness.

ANSWERS

12.1   **B.** There are many risk factors associated with ureteral injury; however the majority are associated with abdominal hysterectomies. Other risk factors include: cancer, extensive adhesions, endometriosis, tubo-ovarian abscess, residual ovaries, interligamentous leiomyomata, and most gynecological procedures. Also, the presentation of fever and flank tenderness after surgery makes the diagnosis of ureteral ligation most likely in comparison to the other options. When the ureter is ligated, the patient is at an increased risk of hydronephrosis and/or hydroureter. Antibiotic treatment and relief of the obstruction should be administered promptly to avoid the situation in this scenario of pyelonephritis. Patients with a bladder perforation injury typically present with gross hematuria, pain, or tenderness in the suprapubic region and difficulty in voiding. Ureters are not typically "dissected out" during a hysterectomy; therefore it would be unlikely for ischemia to occur in this situation.

12.2   **C.** Overdissection of the ureter may lead to devascularization injury because the ureter receives its blood supply from various arteries along its course and flows along its adventitial sheath. Urine is leaked into the abdominal cavity and causes irritation to the intestines and induces nausea and emesis. With a vesicovaginal fistula, urine is continuously leaking out the vagina, but not into the abdominal cavity. Nausea and vomiting are not associated with any of the other answer choices except for bladder perforation. In bladder perforation injuries, patients present with pain in the suprapubic region.

12.3   **A.** Constant urinary leakage after pelvic surgery is a typical history for vesicovaginal fistula (see Case 1). In other words, there is constant connection between the bladder and vagina. Any type of pelvic surgery predisposes to fistula formation. Surgery is necessary to remove the fistula.

12.4   **D.** Thermal injury can spread from cauterized tissue to surrounding structures. As with the patient diagnosed with a ureteral ligation, this patient presents with fever and flank tenderness. The fact that the procedure in this scenario was performed using bipolar cautery, the likelihood that the symptoms deal with thermal injury versus ligation is much higher.

Clinical Pearls

➤ Ureteral injury should be suspected when a patient develops flank tenderness and fever after a hysterectomy or oophorectomy.
➤ Meticulous ureteral dissection can lead to devascularization injury to the ureter since the vascular channels run along the adventitia of the ureter.
➤ A fistula should be considered when there is constant leakage of drainage from the vagina after surgery or radiation therapy.
➤ An intravenous pyelogram (IVP) is the imaging test of choice to assess a postoperative patient with a suspected ureteral injury.

REFERENCES

American College of Obstetricians and Gynecologists. The role of cystourethroscopy in the generalist obstetrician-gynecologist practice. *ACOG Committee Opinion 372.* Washington, DC: 2007.

Gambone JC. Gynecologic procedures. In: Hacker NF, Gambone JC, Hobel CJ, eds. *Essentials of Obstetrics and Gynecology,* 5th ed. Philadelphia, PA: Saunders; 2009:332-344.

Underwood P. Operative injuries to the ureter: prevention, recognition, and management. In: Rock JA, Jones III HW, eds. *TeLinde's Operative Gynecology.* 10th ed. Philadelphia, PA: Lippincott; 2008:960-971.

Case 13

A 66-year-old nulliparous woman who underwent menopause at 55 years complains of a 2-week history of vaginal bleeding. Prior to menopause, she had irregular menses. She denies the use of estrogen replacement therapy. Her medical history is significant for diabetes mellitus controlled with an oral hypoglycemic agent. On examination, she weighs 190 lb, height 5 ft 3 in, blood pressure (BP) is 150/90 mm Hg, and temperature is 99°F (37.2°C). The heart and lung examinations are normal. The abdomen is obese, and no masses are palpated. The external genitalia appear normal, and the uterus seems to be of normal size without adnexal masses.

➤ What is the next step?

➤ What is your concern?

ANSWERS TO CASE 13:
Postmenopausal Bleeding

Summary: A 66-year-old diabetic, nulliparous woman complains of post-menopausal vaginal bleeding. Prior to menopause, which occurred at age 55, she had irregular menses. She denies the use of estrogen replacement therapy. Her examination is significant for obesity and hypertension.

➤ **Next step:** Perform an endometrial biopsy.

➤ **Concern:** Endometrial cancer.

ANALYSIS

Objectives

1. Understand that postmenopausal bleeding requires endometrial sampling to assess for endometrial cancer.
2. Know the risk factors for endometrial cancer.
3. Know that endometrial cancer is staged surgically.

Considerations

This patient has postmenopausal vaginal bleeding, which should always be investigated, because it can indicate malignant or premalignant conditions. The biggest concern should be endometrial cancer. She also has numerous risk factors for endometrial cancer including obesity, diabetes, hypertension, prior anovulation (irregular menses), late menopause, and nulliparity. The endometrial sampling or aspiration can be performed in the office by placing a thin, flexible catheter through the cervix. It is the initial test of choice to assess for endometrial cancer. This patient is not taking unopposed estrogen replacement therapy, which would be another risk factor. If endometrial cancer were diagnosed, the patient would need surgical staging. If the endometrial sampling is negative for cancer, another cause for postmenopausal bleeding, such as atrophic endometrium, is possible. A blind sampling of the endometrium, such as with the endometrial biopsy device, has 90% to 95% sensitivity for detecting cancer. If this patient, who has so many risk factors for endometrial cancer, were to have a negative endometrial sampling, many practitioners would go to a direct visualization of the endometrial cavity, such as hysteroscopy. If the clinician were to elect to observe this patient after the endometrial biopsy, any further bleeding episodes would necessitate further investigation.

APPROACH TO
Postmenopausal Bleeding

DEFINITIONS

ENDOMETRIAL SAMPLING (BIOPSY): A thin catheter is introduced through the cervix into the uterine cavity under some suction to aspirate endometrial cells.

ENDOMETRIAL POLYPS: A growth of endometrial glands and stroma, which projects into the uterine cavity, usually on a stalk; it can cause postmenopausal bleeding.

ATROPHIC ENDOMETRIUM: The most common cause of postmenopausal bleeding is friable tissue of the endometrium or vagina due to low estrogen levels.

ENDOMETRIAL STRIPE: Transvaginal sonographic assessment of the endometrial thickness; a thickness greater than 5 mm is abnormal in a postmenopausal woman.

CLINICAL APPROACH

Postmenopausal bleeding always needs to be investigated because it can indicate malignant disorders and premalignant conditions, such as endometrial hyperplasia. Notably, complex hyperplasia with atypia is associated with endometrial carcinoma in 30% to 50% of cases.

Approximately 20% of postmenopausal women not on hormonal therapy but complaining of vaginal bleeding will have an endometrial carcinoma. The most common etiology of postmenopausal bleeding is atrophic endometritis or vaginitis; also, vaginal spotting can occur in a patient taking hormonal therapy. However, since endometrial malignancy can coexist with atrophic changes or in women taking hormone replacement therapy, **endometrial carcinoma must be ruled out in any patient with postmenopausal bleeding.** Possible methods for assessment of the endometrium include endometrial sampling, hysteroscopy, or vaginal sonography.

Risk factors for endometrial cancer are listed in Table 13–1. They primarily include conditions of estrogen exposure without progesterone. Although endometrial cancer typically affects older women, a woman in her 30s with a history of chronic anovulation, such as polycystic ovarian syndrome, may be affected. When the endometrial sampling is unrevealing, the patient with persistent postmenopausal bleeding, or with numerous risk factors for endometrial cancer, should undergo further evaluation, such as by hysteroscopy. Direct visualization of the intrauterine cavity can identify small lesions that may be

Table 13-1 RISK FACTORS FOR ENDOMETRIAL CANCER

Early menarche
Late menopause
Obesity
Chronic anovulation
Estrogen-secreting ovarian tumors
Ingestion of unopposed estrogen
Hypertension
Diabetes mellitus
Personal or family history of breast or ovarian cancer

missed by the office endometrial sampling device. Additionally, endometrial polyps can be identified by hysteroscopy.

Endometrial carcinoma is the most common female genital tract malignancy. Although endometrial cancer is not the most common cause of postmenopausal bleeding, it is usually the one of most concern. Fortunately because endometrial cancer is associated with an early symptom, postmenopausal bleeding, it is usually detected at an early stage. Once diagnosed, endometrial cancer is staged surgically (Table 13–2). Sometimes endometrial cancer may occur in the atypical patient, such as a thin patient; these cancers tend to be more aggressive.

Table 13-2 STAGING PROCEDURE FOR ENDOMETRIAL CANCER

Total abdominal hysterectomy, bilateral salpingo-ophorectomy
Omentectomy
Lymph node sampling
Peritoneal washings

Comprehension Questions

13.1   A 60-year-old woman presents to her physician's office with post-
        menopausal bleeding. She undergoes endometrial sampling, and is
        diagnosed with endometrial cancer. Which of the following is a risk
        factor for endometrial cancer?
        A. Multiparity
        B. Herpes simplex infection
        C. Diabetes mellitus
        D. Oral contraceptive use
        E. Smoking

13.2   A 48-year-old healthy postmenopausal woman has a Pap smear per-
        formed, which reveals atypical glandular cells. She does not have a his-
        tory of abnormal Pap smears. Which of the following is the best next
        step?
        A. Repeat Pap smear in 3 months
        B. Colposcopy, endocervical curettage, endometrial sampling
        C. Hormone replacement therapy
        D. Vaginal sampling

13.3   A 57-year-old postmenopausal woman with hypertension, diabetes,
        and a history of polycystic ovarian syndrome complains of vaginal
        bleeding for 2 weeks. The endometrial sampling shows a few fragments
        of atrophic endometrium. Estrogen replacement therapy is begun. The
        patient continues to have several episodes of vaginal bleeding 3 months
        later. Which of the following is the best next step?
        A. Continued observation and reassurance
        B. Unopposed estrogen replacement therapy
        C. Hysteroscopic examination
        D. Endometrial ablation
        E. Serum CA-125 testing

13.4   A 52-year-old woman, who has hypertension and diabetes, is diag-
        nosed with endometrial cancer. Her diseases are well controlled. Her
        physician has diagnosed the condition as tentatively stage I disease
        (confined to the uterus). Which of the following is the most impor-
        tant therapeutic measure in the treatment of this patient?
        A. Radiation therapy
        B. Chemotherapy
        C. Immunostimulation therapy
        D. Progestin therapy
        E. Surgical therapy

ANSWERS

13.1   **C.** Diabetes mellitus is associated with endometrial cancer. Other risk factors include early menarche, late menopause, obesity, chronic anovulation, estrogen-secreting ovarian tumors, hypertension, family history, and, the biggest risk factor, ingestion of unopposed estrogen. Taking a combination oral contraceptive decreases the risk of endometrial cancer due to the progestin component in the pill that prevents the endometrium from becoming hyperprolific. Smoking is associated with a lower estrogenic state, which would, therefore, also decrease a patient's risk for endometrial cancer. But this poses a major public health risk, since smoking itself is associated with an overall increase in morbidity and mortality. Multiparity decreases the risk of endometrial cancer as well, and herpes simplex infection does not influence a patient's chance of acquiring endometrial cancer.

13.2   **B.** Atypical glandular cells on the Pap smear may indicate endocervical or endometrial cancer. Therefore, a colposcopic examination of the cervix, curettage of the endocervix, and endometrial sampling are indicated. Because endometrial carcinoma is the most common female genital tract malignancy and is very treatable (as is endocervical cancer) when detected at an early stage, the benefit of using multiple techniques to further examine the cervix and endometrium at a microscopic level is cost effective, specific, and should not be delayed. Delaying further investigation by repeating a Pap smear in 3 months may allow progression of any sort of malignancy the patient might have. Also, an abnormal Pap smear is not very specific, so waiting to repeat the test and retrieving abnormal results again would still not specify whether or not the patient has endometrial cancer, endocervical cancer, or another pathologic process. Vaginal sampling would not give us information as to the patient's likelihood of having an endometrial or cervical malignancy. In addition, vaginal cancer is not nearly as common as endometrial or endocervical cancer and it would not be cost effective if there are no symptoms associated with vaginal carcinoma. Hormone replacement therapy (estrogen) would either worsen the patient's endometrial hyperplasia and atypia or put the patient at an increased risk for endometrial cancer if it is not present already. Unopposed estrogens increase the proliferation of endometrial cells and the likelihood of developing endometrial hyperplasia and eventually endometrial carcinoma.

13.3   **C.** Persistent postmenopausal bleeding, especially in a woman with risk factors for endometrial cancer, must be pursued. Hysteroscopy would be very cost effective in this patient, who, in addition to many risk factors, presents with postmenopausal bleeding. Hysteroscopy is one of the best methods for assessing the uterine cavity since it allows for direct visualization of the uterine cavity. Continued observation and reassurance would not be indicated since there is a high suspicion that this patient may be presenting with endometrial cancer. Any delay in treatment may allow progression of the cancer, making it more difficult to treat, and reassurance would be misleading. Unopposed estrogen replacement therapy would not be indicated for this patient who already has so many risk factors and symptoms for endometrial cancer. Endometrial ablation may be beneficial in stopping bleeding in patients with menorrhagia who no longer wishes to bear children, but it is not a method for diagnosing or treating endometrial carcinoma. This patient would continue to bleed despite an endometrial ablation because of her high estrogenic state, and ablation would delay the diagnosis and treatment. The serum antigen CA-125 is not a specific cancer marker, and is mostly associated with epithelial tumors of the ovary.

13.4   **E.** Surgical treatment is a fundamental aspect of the treatment and staging of endometrial carcinoma. Radiotherapy is used as an adjunctive treatment when the surgery performed for staging shows high suspicion of possible spread. Chemotherapy would be indicated if the surgery revealed metastasis. Progestin therapy is effective in shedding the endometrial lining, but not at inhibiting cellular proliferation. Once the endometrial cells become complex and atypical, progesterone is ineffective.

Clinical Pearls

➤ An endometrial sampling should be performed in a woman with postmenopausal bleeding to assess for endometrial carcinoma.
➤ Unopposed estrogen is generally the biggest risk factor for the development of endometrial cancer.
➤ Endometrial cancer is staged surgically and surgery is a fundamental part of its treatment.
➤ Persistent postmenopausal bleeding warrants further investigation (such as hysteroscopy) even after a normal endometrial sampling.
➤ Endometrial cancer is usually discovered at an early stage due to an early symptom: postmenopausal bleeding.
➤ When endometrial cancer occurs in an atypical patient without a history of anovulation, it tends to be more aggressive.

REFERENCES

American College of Obstetricians and Gynecologists. Management of endometrial cancer. ACOG *Practice Bulletin 65.* August 2005.

Hacker NF. Uterine corpus cancer. In: Hacker NF, Moore JG, Gambone JC, eds. *Essentials of Obstetrics and Gynecology.* 5th ed. Philadelphia, PA: Saunders; 2009: 428-434.

Lu K, Slomovitz BM, Neoplastic diseases of the uterus. In: Katz VL, Lentz GM, Lobo RA, Gersenson DM, eds. *Comprehensive Gynecology.* 5th ed. St. Louis, MO: Mosby-Year Book; 2007:813-839.

Case 14

A 30-year-old G5 P4 woman at 32 weeks' gestation complains of significant bright red vaginal bleeding. She denies uterine contractions, leakage of fluid, or trauma. The patient states that 4 weeks previously, after she had engaged in sexual intercourse, she experienced some vaginal spotting. On examination, her blood pressure is 110/60 mm Hg, and heart rate (HR) is 80 beats per minute (bpm). Temperature is 99°F (37.2°C). The heart and lung examinations are normal. The abdomen is soft and uterus nontender. Fetal heart tones are in the range of 140 to 150 bpm.

➤ What is your next step?

➤ What is most likely diagnosis?

➤ What will be the long-term management of this patient?

ANSWERS TO CASE 14:

Placenta Previa

Summary: A 30-year-old G5 P4 woman at 32 weeks' gestation complains of painless vaginal bleeding. Four weeks previously, she experienced some post-coital vaginal spotting. The abdomen is soft and uterus nontender. Fetal heart tones are in the range of 140 to 150 bpm.

➤ **Next step:** Ultrasound examination.

➤ **Most likely diagnosis:** Placenta previa.

➤ **Long-term management :** Expectant management as long as the bleeding is not excessive. Cesarean delivery at 36 to 37 weeks' gestation.

ANALYSIS

Objectives

1. Know the differential diagnosis of antepartum bleeding. *[handwritten: previa, abruption]*
2. Understand that painless vaginal bleeding is consistent with placenta previa.
3. Understand that the ultrasound examination is a good method for assessing placental location.

Considerations

The patient experiences antepartum vaginal bleeding (bleeding after 20 weeks' gestation). Because of the painless nature of the bleeding and lack of risk factors for placental abruption, this case is more likely to be placenta previa, defined as the placenta overlying the internal os of the cervix. Placenta abruption (premature separation of the placenta) usually is associated with painful uterine contractions or excess uterine tone. The history of postcoital spotting earlier during the pregnancy is consistent with previa, since vaginal intercourse may induce bleeding. The ultrasound examination is performed before a vaginal examination because vaginal manipulation (even a speculum examination) may induce bleeding. Because the patient is hemodynamically stable, and the fetal heart tones are normal, expectant management is the best therapy at 32 weeks' gestation (due to the prematurity risks). If the same patient were at 35 to 36 weeks' gestation, then delivery by cesarean section would be prudent.

APPROACH TO
Antepartum Vaginal Bleeding

DEFINITIONS

ANTEPARTUM VAGINAL BLEEDING: Vaginal bleeding occurring after 20 weeks' gestation.

COMPLETE PLACENTA PREVIA: The placenta completely covers the internal os of the uterine cervix (Figure 14–1).

PARTIAL PLACENTA PREVIA: The placenta partially covers the internal cervical os.

MARGINAL PLACENTA PREVIA: The placenta abuts against the internal os of the cervix.

LOW-LYING PLACENTA: The edge of the placenta is within 2 to 3 cm of the internal cervical os.

PLACENTAL ABRUPTION: Premature separation of a normally implanted placenta.

VASA PREVIA: Umbilical cord vessels that insert into the membranes with the vessels overlying the internal cervical os, thus being vulnerable to fetal exsanguination upon rupture of membranes.

CLINICAL APPROACH

Antepartum hemorrhage is defined as significant vaginal bleeding after 20 weeks' gestation. The two most common causes of significant antepartum bleeding are **placenta abruption** and **placenta previa** (Table 14–1). The classic presentation of previa bleeding is painless vaginal bleeding after the mid–second trimester, whereas placental abruption frequently presents with painful contractions. When the patient complains of antepartum hemorrhage, the physician should first rule out placenta previa by ultrasound even before a speculum or digital examination, since these maneuvers may induce bleeding. Ultrasound is an accurate method of assessing placental location. At times, transabdominal sonography may not be able to visualize the placenta, and transvaginal ultrasound is necessary.

The natural history of placenta previa is such that the first episode of bleeding does not usually cause sufficient concern as to necessitate delivery. Hence, a woman with a preterm gestation and placenta previa is usually observed on bed rest with the hope that time may be gained for fetal maturation. Often, the second or third episode of bleeding forces delivery. The bleeding from previa rarely leads to coagulopathy, as opposed to that of placenta abruption. At or near term (36 to 37 weeks), many practitioners will perform

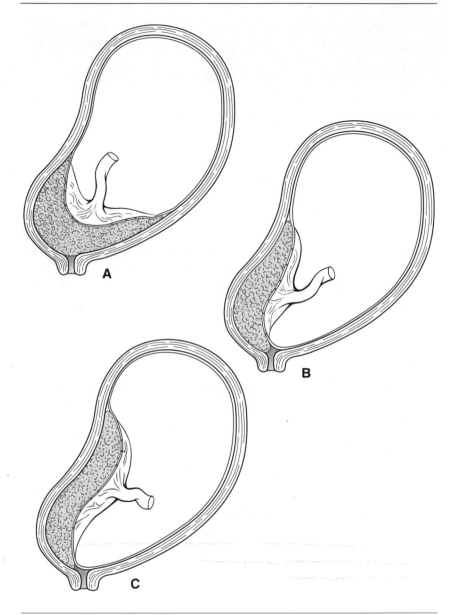

Figure 14–1. **Types of placenta previa.** Complete placenta previa (**A**), marginal placenta previa (**B**), and low-lying placentation (**C**) are depicted.

an amniocentesis to establish fetal lung maturity; if the fetal lungs appear mature, then delivery will be scheduled. The route of delivery as a general rule is by cesarean section. Because the lower uterine segment is poorly contractile, postpartum bleeding may ensue. Also, **placenta accreta** (invasion of the placenta into the uterus) is more common with placenta previa, particularly in the presence of a uterine scar such as a cesarean.

Table 14-1 RISK FACTORS FOR PLACENTA PREVIA

Grand multiparity
Prior cesarean delivery
Prior uterine curettage
Previous placenta previa
Multiple gestation

Comprehension Questions

14.1   A 28-year-old woman at 32 weeks' gestation is seen in the obstetrical (OB) triage area for vaginal bleeding described as significant with clots. She denies cramping or pain. An ultrasound is performed revealing that the placenta is covering the internal os of the cervix. Which of the following is a risk factor for this patient's condition?

A. Prior salpingitis
B. Hypertension
C. Multiple gestations
D. Polyhydramnios

14.2   A 21-year-old patient at 28 weeks' gestation has vaginal bleeding and is diagnosed with placenta previa. Which of the following is a typical feature of this condition?

A. Painful bleeding
B. Commonly associated with coagulopathy
C. First episode of bleeding is usually profuse
D. Associated with postcoital spotting

14.3   A 33-year-old woman at 37 weeks' gestation, confirmed by first-trimester sonography, presents with moderately severe vaginal bleeding. She is noted on sonography to have a placenta previa. Which of the following is the best management for this patient?

A. Induction of labor
B. Tocolysis of labor
C. Cesarean delivery
D. Expectant management
E. Intrauterine transfusion

14.4   A 22-year-old G1 P0 woman at 34 weeks' gestation presents with moderate vaginal bleeding and no uterine contractions. Her blood pressure (BP) is 110/60 mm Hg and heart rate (HR) 103 beats per minute (bpm). The abdomen is nontender. Which of the following sequence of examinations is most appropriate?
   A. Speculum examination, ultrasound examination, digital examination
   B. Ultrasound examination, digital examination, speculum examination
   C. Digital examination, ultrasound examination, speculum examination
   D. Ultrasound examination, speculum examination, digital examination

14.5   An 18-year-old adolescent female is noted to have a marginal placenta previa on an ultrasound examination at 22 weeks' gestation. She does not have vaginal bleeding or spotting. Which of the following is the most appropriate management?
   A. Schedule cesarean delivery at 39 weeks.
   B. Schedule an amniocentesis at 36 weeks and deliver by cesarean if the fetal lungs are mature.
   C. Schedule an MRI examination at 35 weeks to assess for possible percreta involving the bladder.
   D. Reassess placental position at 34 to 35 weeks' gestation by ultrasound.
   E. Recommend termination of pregnancy.

ANSWERS

14.1   **C.** Multiple gestation, with the increased surface area of placentation, is a risk factor for placenta previa. Hypertension is not a risk factor for placenta previa; however it is one of the main risk factors for placenta abruption. Polyhydramnios, due to the excess amount of amniotic fluid in the amniotic sac, is also a risk factor for placenta abruption. Salpingitis involves inflammation and infection of the fallopian tubes and over time may lead to permanent scarring of the tubes. Since this particular process is limited to the tubes, there is not an increased risk of placenta previa; rather there is an increased risk of ectopic pregnancy.

14.2   **D.** Postcoital spotting is a common complaint in a patient with placenta previa. Unlike placenta abruption, placenta previa is not commonly associated with coagulopathy, painful bleeding, or having a profuse first episode of bleeding. The main distinguishing factor between a previa and abruption is the presence or absence of pain. With abruption, painful uterine contractions are typically the chief complaint, whereas previa is painless. Although the first episode of bleeding with a previa usually does not raise enough concern to deliver immediately, the second or third bleeding episodes will send the patient to the operation room (OR) for a cesarean delivery.

14.3   **C.** The best plan for placenta previa at term is cesarean delivery. There is no need to place the patient at risk for hemorrhage when the fetus' lungs are mature enough for life outside the womb, therefore expectant management would not be the best choice for this scenario. A patient with a scheduled cesarean delivery does not need to be induced for labor, nor does she need tocolysis since the status of the patient's labor is typically insignificant in a cesarean delivery. A patient with previa should not deliver vaginally since the lower uterine segment is poorly contractile, and postpartum bleeding may ensue. An intrauterine transfusion is also not indicated for this patient because the baby is going to be delivered and will be independent of the mother's blood supply. Even in the setting of an Rh− mother with an Rh+ fetus, an intrauterine transfusion before delivery would pose a significantly greater risk to the mother and baby than waiting to evaluate the situation after birth.

14.4   **D.** Ultrasound should be performed first to rule out previa, speculum examination second to assess the cervix and look for lacerations, and finally digital examination. Performing either a speculum examination or digital examination before evaluating the patient with ultrasound puts the patient at risk for hemorrhage. In the setting of a previa, the lower uterine segment and cervix are highly vascularized, and varices of the cervix may be visualized on speculum examination in some situations; however, the speculum itself may cause trauma to these varices and induce bleeding. A blind digital examination may result in further separation of the placenta from the uterus, which could also cause significant bleeding.

14.5   **D.** Very often, a marginal or low-lying placenta previa at the early second trimester will resolve by transmigration of the placenta. It is too early to discuss scheduling a cesarean delivery since the placenta previa may resolve and allow for vaginal delivery. At 35 weeks, an ultrasound should be repeated to see whether or not the placenta has migrated. There would be no reason to be concerned about a percreta if the placenta migrates to a more favorable position; therefore scheduling an MRI is not indicated at this time. In addition, an MRI is expensive and only 38% sensitive. If there is suspicion that a percreta exists, a previa has most likely already been diagnosed in the late second trimester or third trimester, so a scheduled cesarean delivery would most likely already be in the plan. During the cesarean, the physician will be able to assess the extent of the previa and base management on how far the placenta has penetrated through the uterine wall. Placenta percreta and increta are usually diagnosed during a cesarean delivery and not radiographically. Again, it would be too early to schedule for an amniocentesis at 36 weeks since the placenta has a chance of transmigrating. Recommending termination of preg-nancy would be inappropriate in this case. Even if the patient has a placenta previa at the time of delivery, both the mother and baby have an excellent prognosis if a cesarean delivery is performed (see Case 8).

Clinical Pearls

➤ Painless antepartum vaginal bleeding suggests the diagnosis of placenta previa.

➤ Ultrasound is the diagnostic test of choice in assessing placenta previa and should be performed before digital or speculum examination.

➤ Cesarean section is the best route of delivery for placenta previa.

➤ Placenta previa, in the face of prior cesarean deliveries, increases the risk of placenta accreta.

➤ When placenta previa is diagnosed at an early gestation, such as second trimester, repeat sonography is warranted since many times the placenta will move away from the cervix (transmigration).

REFERENCES

American College of Obstetricians and Gynecologists. Postpartum hemorrhage. ACOG Practice Bulletin 76. Washington, DC: 2006.

Cunningham FG, Leveno KJ, Bloom SL, Hauth JC, Gilstrap LC III, Wenstrom KD. Obstetrical hemorrhage. In: Williams Obstetrics. 21st ed. New York, NY: McGraw-Hill; 2005:810-823.

Kim M, Hyashi RH, Gambone JC. Obstetrical hemorrhage and puerperal sepsis. In: Hacker NF, Gambone JC, Hobel CJ, eds. Essentials of Obstetrics and Gynecology, 5th ed. Philadelphia, PA: Saunders; 2009:128-138.

Case 15

A 22-year-old G2 P1 woman at 35 weeks' gestation, who admits to cocaine abuse, complains of abdominal pain. She states that she has been experiencing moderate vaginal bleeding, no leakage of fluid per vagina, and has no history of trauma. On examination, her blood pressure is 150/90 mm Hg, and heart rate (HR) is 110 beats per minute (bpm). The fundus reveals tenderness, and a moderate amount of dark vaginal blood is noted in the vaginal vault. The ultrasound examination shows no placental abnormalities. The cervix is 1 cm dilated. The fetal heart tones are in the 160 to 170 bpm range.

➤ What is the most likely diagnosis?

➤ What are complications that can occur due to this situation?

➤ What is the best management for this condition?

ANSWERS TO CASE 15:
Placental Abruption

Summary: A 22-year-old G2 P1 cocaine user at 35 weeks' gestation complains of abdominal pain and moderate vaginal bleeding. On examination, her blood pressure is 150/90 mm Hg, and HR is 110 bpm. The fundus reveals tenderness. The ultrasound is normal. The fetal heart tones are in the 160 to 170 bpm range.

➤ **Most likely diagnosis:** Placental abruption.

➤ **Complications that can occur:** Hemorrhage, fetal to maternal bleeding, coagulopathy, and preterm delivery.

➤ **Best management for this condition:** Delivery (at 35 weeks, the risks of abruption significantly outweigh the risks of prematurity).

ANALYSIS

See also answers to Case 14.

Objectives

1. Understand that placental abruption and placenta previa are major causes of antepartum hemorrhage.
2. Know the clinical presentation of abruptio placentae.
3. Understand that coagulopathy is a complication of placental abruption.

Considerations

The patient complains of painful antepartum bleeding, which is consistent with placental abruption. Also, she has several risk factors for abruptio placentae, such as hypertension and cocaine use (Table 15–1). Because the natural history of placental abruption is extension of the separation, leading to complete shearing of the placenta from the uterus, the best treatment at a gestational age near term (>34 weeks) is delivery. As opposed to the diagnosis of placenta previa, ultrasound examination is a poor method of assessment for abruption. This is because the freshly developed blood clot behind the placenta has the same sonographic texture as the placenta itself.

Table 15–1 RISK FACTORS FOR ABRUPTIO PLACENTAE
Hypertension (chronic and preeclampsia)
Cocaine use
Short umbilical cord
Trauma
Uteroplacental insufficiency
Submucous leiomyomata
Sudden uterine decompression (hydramnios)
Cigarette smoking
Preterm premature rupture of membranes

APPROACH TO
Suspected Placental Abruption

DEFINITIONS

CONCEALED ABRUPTION: When the bleeding occurs completely behind the placenta and no external bleeding is noted; this condition is less common than overt hemorrhage but more dangerous.

FETOMATERNAL HEMORRHAGE: Fetal blood that enters into the maternal circulation.

COUVELAIRE UTERUS: Bleeding into the myometrium of the uterus giving a discolored appearance to the uterine surface.

CLINICAL APPROACH

As compared to placenta previa, **abruptio placentae is more dangerous and unpredictable.** Furthermore, the diagnosis is much more difficult to establish. Ultrasound examination is not helpful in the majority of cases; a normal ultrasound examination does not rule out placental abruption. There is no one test that is diagnostic of placental abruption, but rather the clinical picture must be taken as a whole. Thus, a patient at risk for abruptio placentae (a hypertensive patient or one who has recently been involved in a motor vehicle accident), who complains of vaginal bleeding after 20 weeks' gestation, must be suspected of having a placental abruption. Furthermore, the bleeding is often associated with uterine pain or hypertonus. The blood may seep into the uterine muscle and cause a reddish discoloration also known as the "Couvelaire uterus." Uterine atony and postpartum hemorrhage after delivery may occur. Upon delivery, a blood clot adherent to the placenta is often seen.

Another complication of abruption is coagulopathy. When the **abruption is of sufficient severity to cause fetal death, coagulopathy is found in one-third or more of cases.** The coagulopathy is secondary to hypofibrinogenemia, and clinically evident bleeding is usually not encountered unless the fibrinogen level is below 100 to 150 mg/dL.

The diagnosis of placental abruption is difficult because the clinical presentation is variable. Although painful vaginal bleeding is the hallmark, preterm labor, stillbirth, and/or fetal heart rate abnormalities also may be seen. Ultrasound diagnosis is not sensitive. A concealed abruption can occur when blood is trapped behind the placenta, so that external hemorrhage is not seen. Serial hemoglobin levels, following the fundal height and assessment of the fetal heart rate pattern, are often helpful. Fetal-to-maternal hemorrhage is more common with placental abruption, and some practitioners recommend testing for fetal erythrocytes from the maternal blood. One such test of acid elution methodology is called the Kleihauer–Betke test, which takes advantage of the different solubilities of maternal versus fetal hemoglobin.

The management of placental abruption is dependent on the fetal gestational age, fetal status, and the hemodynamic status of the mother. Delivery is the usual management! In a woman with a premature fetus and a diagnosis of "chronic abruption," expectant management may be exercised if the patient is stable with no active bleeding or signs of fetal compromise. Although there is no contraindication to vaginal delivery, cesarean section is often the chosen route of delivery for fetal indications. In cases of abruptions that are associated with fetal death and coagulopathy, the vaginal route is most often the safest for the mother. In the latter scenario, blood products and intravenous fluids are given to maintain the hematocrit above 25% to 30% and a urine output of at least 30 mL/h. These women generally have very rapid labors. Many of these women will manifest hypertension or preeclampsia following volume replacement and it may be necessary to start magnesium sulfate for seizure (eclampsia prophylaxis).

Comprehension Questions

15.1 An 18-year-old pregnant woman is noted to have vaginal bleeding. She is bleeding from venipuncture sites, IV sites, and from her gums. Which of the following is the most likely underlying diagnosis?

A. Placental abruption
B. Placenta previa
C. Gestational diabetes
D. Multifetal gestation
E. Gestational trophoblastic disease

15.2   A 32-year-old woman is seen in the obstetrical unit at the hospital. She
        is at 29 weeks' gestation, with a chief complaint of significant vaginal
        bleeding. She had a stillbirth with her prior pregnancy due to placental
        abruption. The patient asks the physician about the accuracy of ultra-
        sound in the diagnosis of abruption. Which of the following statements
        is most accurate?
        A. Fetal ultrasound is more accurate in diagnosing placental abrup-
           tion than placenta previa.
        B. Fetal ultrasound is quite sensitive in diagnosing placental abruption.
        C. Ultrasound is sensitive in diagnosing abruption that occurs in the
           lower aspect of the uterus.
        D. Fetal ultrasound is not sensitive in diagnosing placental abruption.

15.3   Which of the following is the most significant risk factor for abruptio
        placentae?
        A. Prior cesarean delivery
        B. Breech presentation
        C. Trauma
        D. Marijuana use
        E. Placenta accreta

15.4   A 35-year-old woman presents with bright red vaginal bleeding at
        30 weeks' gestation. Her urine drug screen is positive. Which of the
        following is most likely to be present in her drug screen?
        A. Marijuana
        B. Alcohol
        C. Barbiturates
        D. Cocaine
        E. Benzodiazepines

ANSWERS

15.1   **A.** Placenta abruption is a common cause of coagulopathy.
        Consumptive coagulopathy, also known as disseminated intravascular
        coagulation (DIC), involves the overactivation of the procoagulant
        pathways and can be a fatal complication of a placenta abruption or
        other causes of hemorrhage. Placenta previa rarely results in consump-
        tive coagulopathy, since there is usually a significantly less amount of
        bleeding involved in comparison with abruption. Gestational diabetes
        is more commonly associated with fetal macrosomia, and places the
        fetus at risk for shoulder dystocia at the time of delivery. Coagulopathy
        is not likely to be seen in gestational diabetes. A multifetal gestation
        puts a patient at a higher risk for a placenta previa due to the larger
        surface area required for the placenta(s), but as mentioned before,
        coagulopathy is not common in previa and the multifetal gestation

itself does not increase maternal risk of coagulopathy either. Gestational trophoblastic disease can be a benign or malignant cancer that develops in a woman's womb and is commonly associated with a molar pregnancy. Bleeding from a site of metastasis may lead to hemorrhagic shock, but this is not very common, and therefore the chance of developing DIC from this complication is even less likely.

15.2   **D.** Sonography is accurate in identifying previa, but not sensitive in diagnosing placental abruption. An ultrasound examination is a poor method for assessment of abruption because the freshly developed blood clot behind the placenta has the same sonographic texture as the placenta itself. High suspicions must be exercised from evaluating the clinical picture as a whole for diagnosing abruption. An extra challenging situation exists in the setting of a concealed abruption in which the bleeding occurs behind the placenta and no external bleeding is noted. This is extremely dangerous since a greater amount of time will most likely pass before the abruption is diagnosed.

15.3   **C.** Trauma is the most significant risk factor for abruption in comparison to the other answer choices. Extreme forces can shear the placenta away from the uterus in these situations. Marijuana, as opposed to cocaine, is not associated with abruption since it does not cause maternal hypertension and vasoconstriction like cocaine. A prior cesarean delivery may predispose a patient to placenta previa with an associated accreta in future pregnancies, but neither a prior cesarean delivery nor an accreta is significant risk factors for abruption. The most significant risk factor of breech presentation of the fetus is cord prolapse, which can lead to significant oxygen deprivation to the fetus. Other risk factors for placental abruption include: uterine leiomyomata (especially submucosal type), hypertension, cocaine use, short umbilical cord, uteroplacental insufficiency, hydramnios, smoking, and preterm premature rupture of membranes (PPROM).

15.4   **D.** Cocaine use is strongly associated with the development of placental abruption.

Clinical Pearls

➤ Painful antepartum bleeding should make one suspicious of placental abruption.

➤ The major risk factors for abruptio placentae are hypertension, trauma, and cocaine use.

➤ A concealed abruption may hide significant bleeding without external hemorrhage.

➤ The most common cause of antepartum bleeding with coagulopathy is abruptio placentae.

➤ Placental abruption may lead to fetal-to-maternal hemorrhage.

REFERENCES

Cunningham FG, Leveno KJ, Bloom SL, Hauth JC, Gilstrap LC III, Wenstrom KD. Obstetrical hemorrhage. In: *Williams Obstetrics*. 22nd ed. New York, NY: McGraw-Hill; 2005:810-823.

Kim M, Hyashi RH, Gambone JC. Obstetrical hemorrhage and puerperal sepsis. In: Hacker NF, Gambone JC, Hobel CJ, eds. *Essentials of Obstetrics and Gynecology*, 5th ed. Philadelphia, PA: Saunders; 2009:128-138.

Case 16

A 50-year-old G5 P5 woman complains of postcoital spotting over the past 6 months. Most recently, she complains of a malodorous vaginal discharge. She states that she has had syphilis in the past. Her deliveries were all vaginal and uncomplicated. She has smoked 1 pack per day for 20 years. On examination, her blood pressure (BP) is 100/80 mm Hg, temperature is 99°F (37.2°C), and heart rate (HR) 80 is beats per minute (bpm). Her heart and lung examinations are within normal limits. The abdomen reveals no masses, ascites, or tenderness. Her back examination is unremarkable and there is no costovertebral angle tenderness. The pelvic examination reveals normal external female genitalia. The speculum examination reveals a 3-cm exophytic lesion on the anterior lip of the cervix. No other masses are palpated.

➤ What is your next step?

➤ What is the most likely diagnosis?

ANSWERS TO CASE 16:
Cervical Cancer

Summary: A 50-year-old G5 P5 woman complains of a 6-month history of postcoital spotting and malodorous vaginal discharge. She has had a prior infection with syphilis, and is a smoker. The speculum examination reveals a 3-cm exophytic lesion on the anterior lip of the cervix.

➤ **Next step:** Biopsy of the cervical lesion.

➤ **Most likely diagnosis:** Cervical cancer.

ANALYSIS

Objectives

1. Understand that a cervical biopsy and not a Pap smear (which is actually a screening test) is the best diagnostic procedure when a cervical lesion is seen.
2. Know that postcoital spotting is a symptom of cervical cancer.
3. Know the risk factors for cervical cancer.

Considerations

This 50-year-old woman presents with postcoital spotting. Abnormal vaginal bleeding is the most common presenting symptom of invasive cervical cancer, and in sexually active women, postcoital spotting is common. This patient's age is close to the mean age of presentation of cervical cancer, 51 years. She also complains of a malodorous vaginal discharge that is because of the large, necrotic tumor. Notably, the woman does not have flank tenderness, which would be a result of metastatic obstruction of the ureter, leading to hydronephrosis. A cervical biopsy and not Pap smear is the best diagnostic test to evaluate a cervical mass. A Pap smear is a screening test and appropriate for a woman with a normal-appearing cervix.

Risk factors for cervical cancer in this woman include multiparity, cigarette smoking, and history of a sexually transmitted disease (syphilis). Other risk factors not mentioned would be early age of coitus, multiple sexual partners, and HIV infection (Table 16–1).

Table 16–1 RISK FACTORS FOR CERVICAL CANCER
Early age of coitus
Sexually transmitted diseases
Early childbearing
Low socioeconomic status
Human papillomavirus
HIV infection
Cigarette smoking
Multiple sexual partners

APPROACH TO
Cervical Cancer

DEFINITIONS

CERVICAL INTRAEPITHELIAL NEOPLASIA: Preinvasive lesions of the cervix with abnormal cellular maturation, nuclear enlargement, and atypia.

HUMAN PAPILLOMAVIRUS: Circular, double-stranded DNA virus that can become incorporated into cervical squamous epithelium, predisposing the cells for dysplasia and/or cancer.

RADICAL HYSTERECTOMY: Removal of the uterus, cervix, and supportive ligaments, such as the cardinal ligament, uterosacral ligament, and proximal vagina.

RADIATION BRACHYTHERAPY: Radioactive implants placed near the tumor bed.

RADIATION TELETHERAPY: External beam radiation where the target is at some distance from the radiation source.

HUMAN PAPILLOMAVIRUS (HPV) VACCINE: Killed virus vaccine, FDA approved, for females aged 9 to 26. The quadrivalent vaccine contains antigens of HPV types 16 and 18 (which are associated with about 50% of cervical cancer and dysplasia) and 6 and 11 (which cause venereal warts).

CLINICAL APPROACH

Cervical Cancer

When a woman presents with postcoital spotting or has an abnormal Pap smear, cervical dysplasia or cancer should be suspected. An abnormal Pap smear is usually evaluated by colposcopy with biopsies, in which the cervix is soaked with 3% or 5% acetic acid solution. The colposcope is a binocular magnifying device that allows visual examination of the cervix. **The majority of cervical dysplasia and cancers arise near the squamocolumnar junction of the cervix.** Many times, cervical intraepithelial lesions will turn white with the addition of acetic acid, the so-called "acetowhite change." Along with the change in color, dysplastic lesions will often have vascular changes, reflecting the more rapidly growing process; in fact, the vascular pattern usually characterizes the severity of the disease. An example of mild vascular pattern is punctations (vessels seen end-on) versus atypical vessels (such as corkscrew and hairpin vessels). A biopsy of the worst-appearing area should be taken during colposcopy for histologic diagnosis. Hence, the next step to evaluate an abnormal Pap smear is colposcopic examinations with directed biopsies.

When a woman presents with a cervical mass, biopsy of the mass, not a Pap smear, is appropriate. Because the Pap smear is a screening test, used for asymptomatic women, it is not the best test when a mass is visible. The Papanicolaou smear test has a false-negative rate and may give false reassurance.

When cervical cancer is diagnosed, then the next step is to stage the severity. Cervical cancer is staged clinically (Table 16–2). Early cervical cancer (contained within the cervix) may be treated equally well with surgery (radical hysterectomy) or radiation therapy. However, advanced cervical cancer is best treated with radiotherapy, consisting of brachytherapy (implants) with teletherapy (whole pelvis radiation) along with chemotherapy, usually platinum-based (*cis*-platinum), to sensitize the tissue to the radiotherapy. Since HPV is the etiologic agent in the vast majority of cervical cancer, the advent of the HPV vaccine promises to prevent much of cervical dysplasia and cancer. The quadrivalent vaccine has been granted FDA approval to be used in females aged 9 to 26. It consists of the antigens of HPV subtypes 6 and 11, which cause the majority of condyloma accuminata (venereal warts), and more importantly subtypes 16 and 18, which cause 50% to 70% of cervical cancer. Clinical research seems to indicate a protection against the acquisition of HPV infection from these subtypes; however, because other subtypes can still cause cervical dysplasia or cancer, regular Pap smears are still required even after vaccination. Ideally, the vaccine should be administered at an age prior to sexual activity. Cervical cancer often spreads through the cardinal ligaments toward the pelvic sidewalls. It can obstruct one or both ureters

---

Table 16–2 STAGING PROCEDURE FOR CERVICAL CANCER

Examination under anesthesia
Intravenous pyelogram
Chest radiograph
Barium enema or proctoscopy
Cystoscopy

leading to hydronephrosis. In fact, bilateral ureteral obstruction leading to uremia is the most common cause of death due to this disease.

Pap Smear and Cervical Cancer Prevention

The purpose of cervical cytology is to detect premalignant conditions, and intervene before it becomes invasive cancer. In general, abnormal Pap smears as a screening test require colposcopy and biopsy to determine the full extent of the dysplasia. Recently, the strategy of cervical cytology has undergone substantial changes due to the availability of HPV testing, and recognition that adolescents often clear the HPV and dysplasia spontaneously.

Cervical cytology is generally begun 3 years after onset of sexual activity, or by age 21 years. Annual Pap smear is then recommended up to age 30 years. If the annual cytology has been negative, then at age 30, the interval of screening can be extended to every 2 to 3 years. Also, after age 30, if cervical cytology and HPV subtype testing are both negative, Pap smear do not need to be performed any sooner than every 3 years. Finally, routine cervical cytology is not recommended in women who have had a total hysterectomy for benign indications, and no history of cervical dysplasia. However, **if hysterectomy is performed for cervical dysplasia (ie, CIN III [cervical intraepithelial neoplasia III]), then Pap smear of the vaginal cuff is still needed.** HPV typing is helpful in triaging cytology showing atypical squamous cells of undetermined significance (ASCUS), but is generally not helpful with any higher dysplasia. Thus, cytology showing low-grade squamous intraepithelial lesion (LSIL) or high-grade squamous intraepithelial lesion (HSIL) generally requires colposcopic examination. Adolescents and pregnant women with ASCUS may be observed instead of immediate colposcopy or even HPV testing.

Comprehension Questions

16.1 A 48-year-old woman who presents with postcoital vaginal bleeding is noted to have a cervical exophytic mass. A biopsy of the mass confirms squamous cell carcinoma. If molecular analysis of the cancer is performed, which of the following HPV subtypes is most likely to be found in the specimen?
A. 6 and 11
B. 16 and 18
C. 55 and 57
D. 89 and 92

16.2   A 39-year-old woman is diagnosed with advanced cervical cancer that appears to have spread to her right pelvic side wall. She has right hydronephrosis as evidenced by the IVP. The biopsy specimen confirms that it is a poorly differentiated carcinoma. Which of the following statements regarding this patient's condition is most accurate?

A. The best therapy for her is surgical excision.

B. Both brachytherapy and teletherapy are important in the treatment of this patient.

C. Radical hysterectomy is an option in the therapy of this patient.

D. The majority of cervical cancers are of adenomatous cell type.

16.3   A 45-year-old woman is diagnosed with an early cervical cancer, noted to be confined to the cervix and about 3 cm in diameter. She asks how she developed this condition. Which of the following is a risk factor for cervical cancer?

A. Early age of coitus

B. Nulliparity

C. Obesity

D. Late menopause

E. Family history of cervical cancer

16.4   A 33-year-old woman has a Pap smear showing moderately severe cervical dysplasia (high-grade squamous intraepithelial neoplasia). She denies a smoking history and does not recall having any sexually transmitted infections. Which of the following is the best next step?

A. Repeat Pap smear in 3 months.

B. Conization of the cervix.

C. Colposcopy-directed biopsies.

D. Radical hysterectomy.

E. CT scan of the abdomen and pelvis.

16.5   A 40-year-old woman is referred for a Pap smear showing high-grade squamous intra-epithelial lesions (HSIL). Which of the following statements is most accurate?

A. If HPV subtyping reveals no high-risk virus present, then routine cytology is recommended.

B. If colposcopy demonstrates the entire transformation zone, then no further analysis is needed.

C. If an endocervical curetting shows cervical dysplasia, then an excisional procedure of the cervix is appropriate.

D. Cervical cancer is highly unlikely due to the Pap smear revealing only HSIL.

16.6   A 47-year-old woman G4 P4 has a Pap smear which shows HGSIL. Colposcopy is performed which is adequate, and reveals CIN III. An endocervical curettage is negative. The patient also has menorrhagia caused by uterine fibroids. Thus, the patient undergoes a total abdominal hysterectomy, including removal of the cervix. The patient asks whether Pap smears need to be performed now that her cervix has been surgically removed. Which of the following is the most accurate statement?

    A. The patient should continue to have annual Pap smears of the vaginal cuff.
    B. The patient should have Pap smears every 2 to 3 years, which may be discontinued if negative after 10 years.
    C. The patient does not need Pap smears any longer.
    D. The patient should have the HPV vaccine.

ANSWERS

16.1   **B.** HPV subtypes 6 and 11 are associated with condylomata acuminata (venereal warts), whereas subtypes 16 and 18 are associated with cervical dysplasia and cancer. The other answer choices are uncommon subtypes and not associated with cervical cancer. Cervical dysplasia or cancer should be suspected when a woman presents with postcoital spotting or an abnormal Pap smear.

16.2   **B.** For patients with advanced cervical cancer, radiotherapy is superior to surgical therapy. Major advantages of radical hysterectomy over radiotherapy are preservation of sexual function (owing to vaginal agglutination caused by the radioactive implants—essentially closes the vagina) and preservation of ovarian function. Radiotherapy can be performed on women who are poor operative candidates and is the best therapy for advanced disease, consisting of brachytherapy and teletherapy. Advanced disease involves spread to the pelvic sidewalls or hydronephrosis. Early-stage cervical cancer can be treated equally well with surgery or radiation therapy. The majority of cervical dysplasia and cancers arise near the squamocolumnar junction of the cervix and are of the squamous, not adenomatous, type.

16.3   **A.** Early age of coitus, a history of STDs, early childbearing, low socioeconomic status, HPV, HIV, cigarette smoking, and multiple sex partners are all risk factors for developing cervical cancer. HPV is the main risk factor, and is usually acquired from sexual exposure. Late menopause, obesity, and nulliparity are risk factors for endometrial cancer, not cervical cancer. Family history is not shown to be a risk factor for cervical cancer.

16.4   **C.** Colposcopic examination with directed biopsies is the next step to evaluate abnormal cytology on Pap smear.

only one you can skip colposcopy
is ASCUS - HPV

16.5   **C.** When high-grade SIL is present, colposcopic examination is important. HPV typing has a role in triaging atypical cells of undetermined significance, but not HSIL. Demonstration of the entire transformation zone during colposcopy allows biopsy of the worst area. A cervical excisional procedure (loop electrosurgical excisional procedure) or cone biopsy are indicated when there is the possibility of endocervical disease.

16.6   **A.** When the patient has a history of cervical dysplasia, even after total hysterectomy (removal of uterine corpus and cervix), annual Pap smears should be performed of the vaginal cuff. This is because vaginal cancer may arise. In contrast, when total hysterectomy is performed for benign reasons, and no history of cervical dysplasia, then no further Pap smears need to be performed.

Clinical Pearls

➤ The main risk factors for cervical cancer are sexually related, especially exposure to human papillomavirus.

➤ Human papilloma virus 16 and 18 are the most commonly isolated subtypes in cervical dysplasia and cancer.

➤ Flank tenderness or leg swelling indicate advanced cervical cancer, which is best treated by radiotherapy with a chemotherapeutic radiosensitizer.

➤ A visible lesion of the cervix should be evaluated by biopsy and not Pap smear.

➤ An abnormal Pap smear is usually evaluated with colposcopy-directed biopsies.

➤ The HPV vaccine is approved for females aged 9 to 26 to reduce the likelihood of cervical dysplasia or cancer, and venereal warts.

➤ Cervical cytology no longer needs to be performed after age 65 to 70 years, and after total hysterectomy for benign reasons and when there is no history of cervical dysplasia .

REFERENCES

American College of Obstetricians and Gynecologists. Diagnosis and treatment of cervical carcinomas. ACOG *Practice Bulletin 35.* May 2002.

American College of Obstetricians and Gynecologists. Evaluation and management of abnormal cervical cytology and histology in the adolescent. ACOG *Committee Opinion 330.* Washington, DC: 2006.

American College of Obstetricians and Gynecologists. Human papillomavirus vaccination. ACOG *Committee Opinion 344.* Washington, DC: 2006.

American College of Obstetricians and Gynecologists. Management of abnormal cervical cytology and histology. ACOG *Practice Bulletin* 99. Washington, DC: 2008.

Hacker NF. Cervical cancer. In: Berek JS, Hacker NF, eds. *Practical Gynecologic Oncology*. 3rd ed. Philadelphia, PA: Lippincott Williams & Wilkins; 2000:345-406.

Hacker NF. Cervical dysplasia and cancer. In: Hacker NF, Gambone JC, Hobel CJ, eds. *Essentials of Obstetrics and Gynecology*, 5th ed. Philadelphia, PA: Saunders; 2009: 402-411.

Jhingran A, Levenback C. Malignant diseases of the cervix. In: Katz VL, Lentz GM, Lobo RA, Gersenson DM, eds. *Comprehensive Gynecology*. 5th ed. St. Louis, MO: Mosby-Year Book; 2007:759-780.

Noller KL. Intraepithelial neoplasia of the lower genital tract (cervix, vulva). In: Katz VL, Lentz GM, Lobo RA, Gersenson DM, eds. *Comprehensive Gynecology*. 5th ed. St. Louis, MO: Mosby-Year Book; 2007:743-754.

Wright TC, Massad S, Dunton CJ, et al. for 2006 American Society for Colposcopy and Cervical Pathology-Sponsored Consensus Conference. 2006 consensus guidelines for the management of women with abnormal cervical cancer screening tests. *Am J Obstet Gynecol.* 2007:197(4);346-355.

Case 17

A 24-year-old G2 P2 woman delivered vaginally 8 months previously. Her delivery was complicated by postpartum hemorrhage requiring curettage of the uterus and a blood transfusion of two units of erythrocytes. She complains of amenorrhea since her delivery. She denies taking medications or having headaches or visual abnormalities. Her pregnancy test is negative. She was not able to breast-feed her baby.

➤ What is the most likely diagnosis?

➤ What are other complications that are likely with this condition?

ANSWERS TO CASE 17:
Amenorrhea (Sheehan Syndrome)

Summary: A 24-year-old G2 P2 woman has had amenorrhea since a vaginal delivery complicated by postpartum hemorrhage and uterine curettage. She was not able to lactate.

➤ **Most likely diagnosis:** Sheehan syndrome (anterior pituitary necrosis).

➤ **Other complications that are likely with this condition:** Anterior pituitary insufficiency, such as hypothyroidism or adrenocortical insufficiency.

ANALYSIS

Objectives

1. Be able to differentiate Sheehan syndrome from intrauterine adhesions (Asherman syndrome).
2. Understand the mechanism of Sheehan syndrome.
3. Know the other tropic hormones that may be affected by anterior pituitary necrosis.

Considerations

This patient developed amenorrhea from the time of her vaginal delivery that was complicated by postpartum hemorrhage. The initial evaluation should be a pregnancy test (which is negative). The patient also underwent a uterine curettage in the treatment of the postpartum bleeding. In this setting, there are two explanations: (1) Sheehan syndrome and (2) intrauterine adhesions (Asherman syndrome). Sheehan syndrome is caused by hypotension in the postpartum period, leading to hemorrhagic necrosis of the anterior pituitary gland. Asherman syndrome is caused by the uterine curettage, which damages the decidua basalis layer, rendering the endometrium unresponsive. The key to differentiating between Sheehan syndrome and intrauterine adhesions is to assess for whether or not the anterior pituitary is functioning, and whether the outflow tract (uterus) is responsive to hormonal therapy. For instance, since this patient's history was "unable to breast-feed after delivery," it would suggest that the anterior pituitary was not functioning (lack of prolactin). Had the patient been able to breast-feed, then the most likely diagnosis would have been intrauterine synechiae. This patient was given a combination oral contraceptive agent, and if the endometrium were responsive to the hormonal therapy, then proliferation of the endometrium should occur followed by stabilization of the endometrium with the progestin component, and then finally bleeding when the placebo pills are taken (days 21-28). Other evidence of anterior pituitary dysfunction may include low thyroid hormones, gonadotropin (FSH and LH), or cortisol levels. A definitive diagnosis of IUA can be made with a hysterosalpingogram.

APPROACH TO
Postpartum Amenorrhea

DEFINITIONS

AMENORRHEA: No menses for 6 months.

SHEEHAN SYNDROME: Anterior pituitary hemorrhagic necrosis caused by hypertrophy of the prolactin-secreting cells in conjunction with a hypotensive episode, usually in the setting of postpartum hemorrhage. The bleeding in the anterior pituitary induces pressure necrosis.

INTRAUTERINE ADHESIONS (ASHERMAN SYNDROME): Scar tissue that forms in the endometrium, leading to amenorrhea caused by unresponsiveness of the endometrial tissue.

POSTPARTUM HEMORRHAGE: Classically defined as bleeding greater than 500 mL for a vaginal delivery and greater than 1000 mL for a cesarean delivery. From a more pathophysiologic standpoint, it is the amount of bleeding that results in, or threatens to result in, hemodynamic instability if left unabated.

CLINICAL APPROACH

Amenorrhea can ensue after a term delivery for 2 to 3 months; breast-feeding may inhibit the hypothalamic function, and lead to a greater duration of amenorrhea. However, in a nonlactating woman, when no menses resumes by 12 weeks after delivery, then pathology must be suspected. Overall, **the most common cause of amenorrhea in the reproductive years is pregnancy.** Hence, a pregnancy test is the appropriate initial test. If the patient does not have a history of postpartum hemorrhage, pursuit of hypothalamic causes, such as hypothyroidism or hyperprolactinemia, is often fruitful. If the patient is somewhat obese, or has a history of irregular cycles, then polycystic ovarian syndrome (PCOS) would be entertained. Findings consistent with PCOS include a positive progestin withdrawal bleed (vaginal bleeding after the ingestion of a progestin, such as medroxyprogesterone acetate or Provera). Polycystic ovarian syndrome is characterized by estrogen excess without progesterone, obesity, hirsutism, and glucose intolerance. Elevated luteinizing hormone to follicle-stimulating hormone ratios are often seen (eg, LH:FSH of 2:1). Polycystic ovarian syndrome should be suspected in patients with obesity, hirsutism, and oligomenorrhea. When women are hypoestrogenic, then two broad categories of causes are common: hypothalamic/pituitary diseases or ovarian failure. The FSH level can distinguish between these two causes, with an elevated FSH indicative of ovarian failure.

The patient in this case had amenorrhea after a vaginal delivery, making Sheehan syndrome or intrauterine adhesions the two most likely causes. Distinguishing between the two entities involves assessing whether the patient has normal or abnormal anterior pituitary function, or some evidence of unresponsiveness of the outflow tract to hormonal treatment (Table 17–1). Treatment of Sheehan syndrome consists of replacement of hormones, such as thyroxine, cortisol, and mineralocorticoid, and estrogen and progestin therapy. Intrauterine adhesions are treated by hysteroscopic resection of the scar tissue.

Table 17–1 DIFFERENCES BETWEEN SHEEHAN SYNDROME AND ASHERMAN SYNDROME

HORMONE FUNCTION	SHEEHAN SYNDROME	INTRAUTERINE ADHESIONS
Thyroid hormone (T_4)	Low	Normal
TSH	Low	Normal
FSH	Low	Normal
Estradiol levels	Low	Normal
LH surge (biphasic basal body temperature chart)	Absent	Normal biphasic
Cortisol levels	Low	Normal
Prolactin levels (able to breast-feed)	Low (unable to lactate)	Normal
Bleeding in response to estrogen and progestin (oral contraceptive)	Yes	No

Comprehension Questions

17.1   A 19-year-old G1 Ab1 woman underwent a uterine curettage after a miscarriage. She has had no menses since and is not pregnant. The physician is suspecting intrauterine adhesions. Which of the following is a feature of intrauterine synechiae (Asherman syndrome)?
       A. Usually occurs after uterine curettage
       B. Associated with low gonadotropin levels
       C. Associated with a monophasic basal body temperature chart
       D. Associated with low cortisol levels

17.2   A 24-year-old G1 P1 woman is seen in the office with secondary amenorrhea after her delivery. She is given a tentative diagnosis of pituitary necrosis (Sheehan syndrome). Which of the following is consistent with her presumed diagnosis?
       A. Usually associated with hypertensive crisis at or soon after a delivery
       B. Is caused by an ischemic necrosis of the posterior pituitary gland
       C. Is associated with decreased prolactin levels
       D. Is often associated with elevated TSH levels

17.3   A 32-year-old G2 P1 Ab1 woman presents to the gynecologist's office with secondary amenorrhea of 8 months' duration. She had normal and regular menses before this time. After an evaluation, she is given a diagnosis of intrauterine adhesions (Asherman syndrome). Which of the following is the best description of the mechanism of intrauterine synechiae (Asherman syndrome)?
       A. Trophoblastic hyperplasia
       B. Pituitary engorgement
       C. Myometrial scarring
       D. Endometrial hypertrophy
       E. Disruption of large segments of the endometrium

17.4   A 25-year-old woman presents with a 6-month history of amenorrhea. Her pregnancy test is negative. She is evaluated for other causes of secondary amenorrhea, and is given a diagnosis of polycystic ovarian syndrome (PCOS). Which of the following is consistent with this disorder?
       A. Estrogen deficiency and vaginal atrophy
       B. Osteoporosis
       C. Endometrial hyperplasia
       D. Hypoglycemia
       E. A history of regular menses each month prior to 6 months

ANSWERS

17.1   **A.** Intrauterine adhesions are associated with a biphasic basal tem-
        perature chart that reflects normal pituitary function and normal ovu-
        lation. This indicates the presence of progesterone, which elevates
        the temperature. Intrauterine adhesions usually occur after curettage
        of the uterus. It is with Sheehan syndrome, and not with Asherman
        syndrome, that due to anterior pituitary hemorrhagic necrosis, the
        patient is unable to breast-feed after delivery, has a monophasic basal
        body temperature chart, and has low cortisol levels. The necrotic
        anterior pituitary is unable to secrete prolactin, FSH/LH, ACTH,
        TSH, or growth hormone, and patients must take hormone replace-
        ments to restore function of the organs and systems these hormones
        acted upon.

17.2   **C.** Sheehan syndrome involves the anterior pituitary undergoing
        hemorrhagic necrosis after a hypotensive episode, usually in the set-
        ting of postpartum hemorrhage. The anterior pituitary is, therefore,
        unable to secrete prolactin among a few other hormones. The poste-
        rior pituitary is not involved because it has a direct arterial supply.
        Hypothyroidism is a result of Sheehan syndrome due to the low or
        absent TSH secretion from the anterior pituitary. A patient may
        have an associated hypotensive episode, and not a hypertensive one,
        in their peripartum period caused by the postpartum hemorrhage.

17.3   **E.** In Asherman syndrome, large patches of endometrium are defec-
        tive because of intrauterine adhesions. The endometrium is unre-
        sponsive, so estrogen exposure will have no effect on the lining of the
        uterus, and therefore cannot pose a risk for endometrial hyperplasia.
        Endometrial, and not myometrial scarring is involved. Pituitary
        engorgement occurs during pregnancy due to the hypertrophy and
        hyperplasia of lactotrophs. There is no associated increase in vascular
        supply, so when postpartum hemorrhage occurs, the anterior pituitary
        is particularly vulnerable to ischemia. Trophoblastic hyperplasia orig-
        inates from placental tissues. It does not directly induce intrauterine
        synechiae; however, if the patient undergoes a D&C for management
        of the trophoblastic disease, Asherman syndrome may develop.

17.4   **C.** PCOS is a condition characterized by chronic anovulation, hyperan-
        drogenism where other causes have been eliminated, and possible evi-
        dence of small ovarian cysts on ultrasound. It is associated with
        unopposed estrogen and estrogen excess. This setting increases the
        patient's risk of endometrial hyperplasia or endometrial cancer.
        Osteoporosis is a risk in hypoestrogenic states, and this patient has estro-
        gen excess, so osteoporosis is not a concern; in fact, bone mineral den-
        sity is usually quite good. Vaginal atrophy is associated with estrogen

deficiency, not excess. Glucose intolerance and diabetes mellitus and a history of oligomenorrhea since menarche are consistent with the diagnosis of PCOS.

Clinical Pearls

➤ The two most common causes of secondary amenorrhea after postpartum hemorrhage are Sheehan syndrome and intrauterine adhesions.

➤ A pregnancy test should be the first test in evaluating a woman with secondary amenorrhea.

➤ Normal function of the anterior pituitary points toward intrauterine adhesions.

➤ Hypothyroidism or a monophasic basal body temperature chart suggests Sheehan syndrome.

➤ The treatment of Sheehan syndrome is replacement of the hormones governed by the anterior pituitary gland.

➤ The most common cause of ovulatory dysfunction in a reproductive-aged woman is polycystic ovarian syndrome (PCOS). PCOS is characterized by obesity, anovulation, hirsutism, glucose intolerance, and estrogen excess.

REFERENCES

Alexander CJ, Mathur R, Laufer LR, Aziz R. Amenorrhea, oligomenorrhea, and hyperandrogenic disorders. In: Hacker NF, Gambone JC, Hobel CJ, eds. *Essentials of Obstetrics and Gynecology*, 5th ed. Philadelphia, PA: Saunders; 2009:355-367.

Lobo RA. Primary and secondary amenorrhea and precocious puberty. In: Katz VL, Lentz GM, Lobo RA, Gersenson DM, eds. *Comprehensive Gynecology*. 5th ed. St. Louis, MO: Mosby-Year Book; 2007:933-962.

Case 18

A 22-year-old G3 P2 at 40 weeks' gestation complains of strong uterine contractions. She denies leakage of fluid per vagina. She denies medical illnesses. Her antenatal history is unremarkable. On examination, the blood pressure (BP) is 120/80 mm Hg, heart rate (HR) is 85 beats per minute (bpm), and temperature is 98°F (36.6°C). The fetal heart rate is in the 140 to 150 bpm range. The cervix is dilated at 5 cm and the vertex is at −3 station. Upon artificial rupture of membranes, fetal bradycardia to the 70 to 80 bpm range is noted for 3 minutes without recovery.

➤ What is your next step?

ANSWER TO CASE 18:

Fetal Bradycardia (Cord Prolapse)

Summary: A 22-year-old G3 P2 at term is in labor with a cervical dilation of 5 cm; the vertex is at −3 station. Upon artificial rupture of membranes, persistent fetal bradycardia to the 70 to 80 bpm range is noted for 3 minutes.

➤ **Next step:** Vaginal examination to assess for umbilical cord prolapse.

ANALYSIS

Objectives

1. Understand that the first step in the evaluation of fetal bradycardia in the face of rupture of membranes should be to rule out umbilical cord prolapse.
2. Understand that the treatment for cord prolapse is emergent cesarean delivery.
3. Know that an unengaged presenting part, or a transverse fetal lie with rupture of membranes, predisposes to cord prolapse.

Considerations

This patient has had two prior deliveries. She is currently in labor and her cervix is 5 cm dilated. The fetal vertex is at −3 station, indicating that the fetal head is unengaged. With artificial rupture of membranes, fetal bradycardia is noted. This situation is very typical for a cord prolapse, where the umbilical cord protrudes through the cervical os. Usually, the fetal head will fill the pelvis and prevent the cord from prolapsing. However, with an unengaged fetal presentation, such as in this case, umbilical cord accidents are more likely. Thus, as a general rule, artificial rupture of membranes should be avoided with an unengaged fetal part. Situations such as a transverse fetal lie or a footling breech presentation are also predisposing conditions. It is not uncommon for a multiparous patient to have an unengaged fetal head during early labor. The lesson in this case is not to rupture membranes with an unengaged fetal presentation. With fetal bradycardia, the next step would be a digital examination of the vagina to assess for the umbilical cord, which would feel like a rope-like structure through the cervical os. If the umbilical cord is palpated and the diagnosis of cord prolapse confirmed, the patient should be taken for immediate cesarean delivery. The physician should place the patient in Trendelenburg position (head down), and keep his or her hand in the vagina to elevate the presenting part, thus keeping pressure off the cord.

APPROACH TO
Fetal Bradycardia

DEFINITIONS

ENGAGEMENT: Largest transverse (biparietal) diameter of the fetal head has negotiated the bony pelvic inlet.

FETAL BRADYCARDIA: Baseline fetal heart rate less than 110 bpm for greater than 10 minutes.

UMBILICAL CORD PROLAPSE: Umbilical cord enters through the cervical os presenting in front of the presenting part.

ARTIFICIAL RUPTURE OF MEMBRANES: Maneuver used to cause a rent in the fetal chorioamniotic membranes.

CLINICAL APPROACH

The onset of fetal bradycardia should be confirmed either by internal fetal scalp electrode or ultrasound, and distinguished from the maternal pulse rate. The initial steps should be directed at improving maternal oxygenation and delivery of cardiac output to the uterus. These maneuvers include (1) placement of the patient on her side to move the uterus from the great vessels, thus improving blood return to the heart; (2) intravenous fluid bolus if the patient is possibly volume depleted; (3) administration of 100% oxygen by face mask; and (4) stopping oxytocin if it is being given (Table 18–1).

Simultaneously with these maneuvers, the practitioner should try to identify the cause of the bradycardia, such as hyperstimulation with oxytocin. With this process, the uterus will be tetanic, or the uterine contractions will be frequent (every 1 minute); often a β-agonist, such as terbutaline, given intravenously will be helpful to relax the uterine musculature. Hypotension due to an epidural catheter is another common cause. Intravenous hydration is the first remedy, and if unsuccessful, then support of the blood pressure with

Table 18–1 STEPS TO TAKE WITH FETAL BRADYCARDIA

Confirm fetal heart rate (vs maternal heart rate)
Vaginal examination to assess for cord prolapse
Positional changes
Oxygen
Intravenous fluid bolus
Discontinue oxytocin

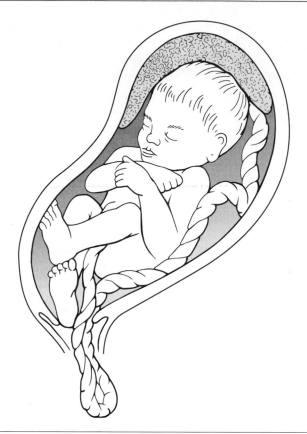

Figure 18-1. Umbilical cord prolapse. A footling breech presentation predisposes to umbilical cord prolapse.

ephedrine, a pressor agent, is often useful. A vaginal examination when the membranes are ruptured is "a must" to identify overt umbilical cord prolapse. A rope-like cord will be palpated, often with pulsations (Figure 18–1). The best treatment is elevation of the presenting part digitally, and emergent cesarean delivery. In women with prior cesarean delivery, uterine rupture may manifest as fetal bradycardia.

Fetal Heart Rate Assessment

The baseline fetal heart rate is normally between 110 and 160 bpm, with fetal bradycardia less than 110 bpm, and tachycardia greater than 160 bpm. The fetal heart rate typically has moderate variability, whereas diminished variability may be caused by sedating medications or more rarely fetal acidosis. Accelerations are abrupt increases in fetal heart rate of at least 15 bpm lasting for 15 seconds, and typically are indicative of adequate fetal oxygenation.

Decelerations may be early, late, or variable depending on its configuration and timing with the uterine contraction (see also Case 6).

Comprehension Questions

18.1 An 18-year-old woman, who had undergone a previous low-transverse cesarean delivery, is admitted for active labor. During labor, an intrauterine pressure catheter displays normal uterine contractions every 3 minutes with intensity up to 60 mm Hg. Fetal bradycardia ensues. Which of the following statements is most accurate?

A. The normal intrauterine pressure catheter display makes uterine rupture unlikely.

B. The most common sign of uterine rupture is a fetal heart rate abnormality.

C. If the patient has a uterine rupture, the practitioner should wait to see whether the heart tones return to decide on route of delivery.

D. The intrauterine pressure catheter has been found to be helpful in preventing uterine rupture.

18.2 A 32-year-old G1 P0 woman is at 42 weeks' gestation and being induced for postterm pregnancy. She has had an uncomplicated pregnatal course. Her BP is 100/60 mm Hg. The fundal height is 40 cm. Her cervix is closed, 3 cm long, and firm on consistency. The obstetrician decides on using a cervical ripening agent with misoprostol in the vagina. Approximately 2 hours after placing the misoprostol, the patient has an episode of fetal prolonged deceleration to the 80 bpm for 6 minutes. Which of the following is the most likely etiology of the prolonged deceleration?

A. Placental abruption   → PGE1

B. Sepsis

C. Umbilical cord prolapse

D. Uterine hyperstimulation

18.3 A 28-year-old G1 P0 at 35 weeks' gestation is in the obstetrical (OB) triage area with spontaneous rupture of membranes. The fetal heart rate baseline is 150 bpm with normal variability. There are accelerations seen, and numerous late decelerations noted. In an effort to improve oxygenation to the fetus, which of the following maneuvers would most likely help in this circumstance?

A. Supine position

B. Epidural anesthesia

C. Morphine sulfate

D. Stop the oxytocin

18.4   A 33-year-old G2 P1 woman at 39 weeks' gestation in active labor is noted to have a 10-minute episode of bradycardia on the external fetal heart rate tracing in the range of 100 bpm, which has not resolved. Her cervix is closed. Which of the following is the best initial step in management of this patient?
A. Fetal scalp pH assessment
B. Emergency cesarean delivery
C. Intravenous atropine
D. Intravenous terbutaline
E. Assess maternal pulse

ANSWERS

18.1   **B.** The most common finding in a uterine rupture is a fetal heart rate abnormality, such as fetal bradycardia, deep variable decelerations, or late decelerations; the intrauterine pressure catheter has not been found to be helpful and sometimes confuses the picture and may delay the diagnosis of uterine rupture. Immediate cesarean section is indicated for suspected uterine rupture.

18.2   **D.** Prolonged fetal decelerations or fetal bradycardia associated with miso-prostol cervical ripening is typically associated with uterine hyperstimulation, defined as greater than five uterine contractions in a 10-minute window. Although any of the prostaglandin cervical ripening agents may induce uterine hyperstimulation, misoprostol generally is associated with a higher risk. Its benefit is the very low cost.

18.3   **D.** The supine position causes uterine compression on the vena cava, which decreases the venous return of blood to the heart, leading to supine hypotension. One important maneuver when encountering fetal heart rate abnormalities is a positional change, such as the lateral decubitus position. Oxytocin and epidural anesthesia both can decrease oxygen delivery to the placental bed. Oxytocin may hyperstimulate the uterus and cause frequent contractions; this then results in frequent vasoconstriction of the uterine vessels which decreases the amount of blood arriving to the placenta and fetus over time. Thus, **stopping the oxytocin may help improve oxygenation.** An epidural can cause hypotension in the mother which may then lead to fetal bradycardia by also decreasing the amount of blood profusing the fetus per given time. Morphine sulfate can cause respiratory depression in the fetus, so it would not be a method of choice for increasing delivery of oxygen to the fetus.

18.4   **E.** The first step in assessment of apparent fetal bradycardia is differentiating the fetal heart rate from the maternal pulse. This may be done with the use of a fetal scalp electrode or ultrasound. A fetal scalp pH is a maneuver to assess whether or not the fetus is receiving sufficient oxygen during labor, but cannot be done with a closed cervix. It requires at least 4 cm dilation to get a sample of blood from the fetal scalp. It is rarely performed today. If fetal bradycardia is confirmed, various maneuvers may be implemented to improve maternal oxygenation (placement of mother on her left side, IV fluid bolus, 100% O_2 face mask, and stopping oxytocin). Simultaneously, IV terbutaline may be given to help relax the uterine musculature in an effort to increase blood flow and O_2 supply to the fetus. If none of these methods work, a vaginal examination may reveal a cord prolapse, in which case the best treatment is elevation of the presenting part digitally and emergent cesarean delivery. Atropine may be used in a nonpregnant patient to treat bradycardia or arrhythmias, but is not indicated for fetal bradycardia.

Clinical Pearls

➤ The first steps in assessing fetal bradycardia after artificial rupture of membranes are distinguishing the heart rate from the maternal pulse rate, and examining the vagina to assess for cord prolapse.

➤ The best therapy for umbilical cord prolapse is elevation of the presenting part and emergency cesarean delivery.

➤ The risk of cord prolapse with a vertex presentation or frank breech presentation is very low; the risk with a footling breech or transverse lie is substantially higher.

➤ The most common finding with uterine rupture is a fetal heart rate abnormality.

➤ The best treatment for suspected uterine rupture is immediate cesarean delivery.

REFERENCES

American College of Obstetricians and Gynecologists. Intrapartum fetal heart rate monitoring. ACOG *Practice Bulletin 70*. Washington, DC: 2005.

Bayshore RA, Koos BJ. Fetal surveillance during labor. In: Hacker NF, Gambone JC, Hobel CJ, eds. *Essentials of Obstetrics and Gynecology*, 5th ed. Philadelphia, PA: Saunders; 2009:119-127.

Cunningham FG, Leveno KJ, Bloom SL, Hauth JC, Gilstrap LC III, Wenstrom KD. Intrapartum assessment. In: *Williams Obstetrics*. 22nd ed. New York, NY: McGraw-Hill; 2005:447-456.

Case 19

A 30-year-old parous woman notes a watery breast discharge of 6 months' duration. Her menses have been somewhat irregular. She denies a family history of breast cancer. The patient had been treated previously with radioactive iodine for Graves disease. Currently, she is not taking any medications. On examination, she appears alert and in good health. The blood pressure (BP) is 120/80 mm Hg, and heart rate (HR) is 80 beats per minute (bpm). The breasts are symmetric and without masses. No skin retraction is noted. A white discharge can be expressed from both breasts. No adenopathy is appreciated. The pregnancy test is negative.

➤ What is the most likely diagnosis?

➤ What is your next step?

➤ What is the likely mechanism for this disorder?

ANSWERS TO CASE 19:
Galactorrhea Due to Hypothyroidism

Summary: A 30-year-old parous woman with irregular menses notes a watery breast discharge of 6 months' duration. She had been treated previously with radioactive iodine for Graves disease. The pregnancy test is negative.

➤ **Most likely diagnosis:** Galactorrhea due to hypothyroidism.

➤ **Next step:** Check serum prolactin and TSH levels.

➤ **Likely mechanism:** Hypothyroidism is associated with an elevated thyroid-releasing hormone (TRH) level, which acts as a prolactin-releasing hormone. The hyperprolactinemia then induces the galactorrhea.

ANALYSIS

Objectives

1. Know the clinical presentation of galactorrhea.
2. Know some of the major causes of hyperprolactinemia.
3. Understand that hyperprolactinemia can induce hypothalamic dysfunction leading to oligo-ovulation and irregular menses.

Considerations

This patient complains of oligomenorrhea and a white, watery breast discharge, which is likely to be milk (galactorrhea). The first investigation should be a pregnancy test. Causes of galactorrhea include a pituitary adenoma, pregnancy, breast stimulation, chest wall trauma, or hypothyroidism. She does not have headaches or visual disturbances. This woman had been treated previously with radioactive iodine for Graves disease and is not taking thyroid replacement. Thus, she likely has hypothyroidism. With primary hypothyroidism, both the thyroid-releasing hormone (TRH) and thyroid-stimulating hormone (TSH) are elevated. TRH acts as a prolactin-releasing hormone. Hence, elevated TSH and prolactin levels will be noted in this patient. The hyperprolactinemia inhibits hypothalamic GnRH pulsations, leading to oligomenorrhea.

APPROACH TO
Galactorrhea

DEFINITIONS

GALACTORRHEA: Nonpuerperal watery or milky breast secretion that contains neither pus nor blood. The secretion can be manifested spontaneously or obtained only by breast examination.

PITUITARY SECRETING ADENOMA: A tumor in the pituitary gland that produces prolactin; symptoms include galactorrhea, headache, and peripheral vision defect (bitemporal hemianopsia).

CLINICAL APPROACH

Galactorrhea is a milky breast secretion that occurs in a nonlactating patient. It is usually bilateral. To determine if the breast discharge is truly galactorrhea, a smear under microscope will reveal multiple fat droplets. Patients with galactorrhea often have associated oligomenorrhea or amenorrhea. See Table 19–1 for the different etiologies for hyperprolactinemia.

Galactorrhea and hyperprolactinemia require a careful diagnostic approach. A thorough history and physical should be done. All medications that can stimulate prolactin production should be discontinued. A magnetic resonance scan is the most sensitive test to detect pituitary adenomas, providing 1-mm resolution; it can detect virtually all microadenomas. The TRH test is useful for patients with mildly elevated hyperprolactinemia (in the range of 20-60 ng/mL). Those with a markedly high prolactin level, or those with neurologic symptoms, should have MRI of the pituitary. Hyperprolactinemia is a common cause of menstrual disturbances. Hence, a woman with galactorrhea, regular

---

Table 19–1 CAUSES OF HYPERPROLACTINEMIA

Drugs (tranquilizers, tricyclic antidepressants, antihypertensives, narcotics, oral contraceptive pills)
Hypothyroidism
Hypothalamic causes (craniopharyngioma, sarcoidosis, histiocytosis, leukemia)
Pituitary causes (microadenoma [<1 cm], macroadenoma [>1 cm])
Hyperplasia of the lactotrophs
Empty sella syndrome
Acromegaly
Renal disease (acute or chronic)
Chest surgery or trauma (breast implants, herpes zoster at the T2 dermatome of the chest)

menses, and normal serum prolactin is at low risk for having a prolactinoma. These patients can be followed with annual serum prolactin tests. However, even in the face of normal prolactin assays, women with oligomenorrhea and galactorrhea should undergo an anteroposterior and lateral coned-down view of the sella turcica. If necessary, a skull MRI will confirm the diagnosis of empty sella. Patients with secondary amenorrhea and low levels of serum estrogen (<40 pg/mL) have a significantly greater risk of having a pituitary adenoma as well as early onset of osteoporosis.

Women with galactorrhea but normal menses and normal serum prolactin levels may be observed. Also, patients with microadenomas, who do not wish to conceive, and without estrogen deficiency may be expectantly managed. Other patients with pituitary adenomas may be offered medical management versus surgery.

Primary hypothyroidism can lead to hyperprolactinemia and should be treated with thyroxine. Patients with hyperprolactinemia and low estrogen levels were once treated with bromocriptine. However, compliance with this medication was low due to the side effects (orthostatic hypotension, fainting, dizziness, and nausea and vomiting) and high cost. Another alternative is exogenous estrogen. Bromocriptine is particularly useful for patients desiring fertility. Another dopamine agonist for patients unresponsive to bromocriptine is cabergolamine, which is also available in depot form. Both bromocriptine and cabergolamine can be given vaginally if the patient does not tolerate the oral form. Patients with hyperprolactinemia, with or without microadenoma, with adequate estrogen levels (>40 pg/mL) and who do not desire pregnancy should be treated with periodic progestin withdrawal.

Surgery involves transsphenoidal microsurgical exploration of the sella turcica with removal of the pituitary adenoma while preserving the functional capacity of the remaining gland. Complications of the surgery include transient diabetes insipidus (occurs in about one-third), hemorrhage, meningitis, cerebrospinal fluid leak, and panhypopituitarism. Cure rate is directly related to the pretreatment prolactin levels (prolactin level of 100 ng/mL has an excellent prognosis, whereas 200 ng/mL has a poor prognosis). It may be preferable to reduce the size of the macroadenoma with bromocriptine before surgical removal of these tumors. Surgery, which is associated with some adverse effects, is usually reserved as secondary management in patients who have a macroadenoma with complete or partial failure of medical treatment or poor compliance.

dopamine agonist → Prolactin
(cabergoline, bromocriptine)

Comprehension Questions

19.1   A 25-year-old woman presents with galactorrhea and irregular menses of 10 months duration. Her pregnancy test is negative. Laboratory tests reveal normal TSH and serum-free T_4 and hyperprolactinemia. Which of the following is most likely to be a cause of her condition?

   A. Posterior pituitary adenoma
   B. Abdominal wall trauma
   C. Psychotropic medication
   D. Hyperthyroidism

19.2   A 38-year-old woman is seen by her physician because of headaches, amenorrhea, and galactorrhea. Her pregnancy test was negative. Her prolactin level was markedly elevated and TSH was normal. The physician makes a presumptive diagnosis of pituitary adenoma and orders an MRI of the brain. Which of the following clinical presentations is consistent with a prolactin-secreting pituitary adenoma?

   A. Diabetes insipidus
   B. Occipital cerebral defect
   C. Central field visual defect
   D. Amenorrhea due to inhibition of gonadotropin-releasing hormone pulsations

19.3   A 47-year-old woman is being evaluated for a possible pituitary tumor. She complains of headaches and has some visual difficulties. The MRI shows a mass in the **posterior** pituitary gland, which the radiologist notes is unusual. Which of the following is a hormone contained in the posterior pituitary gland?

   A. Follicle-stimulating hormone (FSH)
   B. Prolactin
   C. Thyroid-stimulating hormone (TSH)
   D. Oxytocin

19.4   A 33-year-old woman with a microadenoma of the pituitary gland becomes pregnant. When she reaches 28 weeks' gestation, she complains of headaches and visual disturbances. Which of the following is the best therapy?

   A. Craniotomy and pituitary resection
   B. Tamoxifen therapy
   C. Oral bromocriptine therapy
   D. Expectant management
   E. Lumbar puncture

ANSWERS

19.1   **C.** Medications are a common cause of hyperprolactinemia, especially psychotropic medications. Pregnancy is associated with elevated prolactin levels. The anterior, not posterior, pituitary secretes prolactin; an anterior pituitary adenoma is more likely to be a cause of hyperprolactinemia. Symptoms may include galactorrhea, headache, and peripheral vision defect (bitemporal hemianopsia). It is with hypothyroidism that hyperprolactinemia may occur. With primary hypothyroidism, both TRH (secreted by the hypothalamus) and TSH (secreted by anterior pituitary) levels are elevated. TRH acts as a prolactin-releasing hormone in addition to being a thyroid-releasing hormone. Chest wall trauma, and not abdominal wall trauma, can cause hyperprolactinemia.

19.2   **D.** Elevated prolactin levels inhibit GnRH pulsations from the hypothalamus. Without the signal from GnRH, gonadotropins (FSH/LH) are not released from the anterior pituitary and no estrogen (or progesterone) is released from the ovaries; this results in amenorrhea. Pituitary adenomas impinge on the optic chiasm, causing deficits of the peripheral vision (bitemporal hemianopsia) and not the central visual field. The pituitary is located in the anterior half of the cerebrum; therefore an occipital cerebral defect is unlikely to be a clinical presentation relating to a pituitary adenoma. Diabetes insipidus results from a deficiency in antidiuretic hormone (ADH) from the posterior pituitary, and would not be a clinical presentation consistent with an anterior pituitary tumor.

19.3   **D.** Oxytocin and antidiuretic hormone (ADH) are posterior pituitary hormones. The other answer choices are released by the anterior pituitary. Whereas prolactin acts on the breast to produce milk, oxytocin acts on the breast to stimulate ejection of the milk in a lactating woman. Oxytocin is also responsible for uterine contractions during labor. The main function of FSH is to stimulate follicular development and maturity in the ovaries. ADH acts on the kidney to conserve water and is released when the body is dehydrated. TSH causes release of thyroid hormones, T_3 and T_4, which are involved in essential metabolic processes throughout the body.

19.4   **C.** Bromocriptine therapy is indicated during pregnancy if symptoms (eg, headache or visual field abnormalities) arise. No studies have shown bromocriptine to be unsafe to the developing fetus. A craniotomy and pituitary resection is a very high-risk surgery. It is typically reserved for patients with a macroadenoma, who have failed medical treatment. Surgery would not be indicated for this patient who has a microadenoma and has not attempted medical therapy.

Plus, any procedure that may induce hemorrhage in a patient would be considered risky in pregnancy. Tamoxifen is not indicated because it is a selective estrogen receptor modulator (SERM) used in the treatment of breast cancer. It therefore binds to estrogen receptors to inhibit estrogen action, and does not affect the microadenoma or prolactin production and action. A lumbar puncture would not be an option for managing a prolactinoma, but might worsen the patient's headache. Expectant management would not be a good option because a microadenoma can continue to grow during pregnancy from hormonal influences. Therefore, the patient's symptoms would only worsen, and treatment should be initiated promptly.

Clinical Pearls

➤ Galactorrhea in the face of normal menses and a normal prolactin level may be observed. The normal menses indicates normal hypothalamic function.
➤ The first evaluation in a woman with oligomenorrhea and galactorrhea should be a pregnancy test.
➤ Osteoporosis is a danger with hypoestrogenemia due to hyperprolactinemia.
➤ Hypothyroidism can lead to hyperprolactinemia and galactorrhea.
➤ MRI is the most sensitive imaging test to assess pituitary adenomas.

REFERENCES

Alexander CJ, Mathur R, Laufer LR, Aziz R. Amenorrhea, oligomenorrhea, and hyper-androgenic disorders. In: Hacker NF, Gambone JC, Hobel CJ, eds. *Essentials of Obstetrics and Gynecology*, 5th ed. Philadelphia, PA: Saunders; 2009:355-367.

Lobo RA. Hyperprolactinemia, galactorrhea, and pituitary adenomas. In: Katz VL, Lentz GM, Lobo RA, Gersenson DM, eds. *Comprehensive Gynecology*. 5th ed. St. Louis, MO: Mosby-Year Book; 2007:963-978.

Speroff L. Amenorrhea. In: Speroff L, Glass R, Kase N, eds. *Clinical Gynecologic Endocrinology and Infertility*. 6th ed. Philadelphia: Lippincott, Williams and Wilkins; 2005.

Case 20

A 24-year-old G1 P0 at 28 weeks' gestation complains of a 2-week duration of generalized pruritus. She denies rashes, exposures to insects, or allergies. Her medications include prenatal vitamins and iron supplementation. On examination, her blood pressure (BP) is 100/60 mm Hg, heart rate (HR) is 80 beats per minute (bpm), and weight is 140 lb. She is anicteric. The skin is without rashes. The fetal heart tones are in the 140-bpm range.

➤ What is the most likely diagnosis?

ANSWER TO CASE 20:
Pruritus (Cholestasis) of Pregnancy

Summary: A 24-year-old G1 P0 at 28 weeks' gestation complains of a 2-week duration of generalized pruritus. She is anicteric and normotensive. The skin is without rashes. The fetal heart tones are in the 140-bpm range.

➤ **Most likely diagnosis:** Cholestasis of pregnancy.

ANALYSIS

Objectives

1. Know the differential diagnosis of pruritus in pregnancy.
2. Understand the clinical presentation of cholestasis of pregnancy.
3. Know that the first line of treatment of cholestasis of pregnancy is an oral antihistamine.

Considerations

This 24-year-old woman, who is at 28 weeks' gestational age, complains of generalized pruritus. The systemic location of the itching and lack of rash makes a contact dermatitis unlikely. Another cause of pruritus unique to pregnancy is pruritic urticarial papules and plaques of pregnancy (PUPPP), which are erythematous papules and hives beginning in the abdominal area and often spreading to the buttocks. This is unlikely, as the patient does not have a rash. This patient's clinical picture does not resemble herpes gestationis, a condition causing intense itching but associated with erythematous blisters on the abdomen and extremities. Thus, the most likely etiology in this case is intrahepatic cholestasis, a process in which bile salts are incompletely cleared by the liver, accumulate in the body, and are deposited in the dermis, causing pruritus. This disorder usually begins in the third trimester. There are no associated skin rashes, other than excoriations from patient scratching.

DDx Pruritis in Pregnancy

- Cholestasis
- PUPP
- Herpes Gestionis
- Contact Dermatitis

APPROACH TO
Pruritus in Pregnancy

DEFINITIONS

CHOLESTASIS IN PREGNANCY: Intrahepatic cholestasis of unknown etiology in pregnancy whereby the patient usually complains of pruritus with or without jaundice and no skin rash.

PRURITIC URTICARIAL PAPULES AND PLAQUES OF PREGNANCY (PUPPP): A common skin condition of unknown etiology unique to pregnancy characterized by intense pruritus and erythematous papules on the abdomen and extremities.

HERPES GESTATIONIS: Rare skin condition only seen in pregnancy; it is characterized by intense itching and vesicles on the abdomen and extremities.

CLINICAL APPROACH

Jaundice – ?

Pruritus in pregnancy may be caused by many disorders, of which one of the most common is **intrahepatic cholestasis of pregnancy,** a condition that usually begins in the third trimester. It begins as mild pruritus without lesions, usually at night, and gradually increases in severity. The itching is usually more severe on the extremities than on the trunk. It may recur in subsequent pregnancies and with the ingestion of oral contraceptives, suggesting a hormone-related pathogenesis. The disease is common in some ethnic populations such as Swedes, suggesting a genetic basis for the disease process. **Increased levels of circulating bile acids confirm the diagnosis.** Elevated liver function tests are uncommon and there are no hepatic sequelae in the mother. Cholestasis of pregnancy must be distinguished from viral hepatitis and other causes of pruritus or liver disease. **Cholestasis of pregnancy, especially when accompanied by jaundice, is associated with an increased incidence of prematurity, fetal distress, and fetal loss.** There is also an increased incidence of gallstones associated with the pruritus of pregnancy. The first line of treatment has traditionally been antihistamines and cornstarch baths. Other treatments include the bile salt binder, cholestyramine, but it has been associated with vitamin K deficiency. More recently, ursodeoxycholic acid has been shown to decrease pruritus and seems to be better tolerated than cholestyramine.

Herpes gestationis, which has no relationship to herpes simplex virus, is a pruritic bullous disease of the skin. It usually begins in the second trimester of pregnancy and the reported incidence is less than 1 in 1000 pregnancies. The etiology is thought to be autoimmune related. The presence of IgG autoantibody directed at the basement membrane has been demonstrated and may result in activation of the classic complement pathway by autoantibodies directed against the basement membrane zone. The clinical features are characterized by intense pruritus followed by extensive patches of cutaneous erythema and subsequent formation of small vesicles and tense bullae. The limbs are affected more often than the trunk. Definitive diagnosis is made by immuno-fluorescent examination of biopsy specimens. There have been reports of an increased incidence of fetal growth retardation and stillbirth. Transient neonatal herpes gestationis has also been reported at birth. Treatment has primarily been the use of oral corticosteroids.

The lesions of PUPPP usually begin on the abdomen and spread to the thighs and sometimes the buttocks and arms. The lesions, as their name describes, consist of erythematous urticarial plaques and small papules surrounded by a narrow, pale halo. The incidence of PUPPP is less than 1% of pregnant women. Immunofluorescent studies are negative for both IgG and complement. Histologic findings consist of normal epidermis accompanied by a superficial perivascular infiltrate of lymphocytes and histiocytes associated with edema of the papillary dermis. There are no studies to suggest an adverse effect on fetal and maternal outcome. Therapy includes topical steroids and antihistamines.

Comprehension Questions

20.1 A 31-year-old G2 P1001 woman at 28 weeks' gestation presents with generalized pruritus. She has no rashes on her body and is diagnosed as having probable intrahepatic cholestasis of pregnancy. Which of the following is most accurate?
A. Hepatic transaminase levels are usually in the 2000 U/L range.
B. Is associated with hypertension.
C. May be associated with an increased perinatal morbidity.
D. Often is associated with thrombocytopenia.

20.2 A 30-year-old G1 P0 woman presents for her routine prenatal care appointment at 36 weeks' gestation with pruritic skin rash over her abdomen. She is diagnosed as having pruritic urticarial papules and plaques of pregnancy (PUPPP). Which of the following best describes the pregnancy outcome with her diagnosis?
A. Somewhat increased perinatal morbidity and mortality
B. Increased preterm delivery rate
C. Increased preeclampsia
D. No effect on pregnancy

20.3   A 33-year-old woman G1 P0 at 39 weeks' gestation is in labor. She has been diagnosed with herpes gestationis with the characteristic pruritus and vesicular lesions on the abdomen. Which of the following precautions is best advised for this patient?

A. Cesarean delivery is indicated.

B. Neonatal lesions may be noted and will resolve. ⁻

C. Vaginal delivery is permissible if the lesions are not in the introitus region and provided that oral acyclovir is given to the baby.

D. Tocolysis and oral steroid use is advisable until the lesions are healed.

ANSWERS   *Prematurity, Fetal Distress, Fetal loss*

20.1   **C.** Intrahepatic cholestasis in pregnancy may be associated with increased perinatal morbidity, especially when accompanied by jaundice. It is rare for liver enzymes to be elevated or for there to be any hepatic sequelae in the mother; however, every patient who is suspected of having cholestasis of pregnancy should have their liver enzymes checked to avoid fetal morbidity and mortality. Hepatic enzyme levels are less than 3 U/L; women with intrahepatic cholestasis may have slightly elevated levels but almost never in the thousands. On presentation, no rash typically accompanies the pruritus. Thrombocytopenia is not involved in this disorder; however it is involved in a life-threatening condition of pregnancy known as HELLP (hemolysis, elevated liver enzymes, low platelets) syndrome.

20.2   **D.** PUPPP is not thought to be associated with adverse pregnancy outcomes. The diagnosis is made presumptively based on clinical presentation, with the rash almost always beginning with the abdominal striae of the abdomen. They are usually small red "bumps" that are intensely pruritic. The treatment is symptomatic. Interestingly, this condition usually occurs with the first pregnancy and usually does not recur, with the most common onset at 35 to 36 weeks' gestation.

20.3   **B.** Neonatal lesions are sometimes seen with herpes gestationis caused by the IgG antibodies crossing the placenta, and these lesions will resolve. Herpes gestationis is not the same as herpes simplex virus. The latter would necessitate cesarean delivery to avoid infection to the baby.

Clinical Pearls

➤ The most common cause of generalized pruritus in pregnancy in the absence of skin lesions is cholestasis of pregnancy.
➤ Cholestatic jaundice in pregnancy may be associated with increased adverse pregnancy outcomes.
➤ The lesions of PUPPP usually begin on the abdomen and spread to the thighs and sometimes the buttocks and arms.

REFERENCES

Cunningham FG, Leveno KJ, Bloom SL, Hauth JC, Gilstrap LC III, Wenstrom KD. Gastrointestinal disorders In: *Williams Obstetrics*. 22nd ed. New York: McGraw-Hill; 2005:1126-1128.

Castro LC, Ognyemi D. Common medical and surgical conditions complicating pregnancy. In: Hacker NF, Gambone JC, Hobel CJ, eds. *Essentials of Obstetrics and Gynecology*, 5th ed. Philadelphia, PA: Saunders; 2009:191-218.

Case 21

A 23-year-old G0 P0 woman complains of lower abdominal tenderness and subjective fever. She states that her last menstrual period started 5 days previously and was heavier than usual. She also complains of dyspareunia of recent onset. She denies vaginal discharge or prior sexually transmitted diseases. Her appetite has been somewhat diminished. She has urinary urgency or frequency. On examination, her temperature is 100.8°F (38.2°C), blood pressure (BP) 90/70 mm Hg, and heart rate (HR) is 90 beats per minute (bpm). Her heart and lung examinations are normal. The abdomen has slight lower abdominal tenderness. There is no rebound tenderness and no masses. No costovertebral angle tenderness is noted. On pelvic examination, the external genitalia are normal. The cervix is somewhat hyperemic, and the uterus as well as adnexa are bilaterally exquisitely tender. The pregnancy test is negative.

➤ What is the most likely diagnosis?

➤ What are long-term complications that can occur with this condition?

ANSWERS TO CASE 21:

Salpingitis, Acute

Summary: A 23-year-old G0 P0 nonpregnant woman complains of lower abdominal tenderness, subjective fever, heavier menses than usual, and dyspareunia. Her temperature is 100.8°F (38.2°C). The cervix is hyperemic, and the uterus and adnexa are bilaterally exquisitely tender.

➤ **Most likely diagnosis:** Pelvic inflammatory disease (PID).

➤ **Long-term complications that can occur with this condition:** Infertility or ectopic pregnancy.

ANALYSIS

Objectives

1. Understand the clinical diagnostic criteria of salpingitis.
2. Understand that the long-term complications of salpingitis are infertility, ectopic pregnancy, and chronic pelvic pain.
3. Know that one of the outpatient treatment regimens of salpingitis is intramuscular ceftriaxone and oral doxycycline.

Considerations

This nulliparous woman has lower abdominal pain, adnexal tenderness, and cervical motion tenderness. The presence of cervical motion tenderness is indirect, based on the dyspareunia and hyperemic cervix. The patient also has fever. These are the clinical criteria for pelvic inflammatory disease or salpingitis (infection of the fallopian tubes). Salpingitis is most commonly caused by pathogenic bacteria of the endocervix that ascend to the tubes. The fallopian tubes can become damaged by the infection, leading to tubal occlusion and infertility or ectopic pregnancy. The pain occurs around the time of menses, and ascending infection often occurs at the time of menses, during endometrial breakdown. This patient has lower abdominal tenderness, which indicates peritoneal irritation of the pelvis; generalized peritonitis such as involving the entire peritoneal cavity may indicate a more extensive process, such as purulent material throughout the abdominal cavity, or another process. The differential diagnosis of salpingitis includes pyelonephritis, appendicitis, cholecystitis, diverticulitis, pancreatitis, ovarian torsion, and gastroenteritis.

*Fitz Hugh
· Curtis* } RUQ pain; Salpingitis
Perihepatic 183
Adhesions

APPROACH TO
Salpingitis

DEFINITIONS

PELVIC INFLAMMATORY DISEASE: Synonymous with salpingitis, or infection of the fallopian tubes.

CERVICAL MOTION TENDERNESS: Extreme tenderness when the uterine cervix is manipulated digitally, which suggests salpingitis.

ASCENDING INFECTION: Mechanism of upper genital tract infection whereby the offending microorganisms arise from the lower genital tract.

TUBO-OVARIAN ABSCESS (TOA): Collection of purulent material around the distal tube and ovary, which unlike the typical abscess is often treatable by antibiotic therapy rather than requiring surgical drainage.

CLINICAL APPROACH

Pelvic inflammatory disease, or salpingitis, usually involves *Chlamydia*, gonorrhea, and other vaginal organisms, such as anaerobic bacteria. The mechanism is usually by ascending infection. A common presentation would be a young, nulliparous female complaining of lower abdominal or pelvic pain and vaginal discharge. The patient may also have fever, and nausea and vomiting if the upper abdomen is involved. The cervix is inflamed and, therefore, the patient often complains of dyspareunia.

The diagnosis of acute salpingitis is made clinically by abdominal tenderness, cervical motion tenderness, and adnexal tenderness (Table 21–1). Confirmatory tests may include a positive Neisseria gonorrhea or *Chlamydia* culture, or an ultrasound suggesting a tubo-ovarian abscess. Other diseases that must be considered are acute appendicitis especially if the patient has right-sided abdominal pain and ovarian torsion, which usually presents as colicky pain and is associated with an ovarian cyst on ultrasound. Renal disorders, such as pyelonephritis or nephrolithiasis, must also be considered. Right upper quadrant pain may be seen with salpingitis when perihepatic adhesions are present, the so-called Fitz-Hugh and Curtis syndrome. When the diagnosis is in doubt, the best method for confirmation is laparoscopy. The surgeon would look for purulent discharge exuding from the fimbria of the tubes.

The treatment of acute salpingitis depends on whether the patient is a candidate for inpatient versus outpatient therapy. Criteria for outpatient management include low-grade fever, tolerance of oral medication, and the absence of peritoneal signs. The woman must also be compliant. One regimen consists of intramuscular ceftriaxone, as a single injection, and oral doxycycline twice a day for 10 to 14 days. Single agent quinolone therapy had gained

gonorrhea   *Chlamydia*

Table 21–1 SIGNS AND SYMPTOMS OF ACUTE SALPINGITIS
Abdominal tenderness
Cervical motion tenderness
Adnexal tenderness
Vaginal discharge
Fever
Pelvic mass on physical examination or ultrasound

popularity previously, but recent evidence has shown increasing bacterial resistance. It is paramount to reevaluate the patient in 48 hours for improvement. If the patient fails outpatient therapy, or is pregnant, or at the extremes of age, or cannot tolerate oral medication, she would be a candidate for inpatient therapy. One such therapeutic combination is intravenous cefotetan and oral or IV doxycycline. Again, if the patient does not improve within 48 to 72 hours, the clinician should consider laparoscopy to assess the disease.

One important sequelae of salpingitis is **tubo-ovarian abscess.** This disorder generally has anaerobic predominance and necessitates the corresponding antibiotic coverage (clindamycin or metronidazole). The physical examination may suggest an adnexal mass, or the ultrasound may reveal a complex ovarian mass. A devastating complication of TOA is rupture, which is a surgical emergency and one that leads to mortality if unattended. In contrast to most abscesses, TOAs can often be treated with antibiotic therapy without surgical drainage; radiological percutaneous drainage may sometimes be used to hasten resolution.

Long-term complications of salpingitis include chronic pelvic pain, involuntary infertility, and ectopic pregnancy. The risk of infertility due to tubal damage is directly related to the number of episodes of PID. The intrauterine contraceptive device (IUD) places the patient at greater risk for PID, whereas oral contraceptive agents (progestin thickens the cervical mucus) decrease the risk of PID.

Comprehension Questions

21.1 An 18-year-old adolescent female undergoes laparoscopy for an acute abdomen. Erythematous fallopian tubes are noted and a diagnosis of PID is made. Cultures of the purulent drainage would most likely reveal which of the following?

A. Multiple organisms

B. *Neisseria gonorrhoeae*

C. *Chlamydia trachomatis*

D. Peptostreptococcus species

E. *Treponema pallidum*

21.2   An 18-year-old adolescent female presents to the emergency depart-
        ment with a 36-hour history of abdominal pain and nausea. Her tem-
        perature is 100.5°F (38.05°C). Her abdominal examination reveals
        tenderness in the right lower quadrant with some mild rebound ten-
        derness. Pelvic examination shows some cervical motion tenderness
        and adnexal tenderness, and also some right-sided abdominal tender-
        ness. The pregnancy test is negative. In considering the differential
        diagnosis of appendicitis versus PID, which of the following is the
        most accurate method of making the diagnosis?
        A. Following serial abdominal examinations
        B. Sonography of the pelvis and abdomen
        C. Serum leukocyte count and cell differential
        D. Laparoscopy

21.3   A 24-year-old G0 P0 woman is seen at the local sexually transmitted
        disease (STD) clinic. *Chlamydia* is discovered colonizing the endo-
        cervix. The patient is given oral azithromycin therapy and warned
        about the dangers of upper genital tract infection, such as PID. The
        physician notes that the patient is at risk for PID. Which of the fol-
        lowing is a risk factor for developing PID?
        A. Nulliparity
        B. *Candida vaginitis*
        C. Oral contraceptive agents
        D. Depot medroxyprogesterone acetate

21.4   A 33-year-old woman with an intrauterine contraceptive device
        develops symptoms of acute salpingitis. On laparoscopy, sulfur gran-
        ules appear at the fimbria of the tubes. Which of the following is the
        most likely organism?
        A. *C trachomatis*
        B. Nocardia species
        C. *N gonorrhoeae*
        D. *T pallidum*
        E. Actinomyces species

ANSWERS

21.1   **A.** Multiple organisms are most likely encountered in acute salpingitis.
        N gonorrhoeae and *C trachomatis* are the two most common organisms
        involved. Other vaginal organisms, such as anaerobic bacteria, are
        also usually involved in the mix. Peptostreptococci are anaerobic,
        gram-negative bacteria that are natural part of human flora along the
        gastrointestinal (GI) and urinary tracts. They are not involved in
        salpingitis. Syphilis is not a common cause of salpingitis, although it
        is an STD like *Chlamydia* and gonorrhea. In the first stage of syphilis,

chancres may appear on the external genitalia or along the vaginal wall, but not in the endocervix as with *Chlamydia* and gonorrhea.

21.2   **D.** Laparoscopy is considered the "gold standard" for diagnosing salpingitis. The surgeon has direct visualization of the tubes with this method, and looks for purulent discharge exuding from the fimbria of the tubes. Clinical criteria and sonography are not specific enough for this diagnosis. The clinical criteria that may support this diagnosis include: abdominal tenderness, cervical motion tenderness, adnexal tenderness, vaginal discharge, fever, and pelvic mass on physical examination or ultrasound. A pelvic mass, such as a tubo-ovarian abscess, may be visualized using sonography; however, it would still not specify the origin of the mass. Of the imaging tests, CT scan is most helpful when appendicitis is suspected.

21.3   **A.** Nulliparity is associated with an increased risk of PID. IUD use increases the risk of PID. The most typical way this occurs is during the placement of the IUD, since it breaks the endocervical barrier as it enters the uterus and can spread infection from the endocervix into the tubes. Oral contraceptive agents, including depot medroxyprogesterone acetate, decrease the risk of PID by virtue of the progestin thickening the cervical mucus and thinning the endometrium. *Candida vaginitis* is a fungal infection, commonly called a yeast infection, that manifests due to an overgrowth of naturally occurring vaginal flora; fungal infections are typically not involved in the development of PID, and patients typically present with a chief complaint of severe itching and burning of the vagina with curd-like vaginal discharge.

21.4   **E.** Sulfur granules are classic for *Actinomyces*, which occurs more often in the presence of an IUD. *Actinomyces israelii* is a gram-positive anaerobe, which is generally sensitive to penicillin. *Chlamydia* and gonorrhea are the only other answer choices typically involved in the development of acute salpingitis, however neither one of them are associated with sulfur granules.

Clinical Pearls

➤ The organisms responsible for salpingitis are polymicrobial including *N gonorrhea*, *Chlamydia*, anaerobes, and gram-negative rods. Therefore, the antibiotic therapy must be broad spectrum.

➤ The classic clinical triad of PID is lower abdominal tenderness, cervical motion tenderness, and adnexal tenderness.

➤ Laparoscopy is the "gold standard" in the diagnosis of acute salpingitis, by the operator visualizing purulent drainage from the fallopian tubes.

➤ Long-term sequelae of acute salpingitis include chronic pelvic pain, ectopic pregnancy, and involuntary infertility.

REFERENCES

Eckert LO, Lentz GM. Infections of the upper genital tract. In: Katz VL, Lentz GM, Lobo RA, Gersenson DM, eds. *Comprehensive Gynecology.* 5th ed. St. Louis, MO: Mosby-Year Book; 2007:607-632.

McGregor JA, Lench JB. Vulvovaginitis, sexually transmitted infections, and pelvic inflammatory disease. sepsis. In: Hacker NF, Gambone JC, Hobel CJ, eds. *Essentials of Obstetrics and Gynecology,* 5th ed. Philadelphia, PA: Saunders; 2009:265-275.

Case 22

A 19-year-old G1 P0 woman at 20 weeks' gestation complains of the acute onset of pleuritic chest pain and severe dyspnea. She denies a history of reactive airway disease or cough. She has no history of trauma. On examination, her temperature is 98°F (36.6°C), heart rate (HR) 120 beats per minute (bpm), blood pressure (BP) 130/70 mm Hg, and respiratory rate (RR) 40 breaths per minute. The lung examination reveals clear lungs bilaterally. The heart examination shows tachycardia. The fetal heart tones are in the 140- to 150-bpm range. The oxygen saturation level is 82%. Supplemental oxygen is given.

➤ What test would most likely lead to the diagnosis?

➤ What is your concern?

ANSWERS TO CASE 22:
Pulmonary Embolus in Pregnancy

Summary: A 19-year-old G1 P0 woman at 20 weeks' gestation complains of the acute onset of pleuritic chest pain and severe dyspnea. On examination, her HR is 120 bpm and RR 40 breaths per minute. The lung examination reveals clear lungs bilaterally. The oxygen saturation is low.

➤ **Test most likely to lead to the diagnosis:** Spiral computed tomography or magnetic resonance angiography of the lungs.

➤ **Concern:** Pulmonary embolism.

ANALYSIS

Objectives

1. Understand that pleuritic chest pain and severe dyspnea are common presenting symptoms of pulmonary embolism.
2. Know that the pregnant woman is predisposed to deep venous thrombosis due to venous obstruction and a hypercoagulable state.
3. Understand that the spiral CT or MR angiography scan is an initial diagnostic test for pulmonary embolism.

Considerations

This 19-year-old woman at 20 weeks' gestation complains of the acute onset of severe dyspnea and pleuritic chest pain. The physical examination confirms the respiratory distress due to the tachycardia and tachypnea. The lungs are clear on auscultation, which rules out reactive airway disease or significant pneumonia. The patient also does not complain of cough or fever, further making pneumonia unlikely. Clear lungs also speak against pulmonary edema. The patient has significant hypoxia with oxygen saturation of 85%. Thus, the most likely diagnosis and concern is pulmonary embolism. Although many diagnostic tests should be considered in the initial evaluation of a patient with respiratory distress (such as arterial blood gas, chest radiograph, electrocardiograph), in this case a spiral (or helical) CT or MR angiography imaging procedure would likely lead to the diagnosis. Previously ventilation-perfusion (V/Q) scans were recommended in pregnancy; however, recent evidence indicates that V/Q scan exposes the fetus to slightly more radiation and is associated with a high rate of indeterminate cases. If the imaging confirms pulmonary embolism, then the patient should receive anticoagulation to help stabilize the deep venous thrombosis and decrease the likelihood of further embolization. Pregnancy causes venous stasis due to the mechanical effect of the uterus on the vena cava; additionally, the high estrogen level induces a hypercoagulable state due to the increase in clotting factors, particularly fibrinogen.

APPROACH TO
Respiratory Distress in Pregnancy

DEFINITIONS

DEEP VENOUS THROMBOSIS: Blood clot involving the deep veins of the lower extremity, rather than just the superficial involvement of the saphenous system.

PULMONARY EMBOLUS: Blood clot that is lodged in the pulmonary arterial circulation, usually arising from a thrombus of the lower extremity or pelvis.

HELICAL COMPUTED TOMOGRAPHY SCAN: High-resolution imaging using IV contrast with multiple sectors to allow for three-dimensional analysis and examination for vascular filling defects in the pulmonary vasculature.

MAGNETIC RESONANCE ANGIOGRAPHY: Using high-resolution magnetic resonance imaging to assess for vascular defects by intravenous contrast.

VENTILATION-PERFUSION SCAN IMAGING PROCEDURE: Using a small amount of intravenous, radioactively tagged albumin, such as technetium, in conjunction with a ventilation imaging, with inhaled xenon or technetium, in an effort to find large ventilation-perfusion mismatches suggestive of pulmonary embolism.

CLINICAL APPROACH

Respiratory distress is an acute emergency and necessitates rapid assessment and therapy. **Oxygen is the most important substrate for the human body,** and even 5 or 10 minutes of hypoxemia can lead to devastating consequences. Hence, a quick evaluation of the patient's respiratory condition, including the respiratory rate and effort; use of accessory muscles, such as intercostal and supraclavicular muscles; anxiety; and cyanosis; may indicate mild or severe disease. (See Figure 22–1 for one algorithm to evaluate dyspnea in pregnancy). The highest priority is to identify impending respiratory failure, since this condition would require immediate intubation and mechanical ventilation. Pulse oximetry and arterial blood gas studies should be ordered while information is gathered during the history and physical. A cursory and targeted history directed at the pulmonary or cardiac organs, such as a history of reactive airway disease, exposure to anaphylactoid stimuli such as penicillin or bee

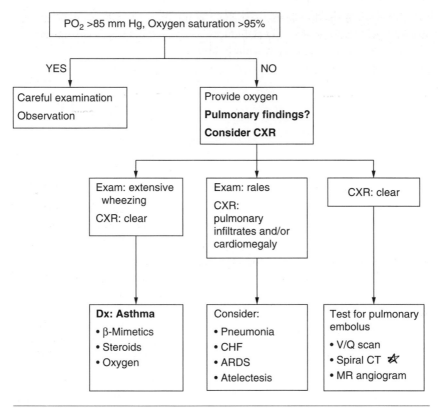

Figure 22–1.   Algorithm for evaluation of dyspnea in pregnancy.

sting, chest trauma, cardiac valvular disease, chest pain, or palpitations, are important. Meanwhile, the physical examination should be directed at the heart and lung evaluation. The heart should be assessed for cardiomegaly and valvular disorders, and the lungs should be auscultated for wheezes, rhonchi, rales, or absent breath sounds. The abdomen, back, and skin should also be examined.

A pulse oximetry reading of less than 90% corresponds to an oxygen tension of less than 60 mm Hg. Supplemental oxygen should immediately be given. An arterial blood gas should be obtained to assess for hypoxemia, carbon dioxide retention, and acid–base status. These findings should be evaluated in the context of the physiological changes in pregnancy (see Table 22–1). A chest radiograph should be performed rather expeditiously to differentiate cardiac versus pulmonary causes of hypoxemia. A large cardiac silhouette may indicate peripartum cardiomyopathy, which is treated by diuretic and inotropic therapy; pulmonary infiltrates may indicate pneumonia or pulmonary edema. A clear chest radiograph in the face of hypoxemia suggests

Table 22–1 NORMAL ARTERIAL BLOOD GAS CHANGES IN PREGNANCY

PARAMETER	NONPREGNANT VALUE	PREGNANT VALUE	COMMENT
pH	7.40	7.45	Respiratory alkylosis with partial metabolic compensation.
Po_2 (mm Hg)	90-100	95-105	Increased tidal volume leads to increased minute ventilation and higher oxygen level.
Pco_2 (mm Hg)	40	28	Higher tidal volume leads to increased minute ventilation and lower Pco_2.
HCO_3 (mEq/L)	24	19	Renal excretion of bicarbonate to partially compensate for respiratory alkylosis, leads to lower serum bicarbonate, making the pregnant woman more prone to metabolic acidosis.

[handwritten annotation: → alk.]

pulmonary embolism, although early in the course of pneumonia, the chest x-ray may appear normal.

The diagnosis of pulmonary embolism may be made presumptively on the basis of the clinical presentation, hypoxemia on arterial blood gas analysis, and a clear chest x-ray. Intravenous heparin may be initiated to stabilize the deep venous thrombosis, which is usually located in the pelvis or lower extremity. Previously ventilation-perfusion nuclear scans were used to diagnose pulmonary emboli; however, more recently, helical CT or MR angiography have emerged as accurate and involving very little radiation to the fetus. Once the diagnosis of acute thromboembolism is confirmed, the pregnant woman is usually placed on full intravenous anticoagulation therapy for 5 to 7 days. Later on, the therapy is generally switched to subcutaneous therapy to maintain the aPTT at 1.5 to 2.5 times control for at least 3 months after the acute event. Low-molecular-weight heparin can also be utilized; its advantages are less bleeding complications and less need for blood tests to assess anticoagulation. After 3 months, either full heparinization or "prophylactic heparinization" can be utilized for the remainder of the pregnancy and for 6 weeks postpartum. Newer imaging tests that are more sensitive for pulmonary embolism include magnetic resonance angiography and spiral computed

[handwritten annotation: Lovenox?]

tomographic evaluation. Usually, the pregnant woman is placed on prophylactic low-dose heparin for the remainder of pregnancy and up to 6 weeks postpartum. Estrogen products, such as oral contraceptive agents, are relatively contraindicated. Prophylactic anticoagulation for future pregnancies is more controversial, but often is used. Although pregnancy itself may induce thrombosis, many experts advise obtaining tests for other causes of thrombosis such as **protein S and protein C levels, antithrombin III activity, Factor V Leiden mutation and hyperhomocysteinemia, and antiphospholipid syndrome** or other thrombophilias.

Comprehension Questions

22.1   A 32-year-old woman pregnant at 29 weeks' gestation is noted to have symptoms concerning for a pulmonary embolism. The evaluation included chest radiograph, arterial blood gas, EKG, and helical CT imaging. A diagnosis of pulmonary embolism is made. Which of the following is most likely to be present in this patient?

   A. Dyspnea
   B. Chest pain
   C. Palpitations
   D. Hemoptysis
   E. Sudden death

22.2   A third-year medical student is assigned to perform a chart review of the cases of maternal mortality of a hospital over the past 20 years. When the cases are collated, the student organizes the deaths by etiology. Which of the following is most likely to be the common underlying mechanism of death?

   A. Uterine atony
   B. Hypercoagulable state
   C. Hypertensive disease
   D. Sepsis
   E. Rupture of pregnancy through the fallopian tube

22.3   A 22-year-old woman at 30 weeks' gestation is noted to have a confirmed pulmonary embolism based on a segmental filling defect on helical CT imaging. An EKG is performed. Which of the following is the most likely finding on the EKG on this patient?

   A. Tachycardia
   B. Right axis deviation
   C. Right bundle branch block
   D. S wave in lead III
   E. QT interval prolongation

22.4 A 28-year-old woman recently underwent cesarean delivery. Which of the following is the most appropriate method to prevent the development of deep venous thrombosis?

A. Unfractionated heparin intravenous infusion

B. Bed rest

C. Early ambulation

D. Depomedroxyprogesterone acetate (Depo-Provera)

22.5 A 29-year-old G1 P0 woman at 14 weeks' gestation is seen in the emergency room for possible diabetic ketoacidosis. The emergency room physician is evaluating the arterial blood gas which has been performed, and the findings are listed below. Based on these findings, which of the following is the most accurate statement?

pH 7.45; Po_2 103 mm Hg; Pco_2 31 mm Hg; HCO_3 18 mEq/L

A. The markedly decreased bicarbonate level indicates that the patient likely has DKA.

B. The decreased Pco_2 indicates that the patient is likely having a panic attack.

C. This arterial blood gas result is normal for pregnancy.

D. The elevated arterial pH reading likely indicates a metabolic alkalosis condition.

22.6 A 19-year-old G1 P0 woman at 29 weeks' gestation has reactive airway disease. She has received two nebulized albuterol inhalant treatments with still some wheezing. Her arterial blood gas findings are listed below. Based on these findings, which of the following is the most accurate statement?

pH 7.40; Po_2 94 mm Hg; Pco_2 35 mm Hg; HCO_3 20 mEq/L

A. The low Po_2 level indicates significant exacerbation of the reactive airway disease.

B. The Pco_2 level indicates significant retained Pco_2 and a worrisome respiratory failure.

C. The arterial blood gas is normal in pregnancy.

D. The serum bicarbonate level is elevated for pregnancy and indicates metabolic alkylosis.

ANSWERS

22.1 **A.** Dyspnea is the most common symptom of pulmonary embolus, whereas tachypnea is the most common sign. Another common symptom is pleuritic chest pain. A person with a pulmonary embolus may also experience palpitation or feel like they are having an anxiety attack and few patients will have hemoptysis. However, these symptoms are not nearly as common as dyspnea. Sudden death is uncommon, but is more likely in a massive embolus. Patients with a preexisting heart or lung condition are at increased risk of mortality. When a patient presents with dyspnea, a focused examination and assessment of oxygenation alert for the possibility of significant hypoxia.

22.2   **B.** Thromboembolism is the most common cause of maternal mortality. Pregnant women are predisposed to deep venous thromboses due to the obstructive effects the growing uterus has on the great vessels (ie, vena cava) and the hypercoagulable state of pregnancy. The hypercoagulable state persists for about 6 weeks postpartum. Hemorrhage typically occurs postpartum, usually due to uterine atony. The readily available blood products decreases the likelihood of death. Hypertensive disease is not typically deadly at the time of diagnosis and can be medically managed before, during, and after pregnancy. Ectopic pregnancies are usually not deadly unless rupture occurs and the patient goes into shock. Though this can occur, it is less common than embolism. Patients usually present with early signs (ie, vaginal bleeding) and symptoms (ie, adnexal pain) of an ectopic pregnancy before rupture occurs. Sepsis can also send a patient into shock, however there are usually signs and symptoms of a bacterial infection (ie, fever, chills, vomiting) that will prompt a patient to see their doctor before there is progression to shock.

22.3   **A.** Although an S wave in lead I, Q wave in lead III, and right-axis deviation may be seen, tachycardia is the most common EKG abnormality associated with pulmonary embolism. These findings typically result from the strain placed on the right side of the heart as it attempts to pump blood to the pulmonary vasculature against increased resistance due to the embolus. These EKG findings are not very specific for a pulmonary embolus. In other words, a normal EKG does not rule out pulmonary embolism.

22.4   **C.** Early ambulation in general is the most important method of preventing deep venous thrombosis after cesarean delivery. Depo-Provera, unlike estrogen-containing oral contraceptives, is a progestin and is not a major cause of a DVT. Bed rest will increase the risk of this patient for developing a DVT. Intravenous heparin is not indicated in a prophylactic regimen but rather is given in this manner in full anticoagulation. Some practitioners will place women, who have undergone cesarean, on sequential compression devices or prophylactic subcutaneous heparin (or low-molecular-weight heparin).

22.5   **C.** This arterial blood gas is normal in a pregnant woman. Pregnancy induces a respiratory alkylosis with partial metabolic compensation. This is the reason the serum bicarbonate level is decreased as compared to the nonpregnant patient.

22.6   **B.** This arterial blood gas reveals a P_{CO_2} of 35 mm Hg, which is elevated. In the face of reactive airway disease, this retained P_{CO_2} is worrisome, and may indicate respiratory failure. Initially, with asthma, hyperventilation should be associated with a decreased P_{CO_2}. When the P_{CO_2} increases, fatigue, ineffective ventilation, or respiratory failure are possibilities.

Clinical Pearls

➤ The diagnosis of pulmonary embolism is suspected in a patient with dyspnea, a clear chest radiograph, and hypoxemia. It is confirmed with imaging tests such as ventilation-perfusion scan or spiral CT scan.

➤ The most common presenting symptom of pulmonary embolism is dyspnea.

➤ The most common cause of maternal mortality is embolism (both thromboembolism and amniotic fluid embolism).

➤ A P_{O_2} of less than 80 mm Hg in a pregnant woman is abnormal.

➤ Anticoagulation is the best treatment of deep venous thrombosis or pulmonary embolism.

REFERENCES

American College of Obstetricians and Gynecologists. Prevention of deep vein thrombosis and pulmonary embolism. ACOG *Practice Bulletin 84*. Washington, DC: 2007.

American College of Obstetricians and Gynecologists. Thromboembolism in pregnancy. ACOG *Practice Bulletin No. 19*. 2000.

Castro LC, Ognyemi D. Common medical and surgical conditions complicating pregnancy. In: Hacker NF, Gambone JC, Hobel CJ, eds. *Essentials of Obstetrics and Gynecology*, 5th ed. Philadelphia, PA: Saunders; 2009:191-218.

Cunningham FG, Leveno KJ, Bloom SL, Hauth JC, Gilstrap LC III, Wenstrom KD. Pulmonary disorders. In: *Williams Obstetrics*. 22nd ed. New York, NY: McGraw-Hill; 2005:1055-1072.

Case 23

A 31-year-old G3 P2 woman at 39 weeks' gestation arrives at the labor and delivery area complaining of strong uterine contractions of 4-hour duration; her membranes ruptured 2 hours ago. She has a history of herpes simplex virus infections. She denies any blisters, and her last herpetic outbreak was 4 months ago. She is taking oral acyclovir. She notes a 1-day history of tingling in the perineal area. On examination, her blood pressure (BP) is 110/60 mm Hg, temperature is 99°F (37.2°C), and heart rate (HR) is 80 beats per minute (bpm). Her lungs are clear to auscultation. Her abdomen reveals a fundal height of 40 cm. The fetal heart rate is 140 bpm, reactive, and without decelerations. The uterine contractions are every 3 minutes. The external genitalia are normal without evidence of lesions. The vagina, cervix, and perianal region are normal in appearance. The vaginal fluid is consistent with rupture of membranes, showing ferning and an alkyotic pH.

➤ What is your next step?

➤ What is the most likely diagnosis?

ANSWERS TO CASE 23:
Herpes Simplex Virus Infection in Labor

Summary: A 31-year-old G3 P2 woman at 39 weeks' gestation is in labor and her membranes ruptured 2 hours ago. She has a history of herpes simplex virus (HSV) infections and is taking oral acyclovir suppressive therapy. She has a 1-day history of tingling in the perineal area.

➤ **Next step:** Counsel patient about risks of neonatal HSV infection and offer a cesarean delivery.

➤ **Most likely diagnosis:** Herpes simplex virus recurrence with prodromal symptoms.

ANALYSIS

Objectives

1. Understand the indications for cesarean delivery due to herpes simplex virus infection in pregnancy.
2. Know that herpes simplex virus may cause neonatal encephalitis.
3. Understand that symptoms of prodromal infection may indicate viral shedding.

Considerations

The patient is in labor and has experienced rupture of membranes. She has a history of herpes simplex virus infections. Although she has no lesions visible and is taking acyclovir suppressive therapy, she complains of tingling of the perineal region. These symptoms are sufficient to suggest an HSV outbreak. With herpes simplex virus shedding of the genital tract, there is risk of neonatal infection, especially encephalitis, which can lead to severe permanent CNS compromise. The patient should be counseled about the neonatal risks, and offered cesarean delivery to decrease the risk of neonatal exposure to the HSV.

APPROACH TO
Herpes Simplex Virus in Pregnancy

DEFINITIONS

HERPES SIMPLEX VIRUS PRODROMAL SYMPTOMS: Prior to the outbreak of the classic vesicles, the patient may complain of burning, itching, or tingling.

NEONATAL HERPES INFECTION: HSV can cause disseminated infection with major organ involvement; be confined to encephalitis, eyes, skin, or mucosa; or be asymptomatic. The vast majority of neonatal herpes infections occur via exposure to virus in fluids and secretions of the genital tract, although 5% to 10% may occur in the antepartum period transplacentally. This is most likely due to primary episodes and significant viremia.

CLINICAL APPROACH

Herpes cultures or polymerase chain reaction (PCR) are not useful in the acute management of pregnant women who present in labor or with rupture of membranes. They are helpful in making the diagnosis during the prenatal course, when the patient may develop lesions and the diagnosis is in question. Once a woman has been diagnosed with herpes simplex virus, the practitioner uses his or her best clinical judgment to assess for the presence of HSV in the genital tract during the time of labor. A meticulous inspection of the external genitalia, vagina, cervix (including by speculum examination), and perianal area should be undertaken for the typical herpetic lesions, such as vesicles or ulcers (Figure 23–1). Additionally, the patient should be queried thoroughly about the presence of prodromal symptoms. When there are no lesions or prodromal symptoms, the patient should be counseled that she is at low risk for viral shedding and likely has a small but possible risk of neonatal herpes infection. Usually, the patient will opt for vaginal delivery under these circumstances. In contrast, **the presence of prodromal symptoms or genital lesions suspicious for HSV is sufficient to warrant a recommendation for cesarean delivery to prevent neonatal infection.**

Acyclovir has activity against both HSV-1 and HSV-2. In a primary herpes outbreak, oral acyclovir reduces viral shedding, pain symptoms, and is associated with faster healing of the lesions. Newer medications such as valacyclovir or famciclovir require less frequent dosing due to their increased bioavailability, but are more expensive. The use of suppressive acyclovir therapy is usually reserved for frequent outbreaks. Some practitioners advocate the use of oral suppressive acyclovir when the woman has her first episode of HSV infection during pregnancy. This therapy may decrease the symptoms during the time of labor, and decrease the need for cesarean delivery.

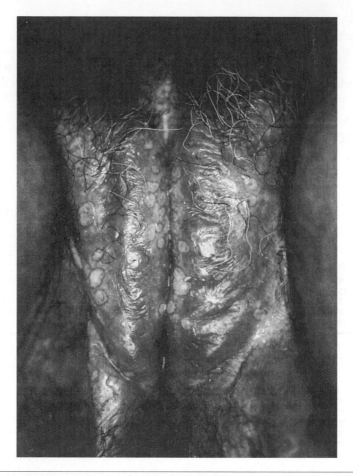

Figure 23–1.   First episode of primary genital herpes simplex virus infection.
*Reproduced with permission from Wendel GD, Cunningham FG. Sexually transmitted diseases in pregnancy. In:*Williams Obstetrics. *18th ed. (Suppl. 13). Norwalk, CT: Appleton & Lange, August/September 1991.*

Comprehension Questions

23.1 A 32-year-old woman G1 P0 at 24 weeks' gestation is seen by her obstetrician for painful vesicles on the vulva. PCR is performed and returns as HSV-2. The obstetrician counsels the patient about the possibility of needing cesarean when she goes into labor. Which of the following is an indication for cesarean section due to maternal herpes simplex virus?

   A. Vesicular lesions noted on the cervix
   B. History of lesions noted on the vagina 1 month previously, now not visible
   C. Lesions noted on the posterior thigh
   D. Tingling of the chest wall with lesions consistent with herpes zoster

23.2 A 29-year-old G2 P1 woman is seen in the office for her pregnancy at 16 weeks' gestation. She complains of some burning of the vulvar area. Two blisters are noted on the labia majora. PCR is performed on the lesions, which returns as HSV-1. Which of the following statements is most accurate in the counseling of this patient?

   A. Because this result is HSV-1, the finding is likely a false-positive result and the patient does not likely have a herpes infection.
   B. Because of the finding of HSV-1, the neonate is not at risk for herpes encephalitis.
   C. The patient should be treated the same whether the infection is HSV-1 or HSV-2.
   D. The patient likely has an HIV infection since HSV-1 was isolated in the vulvar area.

23.3 A 35-year-old healthy G2 P1 woman at 20 weeks' gestation presents with primary episode of herpes simplex virus, confirmed by PCR. Oral acyclovir is given for a 10-day course. Which of the following is the rationale for the acyclovir therapy?

   A. Decrease the likelihood of recurrence and need for cesarean
   B. Decrease the likelihood of transplacental transmission to the fetus
   C. Decrease the duration of viral shedding and duration of the current infection
   D. Increase the patient' immunity and IgG levels to HSV

23.4   A 34-year-old woman is seen at her internist's office complaining of
        vulvar pain. On examination, three ulcers are noted on the right labia
        majora. The lesions have ragged edges, a necrotic base, and there is
        adenopathy noted on the right inguinal region. Which of the follow-
        ing is the most likely diagnosis?
        A. Syphilis
        B. Herpes simplex virus
        C. Chancroid
        D. Squamous cell carcinoma
        E. Bartholin gland abscess

ANSWERS

23.1   **A.** The presence of prodromal symptoms or lesions along the genital
        tract (ie, cervix) suspicious for HSV is sufficient to warrant a
        cesarean delivery to prevent neonatal infection. When there are no
        lesions or prodromal symptoms, the patient should be counseled that
        she is at low risk for viral shedding and has an unknown risk of
        neonatal herpes infection; typically the patient will opt for vaginal
        delivery. The posterior thigh is unlikely to inoculate the baby during
        delivery, and is not an indication for cesarean delivery. Lesions on
        the chest wall consistent with herpes zoster would not necessitate
        cesarean delivery; however, the baby should still not come in contact
        with these lesions and breast-feeding should be avoided. Herpes
        zoster infection in a neonate can have fatal consequences.

23.2   **C.** Although usually HSV-1 is found above the waist and HSV-2
        below the waist, there are often exceptions. PCR is highly sensitive
        and specific, and it is unlikely that the viral subtype is erroneous.
        HSV-1 can also cause neonatal encephalitis, and the patient should
        be counseled and treated the same as if HSV-2 were isolated. A find-
        ing of HSV-1 in the vulvar region does not suggest HIV infection;
        nevertheless, the patient should have screening for sexually trans-
        mitted infections.

23.3   **C.** The rationale for oral acyclovir therapy at the primary outbreak is
        to decrease viral shedding and the duration of infection. The acy-
        clovir does not affect the likelihood of future recurrence and does
        not change the patient's immune response. There is no evidence that
        oral acyclovir alters transplacental transmission to the fetus,
        although reducing the viremia may help.

23.4   **C.** Chancroid is a rare cause of infectious vulvar ulcers in the United
        States, although worldwide it is quite common; thus, cases occurring
        in America are related to ports of entry. HSV is the most common
        cause of infectious vulvar ulcers in the United States, and individuals

are typically infected with the HSV-2 virus that is sexually transmitted. Genital herpes can cause recurrent painful genital sores, and herpes infection can become severe in people who are immunosuppressed. **Syphilis** typically presents during the first stage of the disease as a small, round, and painless chancre in the area of the body exposed to the spirochete. **Chancroid** is an STD caused by the gramnegative bacterium *Haemophilus ducreyi*, and like HSV, is characterized by painful genital lesions. The Bartholin glands, responsible for vaginal secretions, are located at the entrance of the vagina; they may enlarge into painless abscesses when they become clogged and infected. Vulvar carcinoma typically is nontender, ulcerative, and is more common in postmenopausal women.

Clinical Pearls

➤ Cesarean delivery should be offered to a woman with a history of HSV who has prodromal symptoms or suspicious lesions of the genital tract.

➤ Herpes simplex virus is the most common cause of infectious vulvar ulcers in the United States.

➤ Most neonatal herpes infections occur from HSV from genital tract secretions and fluids, although 5% to 10% of neonatal infections are acquired in utero. These are usually due to primary episodes.

➤ The cervix, vagina, and vulva must be inspected carefully for lesions in a patient in labor with a history of herpes simplex virus.

➤ Acyclovir and analogous agents given in pregnancy during primary episodes can decrease the duration of viral shedding and duration of lesions.

➤ Acyclovir suppression, when a primary HSV infection occurs in pregnancy, can decrease the likelihood of recurrence and need for cesarean.

REFERENCES

American College of Obstetricians and Gynecologists. Gynecologic herpes simplex virus infections. ACOG *Practice Bulletin 57*. Washington, DC: 2004.

American College of Obstetricians and Gynecologists. Management of herpes in pregnancy. ACOG *Practice Bulletin No. 82*. Washington, DC: 2007.

Castro LC, Ognyemi D. Common medical and surgical conditions complicating pregnancy. In: Hacker NF, Gambone JC, Hobel CJ, eds. *Essentials of Obstetrics and Gynecology*, 5th ed. Philadelphia, PA: Saunders; 2009:191-218.

Cunningham FG, Leveno KJ, Bloom SL, Hauth JC, Gilstrap LC III, Wenstrom KD. Sexually transmitted diseases. In: *Williams Obstetrics*. 22nd ed. New York, NY: McGraw-Hill; 2005:1307-1310.

Case 24

A 40-year-old G5 P5 woman complains of heavy vaginal bleeding with clots of 2-year duration. She denies bleeding or spotting between periods. She states that several years ago a doctor had told her that her uterus was enlarged. Her records indicate that 1 year ago she underwent a uterine dilation and curettage, with the tissue showing benign pathology. She denies fatigue, cold intolerance, or galactorrhea. She takes ibuprofen without relief of her vaginal bleeding. On examination, her blood pressure (BP) is 135/80 mm Hg, heart rate (HR) 80 beats per minute (bpm), weight 140 lb, and temperature is 98°F (36.6°C). The heart and lung examinations are normal. The abdomen reveals a lower abdominal midline irregular mass. On pelvic examination, the cervix is anteriorly displaced. An irregular midline mass approximately 18 weeks' size seems to move in conjunction with the cervix. No adnexal masses are palpated. Her pregnancy test is negative. Her hemoglobin level is 9.0 g/dL, leukocyte count is 6,000/mm^3, and platelet count is 160,000/mm^3.

➤ What is the most likely diagnosis?

➤ What is your next step?

ANSWERS TO CASE 24:

Uterine Leiomyomata

Summary: A 40-year-old G5 P5 woman with a history of an enlarged uterus complains of menorrhagia and anemia despite ibuprofen. A prior uterine dilation and curettage showed benign pathology. Examination reveals an irregular midline mass approximately 18 weeks' size that is seemingly contiguous with the cervix and there is an anteriorly displaced cervix.

➤ **Most likely diagnosis:** Symptomatic uterine leiomyomata.

➤ **Next step:** Offer the patient hysterectomy.

ANALYSIS

Objectives

1. Understand that the most common reason for hysterectomy in the United States is symptomatic uterine fibroids.
2. Know that hysterectomy is generally reserved for women with symptomatic uterine fibroids that are refractory to an adequate trial of medical therapy.
3. Know that menorrhagia is the most common symptom of uterine leiomyomata.

Considerations

This 40-year-old woman complains of menorrhagia. The physical examination is consistent with uterine fibroids, because of the enlarged midline mass that is irregular and contiguous with the cervix. If the mass were lateral or moved apart from the cervix, another type of pelvic mass, such as ovarian, would be suspected. This patient complains of menorrhagia (excessive bleeding during menses), which is the most common symptom of uterine fibroids. If she had intermenstrual bleeding, the clinician would have to consider other diseases, such as endometrial hyperplasia, endometrial polyp, or uterine cancer, in addition to the uterine leiomyomata. Irregular cycles (menometrorrhagia) may suggest an anovulatory process. The patient has anemia despite medical therapy, which constitutes the indication for intervention, such as hysterectomy. If the uterus were smaller, consideration may be given toward another medical agent, such as medroxyprogesterone acetate (Provera). Also, a gonadotropin-releasing hormone (GnRH) agonist can be used to shrink the fibroids temporarily, to correct the anemia, or make the surgery easier. The maximum shrinkage of fibroids is usually seen after 3 months of GnRH agonist therapy. After the GnRH agonist is stopped, the fibroids would regrow.

APPROACH TO
Suspected Uterine Leiomyomata

DEFINITIONS

whorls.

LEIOMYOMATA: Benign, smooth muscle tumors, usually of the uterus.

LEIOMYOSARCOMA: Malignant, smooth muscle tumor, with numerous mitoses.

SUBMUCOUS FIBROID: Leiomyomata that are primarily on the endometrial side of the uterus and impinge on the uterine cavity (Figure 24–1).

INTRAMURAL FIBROID: Leiomyomata that are primarily in the uterine muscle.

SUBSEROSAL FIBROID: Leiomyomata that are primarily on the outside of the uterus, on the serosal surface. Physical examination may reveal a "knobby" sensation.

PEDUNCULATED FIBROID: Leiomyoma that is on a stalk.

CARNEOUS DEGENERATION: Changes of the leiomyomata due to rapid growth; the center of the fibroid becomes red, causing pain. This is synonymous with red degeneration.

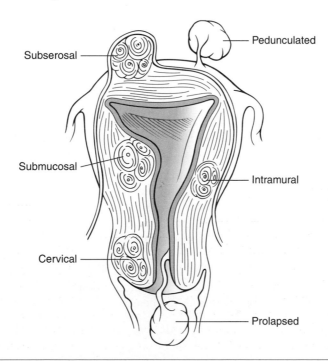

Figure 24–1.   Uterine leiomyomata. Various uterine leiomyomata are depicted, based on their location in the uterus.

CLINICAL APPROACH

Uterine leiomyomata are the most common tumors of the pelvis and the leading indication for hysterectomy in the United States. They occur in up to 25% of women, and have a variety of clinical presentations. The most common clinical manifestation is menorrhagia, or excessive bleeding during menses. The exact mechanism is unclear and may be due to an **increased endometrial surface area** or the **disruption of hemostatic mechanisms during menses** by the fibroids. Another speculated explanation is **ulceration** of the submucosal fibroid surfaces.

Many uterine fibroids are asymptomatic and only need to be monitored. Very rarely, uterine leiomyomata degenerate into leiomyosarcoma. Some signs of this process include rapid growth, such as an increase of more than 6 weeks' gestational size in 1 year. A history of radiation to the pelvis is a risk factor.

If the uterine leiomyomata are sufficiently large, patients may also complain of pressure to the pelvis, bladder, or rectum. Rarely, the uterine fibroid on a pedicle may twist, leading to necrosis and pain. Also, a submucous leiomyomata can prolapse through the cervix, leading to labor-like uterine contraction pain.

The physical examination typical of uterine leiomyomata is an irregular, midline, firm, nontender mass that moves contiguously with the cervix. This presentation is approximately 95% accurate. Most of the time, ultrasound examination is performed to confirm the diagnosis. Lateral, fixed, or fluctuant masses are not typical for fibroids. The differential diagnosis includes ovarian masses, tubo-ovarian masses, pelvic kidney, and endometrioma.

The initial treatment of uterine fibroids is medical, such as with nonsteroidal anti-inflammatory agents or progestin therapy. Gonadotropin-releasing hormone agonists lead to a decrease in uterine fibroid size, reaching its maximal effect in 3 months. After the discontinuation of this agent, the leiomyomata usually regrow to the pretreatment size. Thus, GnRH agonist therapy is reserved for tumor shrinkage or correction of anemia prior to operative treatment. Hysterectomy is considered the proven treatment for symptomatic uterine fibroids when future pregnancy is undesired. **Uterine artery embolization** is a technique performed by cannulizing the femoral artery and catheterizing both uterine arteries directly, and infusing embolization particles that preferentially float to the fibroid vessels. Fibroid infarction and subsequent hyalinization and fibrosis result. Although short-term results appear promising, long-term data does not yet exist. Myomectomy is still considered the procedure of choice for women with symptomatic uterine leiomyomata who desire pregnancy. The indication for surgery is persistent symptoms despite medical therapy. Significant menorrhagia often leads to anemia.

Comprehension Questions

24.1 A 29-year-old woman is noted to have three consecutive first-trimester spontaneous abortions. After an evaluation for the recurrent abortions including karyotype of the parents, hysterosalpingogram, vaginal sonogram, and testing for antiphospholipid syndrome, the obstetrician concludes the uterine fibroids are the etiology. Which of the following types of uterine fibroids would most likely lead to recurrent abortion?

A. Submucosal
B. Intramural
C. Subserous
D. Parasitic
E. Pedunculated

24.2 A 39-year-old woman is diagnosed as having probable uterine fibroids based on a pelvic examination revealing an enlarged irregular uterus. She is currently asymptomatic and expressed surprise that she had "growths" of the uterus. If she were to develop symptoms, which of the following would be the most common manifestation?

A. Infertility
B. Menorrhagia
C. Ureteral obstruction
D. Pelvic pain
E. Recurrent abortion

24.3 A 29-year-old G2 P1 woman at 39 weeks' gestation had a myomectomy for infertility previously. While pushing during the second stage of labor, she is noted to have fetal bradycardia associated with some vaginal bleeding. The fetal head, which was previously at +2 station, is now noted to be at −3 station. Which of the following is the most likely diagnosis?

A. Submucosal myomata
B. Umbilical cord prolapse
C. Uterine rupture
D. Placental abruption
E. Fetal congenital heart block

24.4   A 65-year-old woman is noted to have suspected uterine fibroids on physical examination. Over the course of 1 year, she is noted to have enlargement of her uterus from approximately 12 weeks' size to 20 weeks' size. Which of the following is the best management?
A. Continued careful observation
B. Monitoring with ultrasound examinations
C. Exploratory laparotomy with hysterectomy
D. Gonadotropin-releasing hormone agonist
E. Progestin therapy

ANSWERS

24.1   **A.** Submucous fibroids are the fibroids most likely to be associated with recurrent abortion because of their effect on the uterine cavity. The contours of the endometrium are altered and therefore, less favorable for implantation. There may be insufficient vasculature to provide adequate blood supply to the growing embryo if it were to implant along the side of the endometrium containing a submucosal fibroid. In the second trimester of pregnancy, the other answer choices are not associated with an increased risk of recurrent abortion because they do not alter the integrity of the endometrium.

24.2   **B.** Menorrhagia is the most common symptom of uterine fibroids, and severe menorrhagia often leads to anemia. Infertility and recurrent abortion may occur with submucosal fibroids due to the effects on the uterine cavity, whereas impingement on the ureters is most likely to occur with subserosal fibroids, but these are much less common than menorrhagia. Pelvic pain is not very common, and many uterine fibroids are asymptomatic and only require monitoring. If the uterine leiomyomata are large enough, patients may complain of pressure to the pelvis, bladder, or rectum. Though rare, a uterine fibroid on a pedicle may twist, leading to necrosis and severe pain.

24.3   **C.** Extensive myomectomies sometimes necessitate cesarean delivery because of the risk of uterine rupture. Most practitioners use the rule of thumb that if the endometrial cavity is entered during myomectomy, a cesarean delivery should be performed with pregnancy. As with uterine rupture, fetal bradycardia may also occur if the umbilical cord becomes prolapsed, but cord prolapse is not a risk factor from having a myomectomy. A submucosal myomata is related to problems with fertility and implantation of the embryo, not problems during labor such as uterine rupture. Placental abruption is not associated with fetal bradycardia or as a risk after myomectomy. Myomectomies do not cause congenital anomalies or disease processes to occur in a developing fetus.

24.4 **C.** The rapid growth of the uterus suggests leiomyosarcoma; the diagnosis and treatment are surgical, especially in a woman of non–childbearing age. Also, substantial growth of uterine fibroids in postmenopausal women is unusual due to the lower estrogen levels. In other words, uterine fibroids typically grow in response to estrogen. Once a fibroid degenerates into cancer, progestin therapy and gonadotropin-releasing hormone agonist have no more effect on the tumor and are no longer treatment options for shrinking the mass.

Clinical Pearls

➤ The most common reason for hysterectomy is symptomatic uterine fibroids.

➤ The most common symptom of uterine fibroids is menorrhagia.

➤ The physical examination consistent with uterine leiomyomata is an irregular pelvic mass that is mobile, midline, and moves contiguously with the cervix.

➤ Leiomyosarcoma rarely arises from leiomyoma; rapid growth or a history of prior pelvic irradiation should raise the index of suspicion.

➤ Significant growth in suspected uterine fibroids in a postmenopausal woman is unusual and generally requires surgical evaluation.

➤ Asymptomatic uterine fibroids require surgical intervention in the presence of unexplained rapid growth, ureteral obstruction, or the inability to differentiate the fibroid from other types of pelvic masses.

REFERENCES

American College of Obstetricians and Gynecologists. Alternatives to hysterectomy in the management of leiomyomata. *ACOG Practice Bulletin 96.* Washington, DC: 2008.

Katz VL. Benign gynecologic lesions. In: Katz VL, Lentz GM, Lobo RA, Gersenson DM, eds. *Comprehensive Gynecology.* 5th ed. St. Louis, MO: Mosby-Year Book; 2007:419-470.

Nelson AL, Gambone JC. Congenital anomalies and benign conditions of the uterine corpus and cervix. In: Hacker NF, Gambone JC, Hobel CJ, eds. *Essentials of Obstetrics and Gynecology,* 5th ed. Philadelphia, PA: Saunders; 2009:240-247.

Case 25

A 19-year-old G1 P0 woman at 29 weeks' gestation has severe preeclampsia, with several blood pressure readings of 160/110 mm Hg or greater, and 4+ proteinuria. She denies headaches or visual abnormalities. She notes a 2-day history of severe unremitting epigastric tenderness. The patient's platelet count was 130,000/mL, hemoglobin level is 13 mg/dL, and SGOT is 2100 IU/L. Shortly after admission, she received intravenous magnesium sulfate and was induced with oxytocin. She delivered vaginally. Two hours after delivery, the patient complains of the sudden onset of severe abdominal pain and has a syncopal episode. The patient is found to have a blood pressure of 80/60 mm Hg, a distended abdomen, and heart rate of 140 bpm with a thready pulse.

➤ What is the most likely diagnosis?

➤ What is your next step?

ANSWERS TO CASE 25:
Preeclampsia and Hepatic Rupture

Summary: A 19-year-old G1 P0 woman who delivered at 29 weeks' gestation is noted to have severe preeclampsia, epigastric tenderness, and markedly elevated liver function tests. Shortly after delivery, she develops sudden, severe abdominal pain, abdominal distension, syncope, hypotension, and tachycardia.

➤ **Most likely diagnosis:** Hepatic rupture.

➤ **Next step:** Emergent exploratory laparotomy and blood product replacement.

ANALYSIS

Objectives

1. Know the clinical presentation of preeclampsia.
2. Know the serious sequelae of severe preeclampsia, including hepatic rupture.
3. Understand that immediate laparotomy and massive blood product replacement are important in the management of hepatic rupture.

Considerations

The patient is nulliparous, which is a risk factor for preeclampsia. She has severe preeclampsia based on blood pressure criteria, proteinuria, epigastric tenderness, and elevated liver function tests. The epigastric tenderness occurs because of the ischemia to the liver. Rarely, a hepatic hematoma may form, and if rupture of the hematoma occurs, catastrophic hemorrhage can ensue, leading to rapid exsanguination if immediate exploratory laparotomy is not undertaken.

APPROACH TO
Preeclampsia

DEFINITIONS

CHRONIC HYPERTENSION: Blood pressure of 140/90 mm Hg before pregnancy or at less than 20 weeks' gestation.

GESTATIONAL HYPERTENSION: Hypertension without proteinuria at greater than 20 weeks' gestation.

PREECLAMPSIA: Hypertension with proteinuria (> 300 mg over 24 hour) at a gestational age greater than 20 weeks, caused by vasospasm.

ECLAMPSIA: Seizure disorder associated with preeclampsia.

SEVERE PREECLAMPSIA: Vasospasm associated with preeclampsia of such extent that maternal end organs are threatened, usually necessitating delivery of the baby regardless of gestational age.

SUPERIMPOSED PREECLAMPSIA: Development of preeclampsia in a patient with chronic hypertension.

CLINICAL APPROACH

Hypertensive disorders complicate 3% to 4% of pregnancies and can be organized into several categories: gestational hypertension, mild and severe preeclampsia, chronic hypertension, superimposed preeclampsia, and eclampsia. Gestational hypertensive patients have only increased blood pressures without proteinuria. Chronic hypertension includes preexisting hypertension or hypertension that develops prior to 20 weeks' gestation. A patient with chronic hypertension is at risk for developing preeclampsia and, if this develops, her diagnosis is labeled superimposed preeclampsia. Eclampsia occurs when the patient with preeclampsia develops convulsions or seizures.

Preeclampsia is characterized by hypertension and proteinuria. Although not a criterion, nondependent edema is also usually present. An elevated blood pressure is diagnosed with a systolic blood pressure at or higher than 140 mm Hg or diastolic blood pressure at or higher than 90 mm Hg. Two elevated BPs, measured 6 hours apart (BP taken in the seated position), are needed for the diagnosis of preeclampsia. Proteinuria is usually based on a timed urine collection, defined as equal to or greater than 300 mg of protein in 24 hours. Facial and hand edema would be considered nondependent edema.

Preeclampsia is further categorized into mild and severe. Severe disease is diagnosed with a systolic BP at or higher than 160 mm Hg, diastolic BP of 110 mm Hg or higher, or a 24-hour urine protein level of more than 5 g. If there is no time for a 24-hour urine protein collection (ie, while in labor), a urine dipstick helps estimate proteinuria, with 3+ to 4+ consistent with severe disease and 1+ to 2+ with mild disease. Patients may also be diagnosed with severe disease when symptoms of preeclampsia, such as headache, right upper quadrant or epigastric pain, and vision changes, occur.

The underlying pathophysiology of preeclampsia is vasospasm and "leaky vessels," but its origin is unclear. It is cured only by termination of the pregnancy, and the disease process almost always resolves after delivery. Vasospasm and endothelial damage result in leakage of serum between the endothelial cells and cause local hypoxemia of tissue. Hypoxemia leads to hemolysis, necrosis, and other end-organ damage. Patients are usually unaware of the hypertension and proteinuria, and typically the presence of symptoms indicates severe disease. Hence, one of the important roles of prenatal care is to identify patients with hypertension and proteinuria prior to severe disease. Complications of preeclampsia include placenta abruption, eclampsia (with possible intracerebral hemorrhage), coagulopathies, renal failure, hepatic subcapsular hematoma, hepatic rupture, and uteroplacental insufficiency.

Risk factors for preeclampsia include: nulliparity, extremes of age, African-American race, personal history of severe preeclampsia, family history of preeclampsia, chronic hypertension, chronic renal disease, antiphospholipid syndrome, diabetes, and multifetal gestation. The history and physical examination is focused on end-organ disease (Table 25–1).

It is important to review and evaluate the blood pressures prior to 20 weeks' gestation (to assess for chronic hypertension), evaluate proteinuria, and to document any sudden increase in weight (indicating possible edema). On physical examination serial blood pressures should be checked along with a urinalysis.

Laboratory tests should include a complete blood count (CBC; check platelet count and hemoconcentration), urinalysis and 24-hour urine protein

Table 25–1 CRITERIA FOR SEVERE PREECLAMPSIA

END ORGAN (BY SYSTEM)	SIGNS AND SYMPTOMS OF PREECLAMPSIA
Neurologic	Headache Vision changes Seizures Hyperreflexia Blindness
Renal	Decreased glomerular filtration rate Proteinuria Oliguria
Pulmonary	Pulmonary edema
Hematologic and vascular	Thrombocytopenia Microangiopathic anemia Coagulopathy Severe hypertension (160/110 mm Hg)
Fetal	Intrauterine growth restriction (IUGR) Oligohydramnios Decreased uterine perfusion (ie, late decelerations)
Hepatic	Increased liver enzymes Subcapsular hematoma Hepatic rupture

collection if possible (check for proteinuria), liver function tests, LDH (elevated with hemolysis), and uric acid test (usually increased with preeclampsia). Fetal testing (such as biophysical profile) can also be performed to evaluate uteroplacental insufficiency.

After the diagnosis of preeclampsia is made, the management will depend on the gestational age of the fetus and the severity of the disease (see Figure 25–1 for one management scheme). Delivery is the definitive treatment and the risks of preeclampsia must be weighed against the risk of prematurity. When the pregnancy reaches term, delivery is indicated. When the fetus is premature, severity of the disease needs to be assessed. When severe preeclampsia is diagnosed, delivery is usually indicated regardless of gestational age. In preterm patients, mild preeclampsia can be monitored closely for worsening disease until the risk of prematurity has decreased.

Eclampsia is one of the most feared complications of preeclampsia and the greatest risk for occurrence is just prior to delivery, during labor (intrapartum), and within the first 24 hours postpartum. During labor, the preeclamptic patient should be started on the anticonvulsant **magnesium sulfate.** Since magnesium is excreted by the kidneys, it is important to monitor urine output, respiratory depression, dyspnea (side effect of magnesium sulfate is pulmonary edema), and abolition of the deep tendon reflexes (first sign of toxic effects is hyporeflexia). Hypertension is not affected by the magnesium, but is

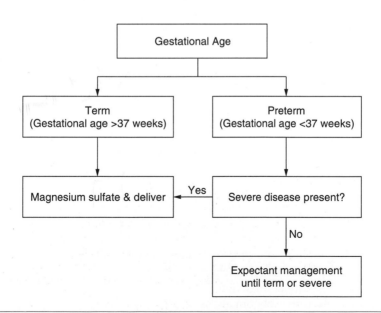

Figure 25–1.   Algorithm for management of preeclampsia.

used to prevent seizures. Severe hypertension needs to be controlled with antihypertensive medications such as hydralazine or labetalol. After delivery, magnesium sulfate is discontinued approximately 24 hours postpartum. The hypertension and proteinuria frequently will resolve. Occasionally, the patient's blood pressure remains high and an antihypertensive medication is needed after delivery. After discharge, the patient usually follows up in 1 to 2 weeks to check blood pressures and proteinuria.

Comprehension Questions

25.1   A 29-year-old G1 P0 woman at 28 weeks' gestation is admitted to the hospital for preeclampsia. Her blood pressure (BP) is 150/100 mm Hg and her protein excretion is 500 mg in 24 hours. On hospital day 7, she is diagnosed with severe preeclampsia and the decision is made to administer magnesium sulfate and deliver the baby. Which of the following findings is most likely present in this patient as criteria for severe preeclampsia?

A. Elevated uric acid levels
B. 5 g of proteinuria excreted in a 24-hour period
C. 4+ pedal edema
D. Platelet count of 115,000/uL

25.2   Which of the following is the best management of an 18-year-old G1 P0 woman at 28 weeks' gestation with a blood pressure of 160/110 mm Hg, elevated liver function tests, and a platelet count of 60,000/uL?

A. Oral antihypertensive therapy
B. Platelet transfusion
C. Magnesium sulfate therapy and induction of labor
D. Intravenous immunoglobulin therapy

25.3   A 19-year-old G1 P0 woman at 39 weeks' gestation is diagnosed with preeclampsia based on blood pressure of 150/90 mm Hg and 2+ proteinuria on urine dipstick. The patient is placed on magnesium sulfate, and develops flushing and fatigue. She asks about the need for the magnesium sulfate. You explain that it is to prevent the seizures that may complicate preeclampsia and may even cause death. The patient asks how seizures associated with preeclampsia can cause mortality. Which of the following is the most common mechanism?

A. Intracerebral hemorrhage
B. Myocardial infarction
C. Electrolyte abnormalities
D. Aspiration

25.4   A 33-year-old woman at 29 weeks' gestation is noted to have blood pressures of 150/90 and 2+ proteinuria. The platelet count and liver function tests were normal. Which of the following is the best management for this patient?

   A. Induction of labor
   B. Cesarean section
   C. Antihypertensive therapy
   D. Expectant management

ANSWERS

25.1   **B.** Severe preeclampsia is associated with a 24-hour urine protein level greater than 5 g; the reason for this is that such severe proteinuria is indicative of widespread and significant renal damage, and if allowed to continue, renal insufficiency may ensue. Other criteria for severe preeclampsia include: blood pressure exceeding 160/110 mm Hg, severe headache, right upper quadrant or epigastric pain, and vision changes. Pedal edema is not pathologic; nondependent edema, such as of the face and hands, may be consistent with preeclampsia but does not indicate severity of disease. Low platelets are associated with HELLP syndrome, a form of hemolytic anemia in pregnancy, and are very worrisome. Uric acid levels are known to be elevated with preeclampsia; however, it is not a criterion for severe preeclampsia. In general, the criteria for severe preeclampsia indicate end-organ threat, and generally require delivery even at a preterm gestation.

25.2   **C.** Although the pregnancy is only 28 weeks, in light of the severe preeclampsia, the best treatment is delivery. When severe preeclampsia is diagnosed, delivery usually is indicated regardless of gestational age. Therefore, none of the other answer choices would be indicated because no type of therapy other than delivery will resolve the patient's severe preeclampsia. Oral antihypertensive therapy, such as labetalol, may be given to the patient to control blood pressure, however should not be used as the "treatment" of severe preeclampsia. The platelet levels are not low enough to require transfusion; intravenous immunoglobulin (IV Ig) is used for various autoimmune diseases, but not indicated in this patient.

25.3   **A.** The most common cause of maternal death due to eclampsia is intracerebral hemorrhage. Eclampsia is one of the most feared complications of preeclampsia, and the greatest risk for occurrence is just prior to delivery, during labor (intrapartum), and within the first 24 hours postpartum. During labor, the patient should be started on the anticonvulsant magnesium sulfate for seizure prophylaxis. Magnesium sulfate has been proven to be superior to other anticonvulsants such as valium, dilantin, or phenobarbital. One dictum that is useful in the emergency room or obstetrical unit is that "a pregnant patient greater than 20 weeks' gestation without a history of epilepsy who presents with seizures has eclampsia until otherwise proven."

25.4   **D.** In the preterm patient with mild preeclampsia, expectant management is generally employed until severe criteria are noted or the pregnancy reaches term. In other words, the risks of prematurity usually outweigh the risks of the preeclampsia until end-organ threat is manifest. Had this patient been at term, the best step in management would be to place her on magnesium sulfate and induce labor; this is because at term, the risks of prematurity are minimal. Severe, but not mild hypertension associated with preeclampsia, should be controlled with hypertensive medication. Antihypertensive agents are useful in chronic hypertension but not preeclampsia unless the BP is in the severe range; lowering these BPs can help avoid stroke. For the patient in this scenario, neither induction nor Cesarean section is indicated since she is not yet at term. It is not a requirement for a preeclamptic patient to deliver by Cesarean.

Clinical Pearls

➤ In general, the treatment of preeclampsia at term is magnesium sulfate and delivery.

➤ The management of preeclampsia in a preterm pregnancy is observation until severe criteria are noted, or term gestation is reached.

➤ The most common cause of significant proteinuria in pregnancy is preeclampsia.

➤ Magnesium sulfate is the best anticonvulsant to prevent eclampsia.

➤ The first sign of magnesium toxicity is loss of deep tendon reflexes.

➤ Chronic hypertension is diagnosed when a pregnant woman has hypertension prior to 20 weeks' gestation, or if the hypertension persists beyond 12 weeks postpartum.

REFERENCES

American College of Obstetricians and Gynecologists. Diagnosis and management of preeclampsia and eclampsia. *ACOG Practice Bulletin No. 33*. Washington, DC: January 2002.

Castro LC. Hypertensive disorders of pregnancy. In: Hacker NF, Gambone JC, Hobel CJ, eds. *Essentials of Obstetrics and Gynecology*, 5th ed. Philadelphia, PA: Saunders; 2009:173-182.

Cunningham FG, Leveno KJ, Bloom SL, Hauth JC, Gilstrap LC III, Wenstrom KD. Hypertensive disorders in pregnancy. In: *Williams Obstetrics*. 22nd ed. New York, NY: McGraw-Hill; 2005:761-808.

Case 26

A 22-year-old woman is seen by her physician for a routine physical examination. She seems to be up to date regarding her immunizations and has received the HPV vaccine. She has no family history of breast cancer. She denies breast leakage or prior medical problems. On examination, her blood pressure (BP) is 100/60 mm Hg. Her physical examination is unremarkable except for 1-cm, right, nontender breast mass. Her neck is supple and the heart and lung examinations are normal. Palpation of her right breast reveals a firm, mobile, nontender, rubbery 1-cm mass in the upper outer quadrant. There are no skin abnormalities noted. No adenopathy is noted. The left breast is normal to palpation.

➤ What is your next step?

➤ What is the most likely diagnosis?

ANSWERS TO CASE 26:

Fibroadenoma of the Breast

Summary: A 22-year-old woman is noted to have a 1-cm breast mass on routine physical examination. Palpation of her right breast reveals a firm, mobile, nontender, rubbery 1-cm mass in the upper outer quadrant. No adenopathy is noted.

➤ **Next step:** Biopsy of the mass (fine needle biopsy or core needle biopsy).

➤ **Most likely diagnosis:** Fibroadenoma of the breast.

ANALYSIS

Objectives

1. Understand that any three-dimensional dominant mass needs a biopsy.
2. Know the characteristic presentation of fibroadenomas of the breast.
3. Understand that the greater the risk of breast cancer, the more tissue that is needed for biopsy.

Considerations

This woman comes in for a health maintenance examination; the approach is generally immunizations, cancer screening, and assessment and prevention for common diseases. On the physical examination, she is found to have a dominant breast mass. The firm, nontender, rubbery description is classic for a fibroadenoma. Fibroadenomas, as opposed to fibrocystic changes, do not change with the menstrual cycle. Although the most likely etiology is a fibroadenoma, this diagnosis needs to be confirmed by biopsy. The three methods of biopsy include fine needle aspiration (FNA), core needle stereotactic biopsy, and excisional biopsy. Both core needle and excisional biopsy remove more tissue but are more prone to bruising and pain; in this case, FNA is acceptable since the patient is at low risk for breast cancer. She has no family history of breast cancer, is of a young age, and her examination does not contain any worrisome features of breast cancer. If the mass were fixed, or if there were nipple retraction or bloody nipple discharge, the better method of biopsy would be excisional biopsy to remove the entire mass for histologic analysis.

APPROACH TO
Breast Masses

DEFINITIONS

CORE NEEDLE BIOPSY: A 14- to 16-gauge needle used to extract tissue from a breast mass, which preserves cellular architecture.

FINE NEEDLE ASPIRATION (FNA): The use of a small-gauge needle with associated vacuum via a syringe to aspirate fluid or some cells from a breast mass and/or cyst. The histology from the FNA would be loose cells (cytology).

FIBROADENOMA: Benign, smooth muscle tumor of the breast, usually occurring in young women.

EXCISIONAL BIOPSY: Surgical procedure to remove the entire lesion.

CLINICAL APPROACH

One of the key skills of any primary care physician is differentiating normal breast changes from abnormal ones, that is, identification of the **dominant breast mass. Fibrocystic changes,** the most common of the benign breast conditions, are described as **multiple, irregular, "lumpiness of the breast."** It is not a disease per se, but rather an exaggerated response to ovarian hormones. Fibrocystic changes are very common in premenopausal women, but rare following menopause. The clinical presentation is cyclic, painful, engorged breasts, more pronounced just before menstruation, and occasionally associated with serous or green breast discharge. Through careful physical examination, fibrocystic changes can usually be differentiated from the three-dimensional dominant mass suggestive of cancer, but occasionally a fine-needle or core biopsy must be performed to establish the diagnosis. Treatment includes decreasing caffeine ingestion, and adding NSAIDs, a tight-fitting bra, oral contraceptives, or oral progestin therapy. With severe cases, danazol (a weak antiestrogen and androgenic compound) or even mastectomy are considered.

In a woman in the adolescent years or in her 20s, the most common cause of a dominant breast mass is a **fibroadenoma.** These tumors are **firm, rubbery, mobile, and solid in consistency.** They typically do not respond to ovarian hormones and do not vary during the menstrual cycle. Since any three-dimensional dominant mass necessitates histologic confirmation, a biopsy should be performed. In a woman less than age 35 years, a fine needle aspiration or core needle biopsy is often chosen. The advantages of FNA are less expense, less pain, but higher nondiagnostic rate; advantages of core needle biopsy include higher sensitivity but higher cost. The concept of the **triple assessment,** that is, clinical examination, imaging (ultrasound or mammography), and histology being concordant (all in agreement) has high reliability with either FNA or core needle biopsy. Nonconcordance usually indicates obtaining more tissue. If the histologic examination supports fibroadenoma (mature smooth muscle cells) and the mass is small and not growing, careful follow-up is possible. Nevertheless, many women choose to have excision of the mass. Most clinicians will excise any dominant three-dimensional mass occurring in a woman over the age of 35 years, or in those with an increased likelihood of mammary cancer (family history).

Comprehension Questions

Match the breast lesion (A-E) to the clinical presentation (26.1-26.4).
    A. Fibroadenoma
    B. Fibrocystic changes
    C. Intraductal papilloma
    D. Breast cancer
    E. Galactocele

26.1   A 34-year-old woman complains of unilateral serosanguineous nipple discharge from the breast, expressed from one duct. No mass is palpated.

26.2   A 27-year-old woman complains of breast pain, which increases with menses. The breast has a lumpy-bumpy sensation.

26.3   A 47-year-old woman has a 1.5-cm right breast mass with nipple retraction and skin dimpling over the mass.

26.4   An 18-year-old adolescent female has an asymptomatic, 1-cm, non-tender, mobile right breast mass.

26.5   A 32-year-old G0 P0 woman complains of a 1-week history of a red and tender breast. She denies trauma, insect bites, pustules, or other lesions. Her family history is negative for breast disease. She denies oral contraceptive use. On examination her temperature is 98°F (36.6°C), heart rate (HR) 80 beats per minute (bpm), and blood pressure (BP) 100/60 mm Hg. Her heart and lung examination is normal. The right breast reveals a 5 × 4 cm area of redness, induration, and tenderness. There is no breast discharge. Her right axillary lymph nodes are mildly tender and enlarged. Which of the following is the best next step for this patient?
    A. Oral antibiotic therapy
    B. Biopsy of the breast
    C. Intravenous antibiotic therapy
    D. Advise the use of a tight fitting bra and avoid caffeine

ANSWERS

26.1 **C.** The most common cause of bloody (serosanguineous) nipple discharge when only one duct is involved and in the absence of a breast mass is intraductal papilloma. These are typically small, benign tumors that grow in the milk ducts. The highest incidence of this condition is in the 35 to 55 age group; causes and risk factors are unknown. The discharge is typically serosanguineous like the woman in this scenario. Because malignancy is also a common cause of bloody nipple charge (Second most common cause!), ductal exploration is required to rule out cancer.

26.2 **B.** A diffuse "lumpy-bumpy" examination suggests fibrocystic changes. They are very common in premenopausal women but rare following menopause. The classic clinical picture includes cyclic, painful, engorged breast, more pronounced just before menstruation, and occasionally associated with breast discharge. Treatment includes decreasing caffeine intake and adding NSAIDs, a tight-fitting bra, oral contraceptives, or oral progestin therapy. With severe cases, danazol (a weak antiestrogen and androgenic compound) or even mastectomy is considered. A patient who presents with painful, engorged breasts may also have a galactocele; however, a galactocele does not have a "lumpy-bumpy" breast examination, nor is it associated with hormonal changes or the menstrual cycle. Galactoceles are mammary gland tumors that are cystic in nature and contain milk or milky fluid. They typically occur when there is any sort of obstruction of milk flow in the lactating breast.

26.3 **D.** Nipple retraction or skin dimpling over a mass is very suggestive of malignancy. In the physical examination, maneuvers to accentuate the skin changes such as "hands on hips" or "arms raised over the head" assist in evaluating for these findings. Most clinicians excise any dominant three-dimensional mass occurring in a woman older than 35 years or in those with an increased likelihood of mammary cancer (family history). Histologic analysis from the excisional biopsy will most likely confirm the diagnosis of cancer.

26.4 **A.** In females in the adolescent years or in their 20s, the most common cause of a dominant breast mass is a fibroadenoma. These tumors are firm, rubbery, mobile, and solid in consistency. The best way to image the breast of a woman less than age 30 is usually ultrasound due to the dense fibrocystic changes that interfere with mammographic interpretation. Ultrasound can differentiate a solid versus a cystic mass, and sometimes can suggest a fibroadenoma; nevertheless, tissue should be obtained to confirm the diagnosis.

26.5   **B.** In a woman who has a "red tender indurated breast" who is nonlactating, inflammatory breast cancer must be ruled out. Biopsy of the breast is critical. Inflammatory breast cancer is aggressive in nature, and the skin changes occur due to the cancer cells within the subdermal lymph channels. Immediate diagnosis and therapy are crucial, whereas delay with various antibiotics would be detrimental. Interestingly, inflammatory breast cancer occurs more in younger patients, although women of any age can be affected.

REFERENCES

American College of Obstetricians and Gynecologists. Breast concerns of the adolescent. ACOG *Committee Opinion 350*. Washington, DC: 2006.

American College of Obstetricians and Gynecologists. Diseases of the Breast. ACOG *Practice Bulletin 42*. Washington, DC: 2003.

Hacker NF, Friedlander ML. Breast disease: a gynecologic perspective. In: Hacker NF, Gambone JC, Hobel CJ, eds. *Essentials of Obstetrics and Gynecology*, 5th ed. Philadelphia, PA: Saunders; 2009:332-344.

Valea FA, Katz VL. Breast diseases. In: Katz VL, Lentz GM, Lobo RA, Gersenson DM, eds. *Comprehensive Gynecology*. 5th ed. St. Louis, MO: Mosby-Year Book; 2007: 327-350.

Case 27

A 31-year-old G1 P1 woman presents with a history of infertility of 2-year duration. She states that her menses began at age 12 years and occurs at 28-day intervals. A biphasic basal body temperature chart is recorded. She denies sexually transmitted diseases, and a hysterosalpingogram shows patent tubes and a normal uterine cavity. Her husband is 34 years old and his semen analysis is normal.

➤ What is the most likely etiology of the infertility?

ANSWER TO CASE 27:

Infertility, Peritoneal Factor

Summary: An infertile couple is evaluated. Her menses are regular, and a biphasic basal body temperature chart is recorded. She denies sexually transmitted diseases, and a hysterosalpingogram shows patent tubes and a normal uterine cavity. The semen analysis is normal.

➤ **Most likely etiology:** Endometriosis (peritoneal factor).

ANALYSIS

Objectives

1. Know the five basic etiologies of infertility.
2. Understand the history and laboratory tests for these five factors.
3. Understand that endometriosis is more common than cervical factor infertility.

Considerations

This 31-year-old woman has secondary infertility. In approaching infertility, there are five basic factors to examine: (1) ovulatory, (2) uterine, (3) tubal, (4) male factor, and (5) peritoneal factor (endometriosis). The patient has regular monthly menses. That by itself argues strongly for regular ovulation; the biphasic basal body temperature chart is further evidence for regular ovulation. The uterine and tubal factors are normal based on the normal hysterosalpingogram, which is a radiologic study in which dye is placed into the uterine cavity via a transcervical catheter. The male factor is not an issue, based on the normal semen analysis. Therefore the remaining factor not addressed is the peritoneal factor. If the patient had prior cryotherapy to the cervix, the examiner might be directed to consider cervical factor (rare); similarly, if the patient complained of the three Ds of endometriosis (dysmenorrhea, dyspareunia, and dyschezia), then the examiner would be pointed toward the peritoneal factor. Since there are no hints favoring one factor over another, the clinician must pick the most common condition, which is endometriosis.

5 etiologies of infertility
1. ovulatory
2. uterine
3. tubal
4. male fx
5. peritoneal fx

3 d's → dysmenorrhea
→ dyspareunia } endometriosis.
→ dyschezia

APPROACH TO
Infertility

DEFINITIONS

INFERTILITY: Inability to conceive after 1 year of unprotected intercourse.
PRIMARY INFERTILITY: A woman has never been able to get pregnant.
SECONDARY INFERTILITY: A woman has been pregnant in the past, but has 1 year of inability to conceive.

CLINICAL APPROACH

Infertility affects approximately 10% to 15% of couples in the reproductive age group. **Fecundability,** defined as the probability of achieving a pregnancy within one menstrual cycle, has been estimated at **20% to 25%** for a normal couple. On the basis of this estimate, approximately 90% of couples should conceive after 12 months. The physician's initial encounter with the couple is very important and sets the tone for further evaluation and treatment. It is extremely important that after the initial evaluation, a realistic plan be established and followed (Table 27–1).

The five main causes of infertility are as follows.

1. **Ovulatory disorders (ovulatory factor).** Ovulatory disorders account for approximately 30% to 40% of all cases of female infertility. A history of regularity or irregularity of the menses is fairly predictive of the regularity of ovulation. The basal body temperature (BBT) chart is the easiest and least expensive method of detecting ovulation (Figure 27–1).

   The temperature should be determined orally, preferably with a basal body thermometer, before the patient arises out of bed, eats, or drinks. The chart documents the rise of temperature of about 0.5°F that occurs after ovulation due to the release of progesterone (a thermogenic hormone) by the ovary. The rise of temperature accounts for the biphasic pattern indicative of ovulation. Midluteal (day 21) serum progesterone level is an indirect method of documenting ovulation. Luteinizing hormone (LH) and, particularly the LH surge, can be detected with self-administered urine test kits. Ovulation occurs predictably about 36 hours after the onset of the LH surge. Other tests include the endometrial biopsy showing secretory tissue, or an ultrasound documenting a decrease in follicular size and presence of fluid in the cul-de-sac, suggesting ovulation.

2. **Uterine problems.** The hysterosalpingogram (HSG) is the initial test for intrauterine shape and tubal patency. It should be performed between days 6 and 10 of the cycle. Hysteroscopy likewise provides direct visualization

Table 27–1 APPROACH TO INFERTILITY

FACTOR	HISTORY	TEST	THERAPY
Ovulatory dysfunction	Irregular menses, obesity	Basal body temperature chart, LH surge, or progesterone level	Clomiphene citrate
Uterine disorder	Uterine fibroids	Hysterosal-pingogram showing abnormal uterine cavity	Hysteroscopic procedure
Male factor	Hernia, varicocele, mumps	Semen analysis	Repair of hernia or varicocele, in vitro fertilization
Tubal disorder	Chlamydial or gonococcal infection	Hysterosal-pingogram	Laparoscopy; in vitro fertilization
Peritoneal factor (endometriosis)	3 Ds: dysmenorrhea, dyspareunia, dyschezia	Laparoscopy (some advocate CA-125)	Ablation of endometriosis, medical therapy

of the uterine cavity when the HSG suggests an intrauterine defect. Uterine abnormalities have been associated with recurrent pregnancy losses. Uterine myomata and, in particular, submucosal myomata may interfere with implantation and fertility.

3. **Tubal factor.** A history of chlamydial or gonococcal cervicitis or salpingitis may point toward tubal disease. The hysterosalpingogram is fairly accurate but not perfect; hence, abnormal findings should be confirmed with laparoscopy, which is considered the "gold standard" for diagnosing tubal and peritoneal disease. In addition, operative laparoscopy can provide for the treatment of tubal and peritoneal disease through a minimally invasive technique.

4. **Abnormalities in the semen (male factor).** The semen analysis is a very basic and noninvasive test and should be one of the initial examinations. Even men who have fathered other children should have a semen analysis.

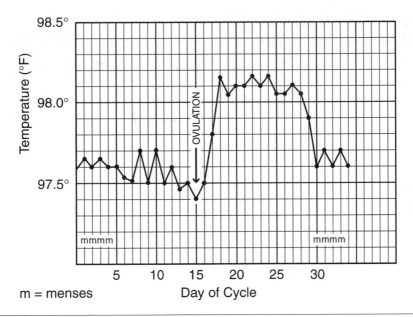

Figure 27–1. Basal body temperature chart. After ovulation, the temperature rises by 0.5°F for 10 to 12 days.

The semen should be evaluated in terms of: volume (nl > 2.0 mL), sperm concentration (nl > 20 million/mL), motility (nl > 50%), and morphology (nl > 30% normal forms). An abstinence period of 2 to 3 days prior to semen collection is recommended. One abnormal test is not sufficient to establish the diagnosis of a male factor abnormality, and the test should be repeated after 2 to 3 months (the process of transforming spermatogonia into mature sperm cells requires 74 days).

5. **Peritoneal factor (endometriosis).** Endometriosis, a common condition associated with infertility, should be suspected in any infertile woman. The suspicion should increase if she complains of dysmenorrhea and dyspareunia, but often is present even in asymptomatic women. Although not completely understood, endometriosis may cause infertility by inhibiting ovulation, inducing adhesions, and, perhaps, interfering with fertilization. Laparoscopy is the gold standard for the diagnosis of endometriosis, and can allow for surgical ablation of the lesions. Lesions can be of various appearances, from clear to red to the classic "powder burn" color.

Note: **Cervical factor** is considered as an **infrequent etiology** and may be suspected with thick viscid cervical mucus before ovulation. Intrauterine insemination, using a catheter to inject washed sperm through the cervix bypasses the cervix.

⤷ isn't there also something like inadequare cervical mucus?

Comprehension Questions

27.1   A 22-year-old G0 P0 woman complains of irregular menses every 30 to
        65 days. The semen analysis is normal. The hysterosalpingogram is nor-
        mal. Which of the following is the most likely treatment for this patient?
        A. Laparoscopy
        B. Intrauterine insemination
        C. In vitro fertilization
        D. Clomiphene citrate

27.2   A 26-year-old G0 P0 woman has regular menses every 28 days. The
        semen analysis is normal. The patient had a postcoital test revealing
        motile sperm and stretchy watery cervical mucus. She has been treated
        for chlamydial infection in the past. Which of the following is the
        most likely etiology of her infertility?
        A. Peritoneal factor
        B. Male factor
        C. Cervical factor
        D. Uterine and tubal factor
        E. Ovulatory factor

27.3   A 28-year-old G1 P1 woman complains of painful menses and pain
        with intercourse. She has menses every month and denies a history of
        sexually transmitted diseases. Which of the following tests would most
        likely identify the etiology of the infertility?
        A. Semen analysis
        B. Laparoscopy
        C. Basal body temperature chart
        D. Hysterosalpingogram
        E. Progesterone assay

27.4   A 34-year-old infertile woman is noted to have evidence of blocked
        fallopian tubes by hysterosalpingogram. Which of the following is the
        best next step for this patient?
        A. FSH therapy
        B. Clomiphene citrate therapy
        C. Laparoscopy
        D. Intrauterine insemination

ANSWERS

27.1   **D.** Irregular menses usually means irregular ovulation, and therefore
        infertility could most likely be attributed to an ovarian factor. The
        three conditions to consider are polycystic ovarian syndrome
        (PCOS), which is most common, hypothalamic disturbances, and

[handwritten margin note: mechanism: niveles estradiol feedback at pit / hypothalamus]

premature ovarian failure (POF). Causes of hypothalamic distur-bances affect pulsatile GnRH, such as hypothyroidism and hyper-prolactinemia. Thus, the evaluation of a woman with irregular ovulation usually includes checking TSH and prolactin levels. Elevated FSH levels would suggest POF. Clomiphene citrate is a treatment for anovulation, particularly polycystic ovarian syndrome (PCOS). The diagnosis of PCOS is a clinical one, with characteris-tics of obesity, anovulation, hirsutism, and possibly glucose intoler-ance. A laparoscopy would be indicated if there was suspicion of a tubal factor causing infertility (such as a prior history (PMH) of chlamydia or gonorrhea) or peritoneal factor (three Ds of endometriosis). Intrauterine insemination is indicated when a cervi-cal factor is thought to be the cause of infertility, such as thick viscid cervical mucus before ovulation. This procedure bypasses the unfa-vorable cervix using a catheter to inject washed sperm. The patient in this scenario does not present with symptoms consistent with cer-vical factor infertility. In vitro fertilization can be considered if the problem was a tubal factor or male factor.

[handwritten margin note: why no hysterosalpingogram to confirm.]

27.2   **D.** The history of chlamydial infection strongly suggests tubal factor infertility. Laparoscopy would be the next step in management and is considered the "gold standard" for diagnosing **tubal and peritoneal dis-**ease. The patient does not present with any of the "three Ds" of peri-toneal factor, and the semen analysis is normal which excludes peritoneal factor and male factor as the cause for infertility. There is no mention of a history of fibroids and she reports regular menses; this eliminates uterine and ovulatory factors as the etiology of her infertility.

27.3   **B.** This patient's history of dysmenorrhea and dyspareunia (two out of the three Ds of peritoneal factor symptoms) suggests endometriosis, which is best diagnosed by laparoscopy. A hysterosalpingogram visu-alizes the inside of the uterus and would not be helpful in the diag-nosis of endometriosis, since it manifests outside the uterus, tubes, and ovaries. She has menses every month; therefore her basal body temperature chart should be normal. A progesterone assay may be used to assess whether ovulation occurs, or the adequacy of the cor-pus luteum (a so-called luteal phase defect).

27.4   **C.** This patient presents with symptoms of tubal factor infertility. The hysterosalpingogram (radiologic study in which dye is injected into the uterus) is not specific and should be followed up with laparoscopy. Laparoscopy can provide for treatment of tubal and peritoneal disease through a minimally invasive technique. Clomiphene is not effective in patients with tubal factor, and is indicated with anovulation. FSH ther-apy and intrauterine insemination would be ineffective for the same reasons.

Clinical Pearls

➤ The five basic factors causing infertility are: ovulatory, uterine, tubal, male, and peritoneal.

➤ Irregular menses usually means irregular ovulation; regular menses usually indicates regular ovulation. In general, ovulatory disorders are fairly amenable to therapy.

➤ A history of salpingitis or chlamydial cervicitis suggests tubal factor infertility.

➤ Laparoscopy is the "gold standard" in diagnosing endometriosis, and lesions may have a variety of appearances.

➤ Surgery is the main therapy for endometrial or tubal abnormalities associated with infertility.

REFERENCES

Lobo RA. Infertility. In: Katz VL, Lentz GM, Lobo RA, Gersenson DM, eds. *Comprehensive Gynecology.* 5th ed. St. Louis, MO: Mosby-Year Book; 2007:1001-1038.

Meldrum DR. Infertilty and assisted reproductive technologies. In: Hacker NF, Gambone JC, Hobel CJ, eds. *Essentials of Obstetrics and Gynecology,* 5th ed. Philadelphia, PA: Saunders; 2009:371-378.

Case 28

A 23-year-old G2 P1 woman at 29 weeks' gestation complains of a 12-hour history of colicky, right lower abdominal pain and nausea with vomiting. She denies vaginal bleeding or leakage of fluid per vagina. She denies diarrhea or eating stale foods. She has a history of an 8-cm ovarian cyst, and otherwise has been in good health. She denies dysuria or fever, and has had no surgeries. Her vital signs include a blood pressure (BP) of 100/70 mm Hg, heart rate (HR) 105 beats per minute (bpm), respiratory rate (RR) 12 breaths per minute, and temperature 99°F (37.2°C). On abdominal examination, her bowel sounds are hypoactive. The abdomen is tender in the right lower quadrant region with significant involuntary guarding. The cervix is closed. The fetal heart tones are in the 140 bpm range.

➤ What is the most likely diagnosis?

➤ What is the best treatment for this condition?

ANSWERS TO CASE 28:
Abdominal Pain in Pregnancy (Ovarian Torsion)

Summary: A 23-year-old G2 P1 woman at 29 weeks' gestation with an 8-cm ovarian cyst complains of a 12-hour history of colicky, right lower abdominal pain and nausea with vomiting. The abdomen is tender in the right lower quadrant region with significant involuntary guarding.

➤ **Most likely diagnosis:** Torsion of the ovary.

➤ **Best treatment for this condition:** Surgery (laparotomy due to the pregnancy).

ANALYSIS

Objectives

1. Know the clinical presentation of some of the common causes of abdominal pain in pregnancy (acute appendicitis, acute cholecystitis, ovarian torsion, placental abruption, and ectopic pregnancy).
2. Understand that surgery is the best treatment for ovarian torsion.
3. Know that oophorectomy does not necessarily need to be performed in ovarian torsion.

Considerations

This woman, who is pregnant at 29 weeks' gestation, has a history of an 8-cm ovarian cyst. The ovarian mass is most likely a dermoid cyst because of her age. The acute onset of colicky, lower abdominal pain and nausea with vomiting are consistent with ovarian torsion, which is the twisting of the ovarian vessels leading to ischemia. Gastrointestinal complaints are common. The treatment for ovarian torsion is surgical. If this woman were not pregnant, laparoscopy would be an option. Sometimes, the size of the mass makes exploratory laparotomy the best choice. Upon opening the abdomen, the surgeon would examine the ovary for viability. Sometimes, untwisting of the ovarian pedicle can lead to reperfusion of the ovary. An ovarian cystectomy, that is, removing only the cyst and leaving the remainder of the normal ovarian tissue intact, is the best treatment. This patient is somewhat atypical regarding the gestational age, since the majority of pregnant women with ovarian torsion present either at 14 weeks' gestation when the uterus rises above the pelvic brim, or immediately postpartum when the uterus rapidly involutes.

APPROACH TO
Abdominal Pain in Pregnancy

CLINICAL APPROACH

Diseases related to and unrelated to the pregnancy must be considered. Additionally, the pregnancy state may alter the risk factors for the different causes of abdominal pain, and change the presentation and symptoms. Common causes of abdominal pain in pregnant women include appendicitis, acute cholecystitis, ovarian torsion, placental abruption, and ectopic pregnancy. Often, it is difficult to differentiate from among these different etiologies, but a careful history and physical and reexamination are the most important steps (Table 28–1).

Table 28–1 DIFFERENTIAL DIAGNOSIS OF ABDOMINAL PAIN IN PREGNANCY

	TIME DURING PREGNANCY	LOCATION	ASSOCIATED SYMPTOMS	TREATMENT
Appendicitis	Any trimester	Right lower quadrant → Right flank	Nausea and vomiting Anorexia Leukocytosis Fever	Surgical
Cholecystitis	After first trimester	Right upper quadrant	Nausea and vomiting Anorexia Leukocytosis Fever	Surgical
Torsion	More commonly at 14 weeks' gestation or after delivery	Unilateral, abdominal, or pelvic	Nausea and vomiting	Surgical
Placental abruption + bleeding	Second and third trimesters	Midline persistent uterine	Vaginal bleeding Abnormal fetal heart tracings	Delivery
Ectopic pregnancy	First trimester	Pelvic or abdominal pain, usually unilateral	Nausea and vomiting Syncope Spotting	Surgical or medical

Acute Appendicitis

The diagnosis of appendicitis can be difficult to make because many of the presenting symptoms are common complaints in pregnancy. Furthermore, a delay in diagnosis (especially in the third trimester) frequently leads to maternal morbidity and perinatal problems, such as preterm labor and abortion. Patients typically present with nausea, emesis, fever, and anorexia. The location of the abdominal pain is not typically in the right lower quadrant (as is classic for nonpregnant patients), but instead is superior and lateral to McBurney point. This is due to the effect of the **enlarged uterus pushing on the appendix to move it upward and outward toward the flank,** at times mimicking pyelonephritis. Diagnosis is made clinically, and because of the morbidity involved in a missed diagnosis, it is generally better to err on the side of overdiagnosing than underdiagnosing this disease. When appendicitis is suspected, the treatment is surgical regardless of gestational age, along with intravenous antibiotics.

Acute Cholecystitis

A common physiologic effect of pregnancy is an increase in gallbladder volume and biliary sludge (especially after the first trimester). The biliary sludge then serves as a precursor to gallstones. While gallstones are often asymptomatic, the most common symptoms are right upper quadrant pain following a meal, nausea, a "bloated sensation," and, possibly, emesis. In the absence of infection or fever, this is called **biliary colic.** Less commonly, when obstruction of the cystic or common bile duct occurs, the pain may be severe and unrelenting, and the patient may become icteric. When fever and leukocytosis are present, the patient with gallstones likely has cholecystitis. Other complications of gallstones include pancreatitis and ascending cholangitis, a serious life-threatening infection. The diagnosis of cholelithiasis is often established by an abdominal ultrasound revealing gallstones and dilation and thickening of the gallbladder wall. Simple biliary colic in pregnancy is usually treated with a low-fat diet and observed until postpartum. However, in the face of **cholecystitis, biliary obstruction, or pancreatitis in pregnancy, surgery is the treatment of choice;** generally, supportive medical management is used initially during the acute phase.

Ovarian Torsion

Patients with known or newly diagnosed large ovarian masses are at risk for ovarian torsion. **Ovarian torsion is the most frequent and serious complication of a benign ovarian cyst.** Pregnancy is a risk factor, especially around 14 weeks and after delivery. Symptoms include unilateral abdominal and pelvic colicky pain associated with nausea and vomiting. **The acute onset of colicky pain is typical.** Treatment is surgical with ovarian conservation if possible. If untwisting the adnexa results in reperfusion, an ovarian cystectomy may be performed. However, if perfusion cannot be restored, oophorectomy is indicated.

Placental Abruption

Abruption is a common cause of third-trimester bleeding and is usually associated with abdominal pain. Risk factors include a history of previous abruption, hypertensive disease in pregnancy, trauma, cocaine use, smoking, or preterm premature rupture of membranes. Patients typically present with vaginal bleeding with persistent crampy midline uterine tenderness and at times abnormal fetal heart tracings. Diagnosis is made clinically and ultrasound is not very reliable. The treatment is generally delivery, often by cesarean.

Ectopic Pregnancy

The leading cause of maternal mortality in the first and second trimesters is ectopic pregnancy. Patients usually have amenorrhea with some vaginal spotting and lower abdominal and pelvic pain. The pain is typically sharp and tearing and may be associated with nausea and vomiting. Physical findings include a slightly enlarged uterus and perhaps a palpable adnexal mass. In case of ectopic ruptures, the patient may experience syncope or hypovolemia. Transvaginal sonography and serum human chorionic gonadotropin (hCG) levels can help with the diagnosis of ectopic pregnancy in more than 90% of cases. Treatment options include surgery (especially with hemodynamically unstable patients) and, in appropriately selected patients, methotrexate.

Comprehension Questions

28.1 A 28-year-old G1 P0 woman at 28 weeks' gestation presents to the hospital with fever, nausea and vomiting, and anorexia of 2 days' duration. On examination, her temperature is 100.7°F (38.16°C), HR 104 bpm, and BP is 100/60 mm Hg. Her abdomen reveals tenderness on the right lateral aspect at the level of the umbilicus. There is mild right flank tenderness. A urinalysis is normal. In consideration of the diagnostic possibilities, which of the following is most accurate regarding this patient?

A. Appendicitis should be considered since the appendix location changes during pregnancy.

B. Cholecystitis is best diagnosed by CT scan of the abdomen.

C. Pyelonephritis commonly presents with normal urinalysis findings.

D. Inflammatory bowel disease should strongly be considered in this patient.

28.2   Upon performing laparoscopy for a suspected ovarian torsion on an 18-year-old nulliparous woman, the surgeon sees that the ovarian vascular pedicle has twisted 1 to 1.5 times and that the ovary appears somewhat bluish. Which of the following is the best management at this point?

A. Oophorectomy with excision close to the ovary

B. Oophorectomy with excision of the vascular pedicle to prevent possible embolization of the thrombosis

C. Unwind the vascular pedicle to assess the viability of the ovary

D. Bilateral salpingo-oophorectomy

E. Intravenous heparin therapy

28.3   A 32-year-old G1 P0 woman at 29 weeks' gestation presents with a 1-day history of severe midepigastric abdominal pain radiating to the back, and multiple episodes of nausea and vomiting. On examination, her BP is 100/60 mm Hg, HR 110 bpm, and temperature is 99°F (36.6°C). Her abdominal examination has tenderness and diffuse rebound. The serum amylase level is markedly elevated. Which of the following is the next step?

A. Initiate a high-protein, low-fat diet

B. Immediate surgical excision of the inflamed aspect of the pancreas

C. Ultrasound imaging of the abdomen

D. Delivery of the infant

28.4   An 18-year-old G1 P0 woman complains of a 2-month history of colicky, right abdominal pain when she eats. It is associated with nausea and emesis. She states that the pain radiates to her right shoulder. The patient has a family history of diabetes. Which of the following is the most likely diagnosis?

A. Peptic ulcer disease

B. Cholelithiasis

C. Appendicitis

D. Ovarian torsion

ANSWERS

28.1   **A.** The growing uterus pushes the appendix superior and lateral. The diagnosis of appendicitis during pregnancy can be difficult since patients frequently present with symptoms common in pregnancy. A delay in diagnosis, on the other hand, can lead to maternal morbidity and perinatal problems. Typically, patients present with nausea, emesis, fever, and anorexia. Abdominal pain is not located in the right lower quadrant as in nonpregnant patients because the growing uterus pushes on the appendix in an upward and outward direction, toward the flank and sometimes mimicking pyelonephritis.

Regardless of gestational age, the treatment is surgical with IV antibiotics. Cholecystitis is also common in pregnancy, but usually presents with right abdominal pain in the subcostal region and may radiate to the right shoulder. Gallstones are best diagnosed with ultrasound rather than CT scan. Pyelonephritis almost always is associated with pyuria (WBC in urine), and usually causes fever and flank tenderness. Inflammatory bowel disease presents in young patients with bloody diarrhea and abdominal pain. This patient does not have diarrhea or loose stools.

28.2   **C.** Unless the ovary appears necrotic, the ovarian pedicle can be untwisted and the ovary observed for viability. An oophorectomy would not be indicated in this patient unless the ovaries were necrotic from the prolonged lack of perfusion, or if after untwisting the ovary, reperfusion cannot be established. It is important to try and conserve the ovary—especially in such a young patient. Previously, it was thought that a torsed ovarian vasculature with thrombus needed excision due to the possibility of embolization. This has been disproved and neither excision of the clotted vessels or heparin is required.

28.3   **C.** With the diagnosis of pancreatitis, the next diagnostic steps include assessing the severity of the condition (such as with Ranson criteria of hypoxia, hemorrhagic complications, renal insufficiency, etc), and looking for an underlying etiology for the pancreatitis. In pregnancy, the most common cause of pancreatitis is gallstones, although alcohol use, hyperlipidemia, and medications are sometimes implicated. Thus, the best next step is ultrasound to assess for gallstones. If gallstones are found, then consideration may be given to eventual cholecystectomy once the patient is stabilized, or ERCP if a common bile duct stone is suspected. A patient with pancreatitis should have nothing by mouth. Surgery on the inflamed pancreas is harmful. Delivery of the pregnancy is not indicated.

28.4   **B.** This patient has a classic presentation of symptomatic cholelithiasis (biliary colic). In pregnancy, this condition is usually treated with a low-fat diet and observed until postpartum. However, if the patient were to develop cholecystitis (gallstones with fever and leukocytosis), biliary obstruction, or pancreatitis in pregnancy, surgery is the treatment of choice; generally, supportive medical management is used initially during the acute phase.

Clinical Pearls

> ➤ In pregnancy, the appendix moves superiorly and laterally from the normal location.
> ➤ The acute onset of colicky abdominal pain is typical of ovarian torsion.
> ➤ With ovarian torsion, the clinician can untwist the pedicle and observe the ovary for viability.
> ➤ Ectopic pregnancy should be suspected in any woman with abdominal pain.
> ➤ Degenerating fibroids can cause intense localized pain and are treated expectantly and with prostaglandin synthetase inhibitors.

REFERENCES

Castro LC, Ognyemi D. Common medical and surgical conditions complicating pregnancy. In: Hacker NF, Gambone JC, Hobel CJ, eds. *Essentials of Obstetrics and Gynecology*, 5th ed. Philadelphia, PA: Saunders; 2009:191-218.

Katz VL. Benign gynecologic lesions. In: Katz VL, Lentz GM, Lobo RA, Gersenson DM, eds. *Comprehensive Gynecology*. 5th ed. St. Louis, MO: Mosby-Year Book; 2007:419-470.

Case 29

A 19-year-old G2 Ab1 woman at 7 weeks' gestation by last menstrual period (LMP) complains of vaginal spotting. She denies the passage of tissue per vagina, any trauma, or recent intercourse. Her past medical history is significant for a pelvic infection approximately 3 years ago. She had used an oral contraceptive agent 1 year previously. Her appetite is normal. On examination, her blood pressure (BP) is 100/60 mm Hg, heart rate (HR) 90 beats per minute (bpm), and temperature is afebrile. The abdomen is nontender with normoactive bowel sounds. On pelvic examination, the external genitalia are normal. The cervix is closed and nontender. The uterus is 4 weeks' size, and no adnexal tenderness is noted. The quantitative beta-human chorionic gonadotropin (β-hCG) is 2300 mIU/mL (Third International Standard). A transvaginal sonogram reveals an empty uterus and no adnexal masses.

➤ What is your next step?

➤ What is the most likely diagnosis?

ANSWERS TO CASE 29:
Ectopic Pregnancy

Summary: A 19-year-old G2 Ab1 woman at 7 weeks' gestation by LMP has vaginal spotting. Her history is significant for a prior pelvic infection. Her BP is 100/60 mm Hg, HR 90 bpm, and her abdomen is nontender. Pelvic examination shows a closed and nontender cervix, a uterus of 4 weeks' size, and no adnexal tenderness. The quantitative β-hCG is 2300 mIU/mL (Third International Standard). A transvaginal sonogram reveals an empty uterus and no adnexal masses.

➤ **Next step:** Laparoscopy.

➤ **Most likely diagnosis:** Ectopic pregnancy.

ANALYSIS

no F/u β hCG
b/c > 1500-2000

Objectives

1. Understand that any woman with amenorrhea and vaginal spotting or lower abdominal pain should have a pregnancy test to evaluate the possibility of ectopic pregnancy.
2. Understand the role of the hCG level and the threshold for transvaginal sonogram.
3. Know that the lack of clinical or ultrasound signs of ectopic pregnancy does not exclude the disease.

Considerations

The woman is at 7 weeks' gestation by last menstrual period and presents with vaginal spotting. Any woman with amenorrhea and vaginal spotting should have a pregnancy test. The physical examination is normal. Notably, the uterus is slightly enlarged at 4 weeks' gestational size. The enlarged uterus does not exclude the diagnosis of an ectopic pregnancy, due to the human chorionic gonadotropin effect on the uterus. The lack of adnexal mass or tenderness on physical examination likewise does not rule out an ectopic pregnancy. The hCG level and transvaginal ultrasound are key tests in the assessment of an extrauterine pregnancy. The ultrasound is primarily used to assess for the presence or absence of an intrauterine pregnancy (IUP), because a confirmed IUP would decrease the likelihood of an ectopic pregnancy significantly (risk 1:10,000 of both an intrauterine and ectopic pregnancy). Also, the presence of free fluid in the peritoneal cavity, or a complex adnexal mass, would make an extrauterine pregnancy more likely. This woman's hCG level of 2300 mIU/mL is greater than the threshold of 1500 mIU/mL (transvaginal sonography); thus, the patient has a high likelihood of an ectopic pregnancy. Although the risk of an extrauterine pregnancy is high, it is not 100%. Therefore, laparoscopy is indicated, and not methotrexate, since the latter would destroy any intrauterine gestation.

↳ b/c you are below the threshold for seeing IUP on TVUS.

APPROACH TO
Possible Ectopic Pregnancy

DEFINITIONS

ECTOPIC PREGNANCY: A gestation that exists outside of the normal endometrial implantation sites.

HUMAN CHORIONIC GONADOTROPIN: A glycoprotein produced by syncytiotrophoblasts, which is assayed in the standard pregnancy test.

THRESHOLD HCG LEVEL: The serum level of hCG where a pregnancy should be seen on ultrasound examination. When the hCG exceeds the threshold and no pregnancy is seen on ultrasound, there is a high likelihood of an ectopic pregnancy.

LAPAROSCOPY: Surgical technique to visualize the peritoneal cavity through a rigid telescopic instrument, known as a laparoscope.

CLINICAL APPROACH

See also Case 7.

The vast majority of ectopic pregnancies involve the fallopian tube (97%), but the cervix, abdominal cavity, and ovary have also been affected. In the United States, 2% of pregnancies are extrauterine. Hemorrhage from ectopic gestation is the most common reason for maternal mortality in the first 20 weeks of pregnancy. Risk factors for ectopic pregnancy are summarized in Table 29–1.

A woman with an ectopic pregnancy typically complains of abdominal pain, amenorrhea of 4 to 6 weeks' duration, and irregular vaginal spotting. In case of ectopic ruptures, the pain becomes acutely worse, and may lead to syncope. Shoulder pain can be a prominent complaint due to the blood irritating the diaphragm. An ectopic pregnancy can lead to tachycardia, hypotension, or orthostasis. Abdominal or adnexal tenderness is common. An adnexal mass is only palpable half the time; hence, the absence of a detectable mass does not exclude an ectopic pregnancy. The uterus may be normal in size, or slightly enlarged. A hemoperitoneum can be confirmed by the aspiration of nonclotting blood with a spinal needle piercing the posterior vaginal fornix into the cul-de-sac (culdocentesis).

HCG grows uterus too

Table 29–1 RISK FACTORS FOR ECTOPIC PREGNANCY

Salpingitis, particularly with *Chlamydia trachomatis*
Tubal adhesive disease
Infertility
Progesterone-secreting IUD
Tubal surgery
Prior ectopic pregnancy
Ovulation induction
Congenital abnormalities of the tube

The diagnosis of an ectopic pregnancy can be a clinical challenge. The differential diagnosis is noted in Table 29–2.

The usual strategy in ruling out an ectopic pregnancy is to try to prove whether an intrauterine pregnancy (IUP) exists. Because the likelihood of a coexisting intrauterine and extrauterine (heterotopic) gestation is so low, in the range of 1 in 10,000, if a definite IUP is demonstrated, the risk of ectopic pregnancy becomes very low. Transvaginal sonography is more sensitive than transabdominal sonography, and can detect pregnancies as early as 5.5 to 6 weeks' gestational age. Hence, the demonstration of a definite IUP by crown–rump length or yolk sac is reassuring. The "identification of a gestational sac" is sometimes misleading since an ectopic pregnancy can be associated with fluid in the uterus, a so-called "pseudogestational sac." Other sonographic findings of an extrauterine gestation include an embryo seen outside the uterus, or a large amount of intra-abdominal free fluid, usually indicating blood.

Often, the quantitative human chorionic gonadotropin level is used in conjunction with transvaginal sonography. **When the hCG level equals or exceeds 1500 to 2000 mIU/mL, an intrauterine gestational sac is usually seen on transvaginal ultrasound; in fact, when the hCG level meets or exceeds this threshold and no gestational sac is seen, the patient has a high**

Table 29–2 DIFFERENTIAL DIAGNOSIS OF ECTOPIC PREGNANCY

Acute salpingitis
Abortion
Ruptured corpus luteum
Acute appendicitis
Dysfunctional uterine bleeding
Adnexal torsion
Degenerating leiomyomata
Endometriosis

likelihood of an ectopic pregnancy. Laparoscopy is usually performed in this situation. When the hCG level is less than the threshold, and the patient does not have severe abdominal pain, hypotension, or adnexal tenderness and/or mass, then a repeat hCG level in 48 hours is permissible. **A rise in the hCG of at least 66% above the initial level is good evidence of a normal pregnancy;** in contrast, a lack of an appropriate rise of the hCG is indicative of an abnormal pregnancy, although the abnormal change does not identify whether the pregnancy is in the uterus or the tube. Some practitioners will use a progesterone level instead of serial hCG levels to assess the health of the pregnancy. A progesterone level of greater than 25 ng/mL almost always correlates with a normal intrauterine pregnancy, whereas a level of less than 5 ng/mL almost always correlates with an abnormal pregnancy.

Treatment of an ectopic pregnancy may be surgical or medical. Salpingectomy (removal of the affected tube) is usually performed for those gestations too large for conservative therapy, when rupture has occurred, or for those women who do not want future fertility. For a woman who wants to preserve her fertility and has an unruptured tubal pregnancy, a salpingostomy can be performed (Figure 29–1).

An incision is carried out along the long axis of the tube, and the pregnancy tissue is removed. The incision on the tube is not reapproximated because suturing may lead to stricture formation. Conservative treatment of the tube is associated with a 10% to 15% chance of persistent ectopic pregnancy. Serial hCG levels are, therefore, required with conservative surgical therapy to identify this condition.

Methotrexate, a folic acid antagonist, is the principal form of medical therapy. It is usually given as a one-time, low-dose, intramuscular injection, reserved for ectopic pregnancies less than 4 cm in diameter. **Methotrexate is highly successful, leading to resolution of properly chosen ectopic pregnancies** in 85% to 90% of cases. Occasionally, a second dose is required because the hCG level does not fall. Between 3 to 7 days following therapy, a patient may complain of abdominal pain, which is usually due to tubal abortion and, less commonly, rupture. Most women may be observed; however, hypotension, worsening or persistent pain, or a falling hematocrit may indicate tubal rupture and necessitate surgery. About 10% of women treated with medical therapy will require surgical intervention.

Rare types of ectopic gestations such as cervical, ovarian, abdominal, or cornual (involving the portion of the tube that traverses the uterine muscle) pregnancies usually require surgical therapy.

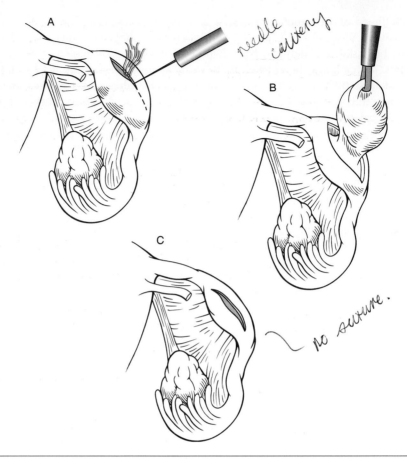

Figure 29–1.   Salpingostomy. Needle-point cautery is used to incise over the ectopic pregnancy (**A**). The pregnancy tissue is extracted (**B**) and heals without closure of the incision (**C**).

Comprehension Questions

29.1   A 22-year-old woman at 8 weeks' gestation has vaginal spotting. Her physical examination reveals no adnexal masses. The hCG level is 400 mIU/mL and the transvaginal ultrasound shows no pregnancy in the uterus and no adnexal masses. Which of the following is the best next step?

A. Laparoscopy

B. Methotrexate

C. Repeat the hCG level in 48 hours

D. Dilatation and curettage

29.2   A 26-year-old G2 P1 woman at 7 weeks' gestation was seen 1 week ago
with crampy lower abdominal pain and vaginal spotting. Her hCG
level was 1000 mIU/mL at that time. Today, the woman does not have
abdominal pain or passage of tissue per vagina. Her repeat hCG level
is 1100 mIU/mL. A transvaginal ultrasound examination today shows
no clear pregnancy in the uterus and no adnexal masses. Which of the
following can be concluded based on the information presented?
    A. The woman has a spontaneous abortion and needs a dilation and
       curettage.
    B. The woman has an ectopic pregnancy.
    C. No clear conclusion can be drawn from this information, and the
       hCG needs to be repeated in 48 hours.
    D. The woman has a nonviable pregnancy, but its location is unclear.

29.3   A 17-year-old woman with lower abdominal pain and spotting comes
into the emergency room. She is noted to have an hCG level of
1000 mIU/mL and a progesterone level of 26 ng/mL. Which of the
following is the most likely diagnosis?
    A. This is most likely a normal intrauterine pregnancy.
    B. This is most likely an ectopic pregnancy.
    C. This is most likely a nonviable intrauterine pregnancy.
    D. No clear conclusion can be drawn form this information.

29.4   Which of the following statements describes the primary utility of the
transvaginal ultrasound in the assessment of an ectopic pregnancy?
    A. Assessment of an intrauterine pregnancy
    B. Assessment of adnexal masses
    C. Assessment of fluid in the peritoneal cavity
    D. Color Doppler flow in the adnexal region

29.5   A 29-year-old woman complains of syncope. She is 6 weeks' pregnant
and on examination has diffuse significant lower abdominal tenderness. The pelvic examination is difficult to accomplish due to guarding. Her hCG level is 400 mIU/mL and the transvaginal ultrasound
shows no pregnancy in the uterus and no adnexal masses. Which of
the following is the best next step?
    A. Follow-up hCG level in 48 hours
    B. Institution of methotrexate
    C. Observation in the hospital
    D. Surgical therapy

ANSWERS

29.1   **C.** When the hCG is *below the threshold* in an asymptomatic patient,
the hCG level may be repeated in 48 hours to assess for viability. If
the hCG level had been above the threshold in this patient, the
chances that an extrauterine pregnancy exists would be even more
likely (close to 100%), laparoscopy would be indicated to confirm suspicion. Since there is still a chance that this is a viable pregnancy,
methotrexate should not be used since it could destroy any intrauterine gestation. Dilation and curettage would also destroy any viable
intrauterine pregnancy, and would not be a good option for treatment
of an ectopic pregnancy since they exist outside the uterus.

[handwritten margin note: It was only 1 day rise, 10% of need 48 hrs.]

29.2   **D.** A plateau in hCG over 48 hours means it is a nonviable pregnancy; this finding does not identify the location of the pregnancy.
Levels of hCG that plateau in the first 8 weeks of pregnancy indicate
an abnormal pregnancy, which may be either a miscarriage or an
ectopic pregnancy. It is unlikely that this patient had an incomplete
or a completed abortion, given that she does not recall any passage of
tissues.

29.3   **A.** A progesterone level greater than 25 ng/mL reflects a normal IUP.
This patient's hCG level is below the threshold of being visible on
ultrasound, so it is a very early pregnancy. Spotting and lower
abdominal pain can be a normal occurrence in pregnancy, especially
very early in the first trimester. Some patients have symptoms of
lower abdominal pain, similar to menstrual cramps, and vaginal spotting during the first few weeks of pregnancy when the embryo
implants into the wall of the uterus.

29.4   **A.** The best use of ultrasound for assessment of an ectopic pregnancy
is to diagnose an IUP, as an IUP and coexisting ectopic pregnancy is
very rare. Color Doppler flow in the adnexal region is typically used
when there is suspicion of ovarian torsion and concern that the ovarian vessels are constricted and unable to perfuse the ovaries.
Assessment of adnexal masses using transvaginal ultrasound is not
very specific. A hemoperitoneum can be confirmed by culdocentesis,
but not typically a transvaginal ultrasound.

29.5   **D.** Surgery is indicated. Although this woman has an hCG level lower
than the threshold, she has an acute abdomen and this is most likely
due a ruptured ectopic pregnancy. If not addressed, the patient may
exsanguinate. Methotrexate requires several days to weeks to act, and
is appropriate in an asymptomatic patient with an ectopic pregnancy
less than 3.5 cm in size.

Clinical Pearls

➤ Levels of hCG that plateau in the first 8 weeks of pregnancy indicate an abnormal pregnancy, which may either be a miscarriage or an ectopic pregnancy.

➤ The classic triad of ectopic pregnancy is amenorrhea, vaginal spotting, and abdominal pain.

➤ When the quantitative hCG exceeds 1500 to 2000 mIU/mL and the transvaginal sonogram does not show an intrauterine gestational sac, then the risk of ectopic pregnancy is high.

REFERENCES

American College of Obstetricians and Gynecologists. Medical management of ectopic pregnancy. ACOG *Practice Bulletin 94*. Washington, DC: 2008.

Lobo VL. Ectopic pregnancy. In: Katz VL, Lentz GM, Lobo RA, Gersenson DM, eds. *Comprehensive Gynecology*. 5th ed. St. Louis, MO: Mosby-Year Book; 2007:389-410.

Shamonki M, Nelson AL, Gambone JC. Ectopic pregnancy. In: Hacker NF, Gambone JC, Hobel CJ, eds. *Essentials of Obstetrics and Gynecology*, 5th ed. Philadelphia, PA: Saunders; 2009:290-297.

Case 30

A 29-year-old woman G2 P1 at 20 weeks' gestation is seen for her second prenatal visit. Her antenatal history is unremarkable except for a urinary tract infection treated with an antibiotic 2 weeks ago. The patient was noted to have an anemia on her prenatal screen with hemoglobin level of 9.5 g/dL, with a mean corpuscular volume (MCV) of 70 fL. On examination, her blood pressure (BP) is 100/60 mm Hg, heart rate (HR) 80 beats per minute (bpm), and she is afebrile. The thyroid gland appears normal on palpation. The heart and lung examinations are unremarkable. The fundus is at the umbilicus. The fetal heart tones are in the 140 to 150 bpm range. The evaluation of the anemia includes: ferritin level: 90 mcg/L (normal 30-100); serum iron 140 mcg/dL (normal 50-150); hemoglobin electrophoresis: Hb A1 95% and Hb A2 5%.

➤ What is the most likely diagnosis?

➤ What is the underlying mechanism?

ANSWERS TO CASE 30:

Anemia in Pregnancy (Thalassemia)

Summary: A 29-year-old woman G2 P1 at 20 weeks' gestation is being seen for prenatal care. On examination, her BP is 100/60, HR 80 bpm, and temperature is normal. Her hemoglobin level is 9.5 g/dL.

➤ **Most likely diagnosis:** Anemia due to β-thalassemia minor.

➤ **Underlying mechanism:** Decreased β-globin chain production.

ANALYSIS

Objectives

1. Know that iron deficiency and thalessemia are common causes of micro-cytic anemia.
2. Understand that deficiency of folate and vitamin B_{12} are causes of anemia.
3. Know the diagnostic approach to anemia in pregnancy.

Considerations

This pregnant patient has a mild anemia, since the hemoglobin level is less than 10.5 g/dL. The red blood cell (RBC) indices give an indication of the etiology. In this case, the MCV is low, microcytic. The most common cause of microcytic anemia is iron deficiency. Typically, with a mild microcytic anemia in the absence of risk factors for thalassemia (such as Southeast Asian ethnicity), a trial of iron supplementation and recheck of the hemoglobin in 3 weeks would be the next step. This is called a therapeutic trial of iron. If the hemoglobin level improves, the evidence supports iron deficiency. If the hemoglobin level does not improve, then iron studies and a hemoglobin electrophoresis would be the next step. In this case, iron studies were performed which were normal/high normal, thus eliminating iron deficiency as a cause. The hemoglobin electrophoresis studies strongly suggest β-thalassemia trait (heterozygous for β-thalassemia) with the elevated A2 hemoglobin. If the patient had β-thalassemia homozygous disease, there would have been complications and clinical manifestations since childhood. The patient should now be counseled about her laboratory findings, referral to genetic counseling, and instructed that her baby has a 1 in 4 risk for β-thalassemia disease if the father of the baby also has β-thalassemia trait. Extra iron should not be given, since these patients can be prone to iron overload.

APPROACH TO
Anemia in Pregnancy

DEFINITIONS

ANEMIA: A hemoglobin level of less than 10.5 g/dL in the pregnant woman.

IRON DEFICIENCY ANEMIA: A fall in hemoglobin level that is due to insufficient iron to meet the increased iron requirements in pregnancy.

THALASSEMIA: A decreased production of one or more of the peptide chains (most common are the α and β chains) that make up the globin molecule. This process may result in ineffective erythropoiesis, hemolysis, and varying degrees of anemia.

HEMOLYTIC ANEMIA: An abnormally low hemoglobin level due to red blood cell destruction, which may be divided into congenital causes and acquired causes.

GLUCOSE-6-PHOSPHATE DEHYDROGENASE DEFICIENCY: An X-linked condition whereby the red blood cells may have a decreased capacity for anaerobic glucose metabolism. Certain oxidizing agents, such as nitrofurantoin, can lead to hemolysis.

What decreases w/ rapid RBC turnover?
↳ MbA1c ↓

CLINICAL APPROACH

Physiology of Pregnancy

Anemia is a common complication in the pregnant woman. It is **most often due to iron deficiency,** partially because of decreased iron stores prior to pregnancy, and increased demands for iron (due to fetus' need and expanded maternal blood volume). A hemoglobin level below 10.5 g/dL is usually considered a sign of anemia in the pregnant woman, with a mild anemia between 8 to 10 g/dL and severe as less than 7g/dL.

Iron Deficiency

A gravid woman who presents with mild anemia and no risk factors for hemoglobinopathies (African American, Southeast Asian, or Mediterranean descent) may be treated with supplemental iron and the hemoglobin level reassessed in 3 to 4 weeks. Persistent anemia necessitates an evaluation for iron stores, such as ferritin level (low with iron deficiency) and hemoglobin electrophoresis.

Hemoglobinopathies

The size of the red blood cell may give a clue about the etiology. A microcytic anemia is most commonly due to iron deficiency, although thalassemia may also be causative. Results from a **hemoglobin electrophoresis** can differentiate between the two, and may also indicate the presence of sickle cell trait or sickle cell anemia. The different types of **thalassemias** are classified according to the peptide chain that is deficient. In β-thalassemia minor, for example, there is a decreased production of the β-globin chain. This particular thalassemia during pregnancy is usually safe for both the mother and fetus, and there is no specific therapy given other than prophylactic folic acid. A patient may go their whole lives and not know they have β-thalassemia minor; patients may remain asymptomatic throughout their lives. Genetic counseling in a patient with a known hemoglobinopathy is important because if the baby inherits a recessive trait from both parents, they will typically be born with a more serious or fatal disease (ie, β-thalassemia major). A neonate born with β-thalassemia major may appear healthy at birth, but as the hemoglobin F level falls (and no β-chains are able to replace the diminishing γ-chains of the fetal hemoglobin), the infant may become severely anemic and fail to thrive if not adequately transfused. The life expectancy with transfusions is somewhere in the third decade.

Whereas the thalassemias are *quantitative* defects in a hemoglobin chain production, sickle cell disease involves a *qualitative* defect that results in a sickle-shaped and rigid hemoglobin molecule. **Sickle cell anemia** is a recessive disorder caused by a point mutation in the β-globin chain in which the amino acid glutamic acid is replaced with valine. This results is improper folding of the hemoglobin molecule which results in either sickle cell disease (HbSS) or sickle cell trait, (HbS), when only the sickle cell trait is inherited. A patient with **sickle cell trait** should not be discouraged to get pregnant as far as risk to her is concerned; however, her baby has a 1:4 chance of inheriting sickle cell disease if the father also has the sickle cell trait. Infants born with sickle cell disease typically do not show signs of being affected until about 4 months. Patients with sickle cell disease usually deal with symptoms related to anemia (ie, fatigue and shortness of breath) and pain. In pregnancy, women with sickle cell disease often have a more intense anemia, more frequent bouts of **sickle cell crisis** (painful vasoocclusive episodes), and more frequent infections and pulmonary complications. Careful attention must be taken when a pregnant sickle cell patient presents in crisis because some of the symptoms may mimic other common occurrences during pregnancy (ectopic pregnancy, placental abruption, pyelonephritis, appendicitis, or cholecystitis), and they may be missed. All causes of fever, pain, and low Hg laboratory value should be considered before attributing it to a pain crisis. Also, these patients have a higher incidence of fetal growth retardation and perinatal mortality; therefore, serial ultrasonography is recommended.

G6PD deficiency + Sulfonamides, Nitrofurantoin, Antimalarial

Macrocytic Anemia

Macrocytic anemias may be due to vitamin B_{12} and folate deficiency. Because vitamin B_{12} stores last for many years, megaloblastic anemias in pregnancy are much more likely to be caused by folate deficiency.

Other Conditions

Less commonly, a woman with glucose-6-phosphate dehydrogenase deficiency (G6PD) may develop hemolytic anemia triggered by various medications such as sulfonamides, nitrofurantoin, and antimalarial agents. Nitrofurantoin is a common medication utilized for uncomplicated urinary tract infections. Affected women usually have dark-colored urine due to the bilirubinuria, jaundice, and fatigue due to the anemia. G6PD deficiency is more commonly seen in the African American population.

In the pregnant woman with anemia, jaundice, and thrombocytopenia, the examiner must also consider other hemolytic processes, such as HELLP syndrome (hemolysis, elevated liver enzymes, low platelets), which is a life-threatening condition best treated by delivery. In evaluating anemia, if other hematologic cell lines are also decreased, such as the white blood cell count or platelet count, a bone marrow process, such as leukemia or tuberculosis infection of the marrow, should be considered. Bone marrow biopsy may be indicated in these circumstances.

Comprehension Questions

30.1   A 30-year-old G1 P0 woman complains of nausea and vomiting for the first 3 months of her pregnancy. She is noted to have a hemoglobin level of 9.0 g/dL and the mean corpuscular volume was 110 fL (normal 90-105). Which of the following is the most likely etiology of the anemia?

    A. Iron deficiency
    B. Folate deficiency
    C. Vitamin B_{12} deficiency
    D. Physiologic anemia of pregnancy

30.2   A 29-year-old G2 P1 at 28 weeks' gestation, who had normal hemoglobin level 4 weeks ago at her first prenatal visit complains of 1 week of fatigue and now has hemoglobin level of 7.0 g/dL. She noted dark-colored urine after taking an antibiotic for a urinary tract infection. Which of the following is the most likely diagnosis?

    A. Iron deficiency anemia
    B. Thalassemia
    C. Hemolysis
    D. Folate deficiency
    E. Vitamin B_{12} deficiency

30.3   A 33-year-old African American G1 P0 at 16 weeks' gestation is diag-
nosed with sickle cell trait. Her husband also is a carrier for the sickle
cell gene. Which of the following best describes the likelihood that
their unborn baby will have sickle cell disease?
A. 1/100
B. 1/50
C. 1/10
D. 1/4

30.4   A 36-year-old G2 P1 at 24 weeks' gestation is noted to have fatigue of
4 weeks' duration. Her hemoglobin level is 8.0 g/dL, leukocyte count
is 2.0 cells/uL, and platelet count is 20,000/uL. Which of the follow-
ing is the most likely diagnosis?
A. Iron deficiency anemia
B. HELLP syndrome
C. Severe preeclampsia
D. Acute leukemia

ANSWERS

30.1   **B.** This is a macrocytic anemia, since the mean corpuscular volume
is above normal. Macrocytic anemias include folate deficiency and
vitamin B_{12} deficiency; however, folate deficiency is more commonly
seen in pregnancy than vitamin B_{12} deficiency. Iron deficiency is a
microcytic anemia (MCV below normal), and it is the most common
cause of anemia in pregnancy. Physiologic anemia of pregnancy is a
result of the physiologic hemodilution that occurs in the vasculature.
There is a disproportionate increase in plasma volume over the
increased RBC volume, and this "diluted state" also gives the appearance of a fall in the laboratory values of hemoglobin and hematocrit.

30.2   **C.** This 29-year-old woman at 28 weeks' gestation complains of fatigue.
She took an antibiotic for a urinary tract infection and then developed
dark-colored urine. She was also probably icteric. Currently, her hemoglobin level is low, reflecting an anemia. This constellation of symptoms likely reflects a hemolytic process. The dark urine suggests
bilirubinuria. Other causes of hemolysis could include malaria, HELLP
(hemolysis, elevated liver enzymes, low platelets) syndrome, autoimmune hemolytic anemia, or sickle cell crisis. In this case, the woman
ingested an antibiotic, which likely was nitrofurantoin, a commonly
prescribed medication for pregnant women. She does not have hypertension, symptoms of systemic lupus erythematosus or other autoimmune diseases, or pain suggestive of sickle cell disease.

30.3   **D.** With autosomal recessive disorders, when both parents are heterozygous for the gene (gene carriers), then there is a 1:4 chance that
the offspring will be affected by the disease or will be homozygous for
the gene. It is important for expectant mothers, who are at high risk for
having the sickle cell disease or trait, to get a hemoglobin electrophoresis in addition to the other prenatal laboratory tests. They
need to know what risks they may have during pregnancy and be counseled on how to have a healthy pregnancy with sickle cell disease. They
should also know what kinds of risks they may have in either passing
the disease or trait to their children and may seek genetic counseling
for this reason. During pregnancy, pain crisis may be more severe, so it
is especially important for these women to stay well hydrated and avoid
dehydration. There is an increased rate of preterm labor and having a
low-birthweight baby in a sickle cell patient, but with proper prenatal
care, these women can have perfectly normal pregnancies.

30.4   **D.** Pancytopenia, a reduction in the number of RBCs, WBCs, and platelets
circulating throughout the body, suggests a bone marrow process. None of
the other answer choices involve low leukocyte counts (leucopenia). Low
platelets (thrombocytopenia) may also be a manifestation of severe
preeclampsia, and is part of the criteria for HELLP (<u>hemolytic anemia</u>, elevated liver enzymes, and <u>low platelets</u>) syndrome as well. Iron deficiency
anemia involves low hemoglobin levels and is common in pregnancy due
to decreased iron stored prior to pregnancy, and increased demands for iron
during pregnancy. Since this patient's blood work showed low WBCs, a
bone marrow biopsy should be done. A pregnant woman with leukemia
may require chemotherapy, which poses a risk to the developing fetus of
IUGR. Acute leukemia itself carries a risk for preterm labor, spontaneous
abortion, and stillbirth.

but not leukopenia

Clinical Pearls

➤ The most common cause of anemia in pregnancy is iron deficiency.
➤ The two most common causes of microcytic anemia are iron deficiency
  and thalassemia.
➤ An elevated A2 hemoglobin level is suggestive of β-thalassemia disorder,
  whereas an elevated hemoglobin F level is suggestive of α-thalassemia.
➤ For mild anemias, it is acceptable to initiate a trial of iron supplementation
  and reassess the hemoglobin level.
➤ The most common cause of megaloblastic anemia in pregnancy is folate
  deficiency.
➤ Hemolysis in individuals with glucose-6-phosphate dehydrogenase deficiency may be triggered by sulfonamides, nitrofurantoin, or antimalarial
  agents.

REFERENCES

American College of Obstetricians and Gynecologists. Anemia in pregnancy. ACOG *Practice Bulletin 95*. Washington, DC: 2008.

Castro LC, Ognyemi D. Common medical and surgical conditions complicating pregnancy. In: Hacker NF, Gambone JC, Hobel CJ, eds. *Essentials of Obstetrics and Gynecology*, 5th ed. Philadelphia, PA: Saunders; 2009:191-218.

Cunningham FG, Leveno KJ, Bloom SL, Hauth JC, Gilstrap LC III, Wenstrom KD. Hematological disorders. In: *Williams Obstetrics*. 22nd ed. New York, NY: McGraw-Hill; 2005:1043-1167.

Cunningham FG, Leveno KJ, Bloom SL, Hauth JC, Gilstrap LC III, Wenstrom KD. Teratology, drugs, and medications. In: *Williams Obstetrics*. 22nd ed. New York, NY: McGraw-Hill; 2005:1021.

Case 31

A healthy 19-year-old G1 P0 at 29 weeks' gestation presents to the labor and delivery area complaining of intermittent abdominal pain. She denies leakage of fluid or bleeding per vagina. Her antenatal history has been unremarkable. She has been eating and drinking normally. On examination, her blood pressure (BP) is 110/70 mm Hg, heart rate (HR) 90 beats per minute (bpm), and temperature 99°F (37.2°C). The fetal heart rate tracing reveals a baseline heart rate of 120 bpm and a reactive pattern. Uterine contractions are occurring every 3 to 5 minutes. On pelvic examination, her cervix is 3 cm dilated, 90% effaced, and the fetal vertex is presenting at −1 station.

➤ What is the most likely diagnosis?

➤ What is your next step in management?

➤ What test of the vaginal fluid prior to digital examination may indicate risk for preterm delivery?

ANSWERS TO CASE 31:

Preterm Labor

Summary: A healthy 19-year-old G1 P0 at 29 weeks' gestation complains of intermittent abdominal pain. Her vital signs are normal. The fetal heart rate tracing reveals a baseline heart rate of 120 bpm and is reactive. Uterine contractions are noted every 3 to 5 minutes. Her cervix is 3 cm dilated, 90% effaced, and the fetal vertex is presenting at −1 station.

➤ **Most likely diagnosis:** Preterm labor.

➤ **Next step in management:** Tocolysis, try to identify a cause of the preterm labor, antenatal steroids, and antibiotics for GBS prophylaxis.

➤ **Test of vaginal fluid:** Fetal fibronectin assay.

ANALYSIS

Objectives

1. Understand how to diagnose preterm labor.
2. Understand that the basic approach to preterm labor is tocolysis, identification of an etiology, and steroids (if appropriate).
3. Know the common causes of preterm delivery.

Considerations

This 19-year-old nulliparous woman is at 29 weeks' gestation and complains of intermittent abdominal pain. The monitor indicates uterine contractions every 3 to 5 minutes, and her cervix is dilated at 3 cm and effaced at 90%. This is sufficient to diagnose preterm labor in a nulliparous woman. If she had a previous vaginal delivery, the diagnosis may not be as clear-cut. Because of the significant prematurity, many practitioners may elect to treat for preterm labor. A single examination revealing 2 cm dilation and 80% effacement in a nulliparous woman would be sufficient to diagnose preterm labor. Prior to digital examination, swabbing the posterior vaginal fornix for fetal fibronectin (ffn), which if positive may indicate risk of preterm birth. In contrast, a negative ffn assay is strongly associated with no delivery within 1 week. Another objective test for preterm delivery risk is transvaginal cervical length ultrasound measurements. A shortened cervix, especially with lower uterine segment changes (funneling or beaking of the amniotic cavity into the cervix), are worrisome. Tocolysis should be initiated, unless there is a contraindication (such as intra-amniotic infection or severe preeclampsia). Also, since the pregnancy is less than 34 weeks' gestation, intramuscular antenatal steroids should be given to enhance fetal pulmonary maturity. A careful search should also be undertaken to identify an underlying cause, such as urinary tract infection, cervical infection, bacterial vaginosis, generalized infection, trauma or abruption, hydramnios, or multiple gestations. Finally, intravenous antibiotics, such as penicillin, are helpful in case the tocolysis is unsuccessful, to reduce the likelihood of GBS sepsis in the neonate.

APPROACH TO
Preterm Labor

DEFINITIONS

PRETERM LABOR: Cervical change associated with uterine contractions prior to 37 completed weeks and after 20 weeks' gestation. In a nulliparous woman, uterine contractions and a single cervical examination revealing 2-cm dilation and 80% effacement or greater is sufficient to make the diagnosis.

TOCOLYSIS: Pharmacologic agents used to delay delivery once preterm labor is diagnosed. The most commonly used agents are indomethacin, nifedipine, terbutaline, and ritodrine. Recent evidence has indicated that magnesium sulfate may be ineffective.

ANTENATAL STEROIDS: Betamethasone or dexamethasone given intramuscularly to the pregnant woman in an effort to decrease some of the complications of prematurity, particularly respiratory distress syndrome (intraventricular hemorrhage in the more extremely premature babies).

FETAL FIBRONECTIN ASSAY: A basement membrane protein that helps bind placental membranes to the decidua of the uterus. A vaginal swab is used to detect its presence. Its best utility is a negative result, which is associated with a 99% chance of not delivering within 1 week.

CERVICAL LENGTH ASSESSMENT: Transvaginal ultrasound to measure the cervical length. Cervical length less than 25 mm results in an increased risk of preterm delivery. Also an impinging of the amniotic cavity into the cervix, so-called funneling, increases the risk of preterm delivery.

CLINICAL APPROACH

Preterm labor is defined as cervical change in the midst of regular uterine contractions occurring between 20 and 37 weeks' gestation. The incidence in the United States is approximately 11% of pregnancies, and it is the cause of significant perinatal morbidity and mortality. There are many risk factors associated with preterm delivery (Table 31–1).

Table 31–1 RISK FACTORS FOR PRETERM LABOR

Preterm premature rupture of membranes
Multiple gestations
Previous preterm labor or birth
Hydramnios
Uterine anomaly
History of cervical cone biopsy
Cocaine abuse
African American race
Abdominal trauma
Pyelonephritis
Abdominal surgery in pregnancy

The main symptoms of preterm labor are uterine contractions and abdominal tightening. Sometimes, pelvic pressure or increased vaginal discharge may also be present. The diagnosis is established by confirming cervical change over time by the same examiner, if possible, or finding the cervix to be 2 cm dilated and 80% effaced in a nulliparous woman. Once the diagnosis has been made, then an etiology should be sought. Tocolysis is considered if the gestational age is less than 34 to 35 weeks, and steroids are administered if the gestational age is less than 34 weeks. The work-up for preterm labor is summarized in Table 31–2.

Recent randomized controlled trials have suggested that magnesium sulfate is not effective as a tocolytic agent. Other medications include terbutaline, ritodrine, nifedipine, and indomethacin. The speculated mechanism of action of magnesium is competitive inhibition of calcium to decrease its availability for actin-myosin interaction, thus decreasing myometrial activity (see Table 31–3).

Nifedipine reduces intracellular calcium by inhibiting voltage-activated calcium channels. Side effects include pulmonary edema, respiratory depression,

Table 31–2 WORKUP FOR PRETERM LABOR

History to assess for risk factors
Physical examination with speculum examination to assess for ruptured membranes
Serial digital cervical examinations
Complete blood count
Urine drug screen (especially for cocaine metabolites)
Urinalysis, urine culture, and sensitivity
Cervical tests for gonorrhea (possibly *Chlamydia*)
Vaginal culture for group B streptococcus
Ultrasound examination for fetal weight and fetal presentation

Table 31–3 COMMON TOCOLYTIC AGENTS

TOCOLYTIC AGENTS	DRUG CLASS	METHOD OF ACTION	SIDE EFFECTS/COMPLICATIONS	CONTRAINDICATIONS
Magnesium sulfate	Minerals	Competitively inhibits calcium	**Pulmonary edema,** respiratory depression Neonatal depression, osteoporosis (when used long term)	Myocardial damage, heart block, diabetic coma (don't use with calcium channel blockers)
Terbutaline Ritodrine	β-agonists	Selective for β_2 receptors; Relaxes smooth muscles	**Pulmonary edema, increased pulse pressure, *hyperglycemia*, *hypokalemia*, and tachycardia**	Arrhythmia, hypertension, seizure disorder
Nifedipine	Calcium channel blocker	Inhibits calcium ion influx into vascular smooth muscle	CHF, MI, pulmonary edema, and severe hypotension	**Hypotension; *do not give* with magnesium sulfate (both act on calcium channels)**
Indomethacin	NSAID	Decreased prostaglandin synthesis	**Closure of fetus' ductus arteriosus which would lead to pulmonary hypertension,** oligohydramnios → could compromise	3rd trimester of pregnancy due to possible effects on ductus arteriosus
17-α-hydroxyprogesterone caproate	Synthetic progesterone, hormone replacement therapy	Inhibits pituitary gonadotropin release; maintains a pregnancy	Breast pain and tenderness, dizziness, abdominal pain, intermittent bleeding	Undiagnosed vaginal bleeding

neonatal depression, and if given long term, osteoporosis. **Pulmonary edema** is often the most serious side effect, and is seen more often with the β-agonist agents. A complication of indomethacin is closure of the ductus arteriosus, leading to severe neonatal pulmonary hypertension.

Antenatal steroids are given between 24 and 34 weeks' gestation when there is no evidence of infection. Only one course of corticosteroids is utilized. In other words, they are not repeated for recurrent threatened preterm delivery. In the early gestational ages, the effect is to lower the risk of intraventricular hemorrhage; at gestations greater than 28 weeks, the primary goal is to lower the incidence of respiratory distress syndrome. Weekly injections of 17 α-hydroxyprogesterone caproate from 20 weeks' gestation until 36 weeks' gestation has been shown to help prevent preterm birth in women at high risk. These include a history of previous spontaneous preterm delivery.

Comprehension Questions

31.1   A 26-year-old woman is noted to be at 29 weeks' gestation. Her last pregnancy ended in delivery at 30 weeks' gestation. In screening for various types of infection, which of the following is most likely to be associated with preterm delivery?

A. Herpes simplex virus
B. *Candida vaginitis*
C. *Chlamydia cervicitis*
D. Gonococcal cervicitis
E. Group B streptococcus of the vagina

31.2   A 25-year-old G1 P0 woman is noted to be 28 weeks' gestation. She is noted to have regular uterine contractions, and is dilated at 2 cm, and 80% effaced. Preterm labor is diagnosed. The physician reviews the record and notes that the patient should not have tocolytic therapy. Which one of the following is a contraindication for tocolysis?

A. Suspected placental abruption
B. Group B streptococcal bacteriuria
C. Recent laparotomy
D. Uterine fibroids

31.3   A 35-year-old G1 P0 woman at 32 weeks' gestation is noted to be seen in the obstetric (OB) triage unit the previous day with uterine contractions. On admission, the fetal heart rate is 140 bmp with accelerations and no decelerations. A fetal fibronectin assay is performed which is positive. Over the course of the next 24 hours, the patient was examined and noted to have cervical dilation from 1 to 2 cm and effacement from 30% to 90%. A tocolytic agent is used. A repeat fetal heart rate pattern reveals a baseline of 140 bpm with moderate repetitive variable decelerations. Which of the following is the most likely tocolytic agent used?

A. Nifedipine
B. Indomethacin
C. Magnesium sulfate
D. Terbutaline

31.4   A 28-year-old woman G1 P0 at 29 weeks' gestation is treated with terbutaline for preterm labor. Her cervix had dilated to 3 cm and 90% effaced. She also received betamethasone intramuscularly to enhance fetal lung maturity. The following day, the patient develops dyspnea, tachypnea, and an oxygen saturation level of 80%. Oxygen is given. Which of the following is the best therapeutic agent?

A. IV antibiotic therapy for probably pneumonia
B. IV heparin therapy for probable deep venous thrombosis
C. IV furosemide for probable pulmonary edema
D. Oral digoxin for probable cardiomyopathy

ANSWERS

31.1   **D.** Infections of various types are associated with preterm delivery. Gonococcal cervicitis is strongly associated with preterm delivery, whereas chlamydial infection is not as strongly associated. Urinary tract infections, particularly pyelonephritis, are associated with preterm delivery. Bacterial vaginosis may be linked with preterm delivery, although treatment of this condition does not seem to affect the risk.

31.2   **A.** Suspected abruption is a relative contraindication for tocolysis because the abruption may extend. The natural history of abruption is extension of the separation, leading to complete shearing of the placenta from the uterus. If this happens, delivery would be the best treatment with the administration of antenatal steroids to decrease the chance of respiratory distress syndrome in the preterm baby; expectant management may be exercised if the patient is stable with no active bleeding or sign of fetal compromise since this is a premature fetus. Nevertheless, giving tocolytics would increase the mother's chance of hemorrhage after delivery because it will be more difficult to get the uterus to contract on itself, since tocolytics also act as uterine relaxant. Infection with Group B streptococcal bacteriuria is not a contraindication for tocolysis; however the mother should be placed on antibiotic prophylaxis in the event that she delivers or has preterm premature rupture of membranes (PPROM). A recent laparotomy and uterine fibroid may increase the risk of preterm labor, but would not be a contraindication for administration of tocolytics, assuming both the mother and fetus are stable.

31.3   **B.** This patient has a change in her fetal heart rate tracing after tocolysis is used. Now, she has significant variable decelerations, which is caused by cord compression. A sudden change increasing variable decelerations can include oligohydramnios (less amniotic fluid to buffer the cord from compression), rupture of membranes, or descent of the fetal head, such as in labor, so that a nuchal cord (around the neck) may tighten. Indomethacin is associated with decreased amniotic fluid and oligohydramnios, and this is the most likely etiology.

31.4   **C.** In a patient on tocolytic therapy, pulmonary edema is a hazard, particularly when on β-agonists. The tachycardia that often occurs decreases the diastolic filling time, leading to increased end-diastolic pressure. Besides oxygen, IV furosemide is effective in decreasing intravascular fluid and thus decreasing hydrostatic pressure, hopefully relieving the fluid from the interstitial spaces of the lungs. The terbutaline of course also should be discontinued. A β-agonist therapy is associated with an increased pulse pressure, hyperglycemia, hypokalemia, and tachycardia.

Clinical Pearls

➤ Dyspnea occurring in a woman with preterm labor and tocolysis is usually due to pulmonary edema.

➤ The goal in treating preterm labor is to identify the cause, give steroids (if gestation is at 24 to 34 weeks), and tocolysis.

➤ The most common cause of neonatal morbidity in a preterm infant is respiratory distress syndrome.

➤ β-Agonist therapy has multiple side effects including tachycardia, widened pulse pressure, hyperglycemia, and hypokalemia.

➤ A negative cervical fetal fibronectin assay virtually guarantees no delivery within 1 week.

➤ Transvaginal sonography indicating a shortened cervix especially with funneling and/or beaking is suggestive of risk for preterm delivery.

REFERENCES

American College of Obstetricians and Gynecologists. Management of preterm labor. *ACOG Practice Bulletin 43.* 2003.

American College of Obstetricians and Gynecologists. Use of progesterone to reduce preterm birth. ACOG *Committee Opinion 419.* 2008.

Cunningham FG, Leveno KJ, Bloom SL, Hauth JC, Gilstrap LC III, Wenstrom KD. Preterm birth. In: *Williams Obstetrics.* 22nd ed. New York, NY: McGraw-Hill; 2005:855-880.

Hobel CJ. Obstetrical complications: preterm labor, PROM, IUGR, postterm pregnancy, and IUFD. In: Hacker NF, Gambone JC, Hobel CJ, eds. *Essentials of Obstetrics and Gynecology,* 5th ed. Philadelphia, PA: Saunders; 2009:146-159.

Case 32

A 29-year-old woman complains of a 2-day history of dysuria, urgency, and urinary frequency. She denies the use of medications and has no significant past medical history. On examination, her blood pressure (BP) is 100/70 mm Hg, heart rate (HR) 90 beats per minute, and temperature 98°F (36.6°C). The thyroid is normal on palpation. The heart and lung examinations are normal. She does not have back tenderness. The abdomen is nontender and without masses. The pelvic examination reveals normal female genitalia. There is no adnexal tenderness or masses.

➤ What is the most likely diagnosis?

➤ What is the next step in the diagnosis?

➤ What is the most likely etiology of the condition?

ANSWERS TO CASE 32:
Urinary Tract Infection (Cystitis)

Summary: A 29-year-old woman complains of a 2-day history of dysuria, urgency, and urinary frequency. Her temperature is 98°F (36.6°C). She does not have back tenderness. The abdomen is nontender and without masses. The pelvic examination is normal.

➤ **Most likely diagnosis:** Simple cystitis (bladder infection).

➤ **Next step in the diagnosis:** Urinalysis and/or urine culture.

➤ **Most likely etiology of the condition:** *Escherichia coli.*

ANALYSIS

Objectives

1. Know the symptoms of a urinary tract infection (cystitis).
2. Know that the most common bacteria causing cystitis is *E coli.*
3. Be familiar with some of the antibiotic therapies for cystitis.

Considerations

This 29-year-old woman has a 2-day history of urinary urgency, frequency, and dysuria, all which are very typical symptoms of a urinary tract infection. Because she does not have fever or flank tenderness, she most likely has a bladder infection or cystitis. Other symptoms of cystitis include hesitancy or hematuria (hemorrhagic cystitis). Urinalysis and/or urine culture and sensitivity would be the appropriate test to confirm the diagnosis. Since *E coli* is the most common etiologic agent, the antibiotic treatment should be aimed at this organism. Sulfa agents, cephalosporins, quinolones, or nitrofurantoin are all acceptable. If the urine culture returns showing no organism and the patient still has symptoms, urethritis is a possibility (often caused by *Chlamydia trachomatis*). In this setting, urethral swabbing for chlamydial testing is advisable. Another possibility is candidal vulvovaginitis. Finally, some women with symptoms of bladder discomfort with negative urine culture and urethral culture may have a chronic condition of urethral syndrome.

APPROACH TO
Urinary Tract Infections

DEFINITIONS

CYSTITIS: Bacterial infection of the bladder defined as having greater than 100,000 colony-forming units of a single pathogenic organism on a midstream-voided specimen.

URETHRITIS: Infection of the urethra commonly caused by *C trachomatis*.

URETHRAL SYNDROME: Urgency and dysuria caused by urethral inflammation of unknown etiology; urine cultures are negative.

CLINICAL APPROACH

Urinary tract infections (UTI) may involve the kidneys (pyelonephritis), bladder (cystitis), and urethra (urethritis). One in five women will acquire a UTI sometime in her life. The shorter urethra and its proximity to the rectum are the most commonly stated reasons for the increased incidence in women. Pregnancy further predisposes women to UTIs due to incomplete emptying of the bladder, ureteral obstruction, and immune suppression. Pathogenic bacteria include *E coli* (isolated 80% of the time) followed by *Enterobacter*, *Klebsiella*, *Pseudomonas*, *Proteus*, group B streptococcus, *Staphyloccoccus saprophyticus*, and *Chlamydia*.

The most common symptoms of lower tract infection (cystitis) are dysuria, urgency, and urinary frequency. Occasionally, the infection may induce a hemorrhagic cystitis and the patient will have gross hematuria. Nevertheless, **gross hematuria should raise the suspicion of nephrolithiasis.** Fever is uncommon unless there is kidney involvement, which is usually reflected by flank tenderness. The diagnosis of cystitis hinges on identification of pathogenic bacteria in the urine; bacteriuria is defined as greater than 100,000 colony-forming units per milliliter of a single uropathogen obtained from a midstream voided urine on culture. In symptomatic patients, as few as 1000 colony-forming units per milliliter may be significant. On a catheterized specimen, 10,000 colony-forming units per milliliter is considered bacteriuria. The presence of leukocytes in the urine is presumptive evidence of infection in a patient with symptoms.

Simple cystitis is the most common form of UTI and is diagnosed by the symptoms in the absence of fever or flank tenderness. Oral antimicrobial therapy is effective, and varies from one dose to 3 days, to 7 days, or even 10 days. Trimethoprim/sulfa (Bactrim), nitrofurantoin, norfloxacin, ciprofloxacin, and cephalosporins, such as cephalothin, are effective. Ampicillin is generally not used due to the widespread resistance of *E coli*. The utility of urine cultures in the first episode of simple cystitis is unclear. Some practitioners will routinely obtain cultures, whereas others will reserve these studies for recurrences, persistent symptoms, or in pregnancy. In the pregnant woman, **asymptomatic bacteriuria (ASB) leads to acute infection in up to 25% of untreated women and thus it should always be treated.**

A patient with urethritis has similar complaints to one with cystitis (ie, urgency, frequency, and dysuria). Sometimes, the urethra may be tender on palpation and purulent drainage expressed on examination. The most commonly isolated organisms are *Chlamydia*, *Gonococcus*, and *Trichomonas*. Urethritis should be suspected in a woman with typical symptoms of UTI yet with sterile culture and no response to the standard antibiotics. Cultures of the urethra for *Gonococcus* and *Chlamydia* should be performed. Treatment may be initiated empirically for *Chlamydia* with doxycycline; if *Neisseria gonorrhea* is suspected, intramuscular ceftriaxone with oral doxycycline is usually curative. Doxycycline should be avoided in pregnant women.

Women with pyelonephritis usually present with fever, chills, flank pain, and nausea and vomiting. Mild cases in the nonpregnant female may be treated with oral trimethoprim/sulfa or a fluoroquinolone for a 10- to 14-day course; these women should be reexamined within 48 hour. Sulfa agents are generally the most cost-effective. Those who are more ill, unable to take oral medications, pregnant, or immunocompromised should be hospitalized and treated with intravenous antibiotics, such as ampicillin and gentamicin, or a cephalosporin, such as cefazolin, cefotetan, or ceftriaxone. Following resolution of fever and symptoms, pregnant women with acute pyelonephritis are often treated with suppressive antimicrobial therapy (such as nitrofurantoin macrocrystals 100 mg once daily) for the remainder of pregnancy.

Comprehension Questions

32.1   A 29-year-old G1 P0 at 19 weeks' gestation is noted to have dysuria, urinary frequency, and urgency. A urine culture is performed, and growth is noted, which the microbiology laboratory notes, is not *E coli*. Which of the following is the most likely causative organism of cystitis?

A. *Chlamydia trachomatis*
B. *Klebsiella* species
C. Peptostreptococcus
D. *Bacteroides* species

32.2 A 19-year-old G2 P1 woman at 13 weeks' gestation comes in for her first prenatal visit. Among other tests, a urine culture is performed showing 100,000 cfu/mL of *E coli*. The patient has no symptoms, and has not had pyelonephritis, dysuria, or fever. Which of the following is best next step for this patient?

A. Observation, as no therapy is needed
B. No therapy needed unless the patient develops symptoms
C. Initiation of antibiotic therapy
D. No therapy needed at this time, but antibiotics should be given during labor

32.3 A 30-year-old G1 P0 woman at 29 weeks' gestation is noted to have a urinary tract infection with 100,000 cfu/mL of *E coli* growing on culture. Her obstetrician notes that an upper urinary tract infection leads to increased complications. Which of the following is a common manifestation of upper urinary tract infection rather than simple cystitis?

A. Fever
B. Urgency
C. Hesitancy
D. Dysuria

ANSWERS

32.1 **B.** The most common cause of UTIs in women is *E coli*. Other causes include *Enterobacter*, *Klebsiella*, *Pseudomonas*, and *Proteus*. *Chlamydia trachomatis* is a common cause of urethritis along with *Gonococcus* and *trichomonas*. *Peptostreptococcus* is a gram-positive anaerobe that is a commensal organism with humans and usually does not cause pathology except in immunosuppressed individuals. Along with *Peptostreptococcus*, *Bacteroides* species live as gut flora in humans. *Bacteroides* is a gram-negative anaerobe and, along with other anaerobes, rarely causes cystitis.

32.2 **C.** This patient has asymptomatic bacteriuria, which should be treated even without symptoms. If untreated, the patient has a 25% risk of developing pyelonephritis during the pregnancy. Asymptomatic bacteriuria (ASB) complicates approximately 8% to 10% of pregnant patients. Providing treatment of ASB at the first prenatal visit reduces the risk of pyelonephritis markedly.

32.3 **A.** Upper UTIs (including pyelonephritis) usually present with fever, costovertebral tenderness, chills, malaise, and often ill-appearing individual. They are at increased risk for septicemia, kidney dysfunction, or preterm labor. In severe cases, patient should be hospitalized and started on intravenous antibiotics. Presenting symptoms of urgency, hesitancy, and dysuria are symptoms for a simple cystitis or urethritis.

Urethritis can be differentiated from cystitis by a sterile culture and no response to antibiotics. Doxycycline (covers *Chlamydia*) with ceftriaxone (gonorrhea) is a good choice for suspected urethritis. Doxycycline should be avoided in pregnant women.

Clinical Pearls

➤ The most common cause of cystitis is *E coli.*
➤ Bacteriuria caused by group B streptococcus in pregnancy necessitates the use of intravenous penicillin or ampicillin in labor to decrease the risk of neonatal GBS sepsis.
➤ Pyelonephritis presents with flank tenderness and fever.
➤ Urethritis, commonly caused by *Chlamydia* or *N gonorrhea,* should be suspected with negative urine cultures and symptoms of a UTI.
➤ Asymptomatic bacteriuria has a high incidence in women with sickle cell trait.

REFERENCES

American College of Obstetricians and Gynecologists. Treatment of urinary tract infections in nonpregnant women. *ACOG Practice Bulletin 91.* Washington, DC: 2008.

Lentz GM. Urogynecology. In: Katz VL, Lentz GM, Lobo RA, Gersenson DM, eds. *Comprehensive Gynecology.* 5th ed. St. Louis, MO: Mosby-Year Book; 2007:537-567.

Tarnay CM, Bhatia NN. Genitourinary dysfunction, pelvic organ prolapse, urinary incontinence, and infections. In: Hacker NF, Gambone JC, Hobel CJ, eds. *Essentials of Obstetrics and Gynecology,* 5th ed. Philadelphia, PA: Saunders; 2009:276-289.

⭐Case 33

A 25-year-old G2 P2002 desires contraception for the next 3 years. She reports that she had a deep venous thrombosis when she took the combination oral contraceptive pill 2 years ago. She cannot remember to take the pill every day and wants contraception that will allow her to be spontaneous. She does not take any medications and has no known allergies to medications. Menarche was age 13. Menstrual cycle is every 28 days, lasting for 7 days. She has quarter-size clots the first 3 days of her menstrual cycle. She has been married for 3 years and denies any sexually transmitted infections. Her blood pressure is 120/70 mm Hg, heart rate 80 beats per minute (bpm), and temperature 99°F (37.2°C). Heart and lung examinations are normal. The abdomen is nontender and without masses. Pelvic examination reveals a normal anteverted uterus and no adnexal masses.

➤ What would be the best contraceptive agent for this patient?

➤ What would be contraindications to the proposed contraceptive agent?

ANSWERS TO CASE 33:
Contraception

Summary: A 25-year-old multiparous woman, in a stable monogamous relationship, desires long-term contraception. She has had a DVT while taking a combination oral contraceptive pill, is forgetful about taking pills everyday, and wants contraception that will allow spontaneity. She reports heavy menses. Physical examination is within normal limits.

➤ **Best contraceptive agent for this patient:** The levonorgestrel releasing intrauterine device.

➤ **Contraindications to the proposed contraceptive agent:** Contraindications for an IUD include recent sexually transmitted infection, behavior that increases risk for sexually transmitted infections, abnormal size and shape of the uterus.

ANALYSIS

Objectives

1. Know the various types of contraceptive agents including indications and contraindications, mechanisms of action, and efficacy.
2. Know benefits, risks, and contraindications for the combination oral contraceptive pill.
3. Know about intrauterine devices.
4. Know about emergency contraception.

Considerations

Each form of contraception has advantages and disadvantages, and the individual patient situation should be evaluated to find the best contraceptive choice. Factors that assist the physician in the counseling of the patient include agents requiring more patient action, such as remembering to take a pill each day, or putting on a barrier device (diaphragm or condom), duration of contraception desired, history of sexually transmitted infections, amount of vaginal bleeding, and medical complications. Because of the history of DVT, estrogen-containing contraception agents would be contraindicated. The desire for spontaneity would make barrier methods less desirable. Options for this patient would include depomedroxyprogesterone acetate or the levonorgestrel IUD. Because of the heavy menses, this 25 year old would most benefit from a levonorgestrel-releasing intrauterine device, since the progestin would cause the endometrial lining to be thinner and decrease the

→ misoprostal →PGoE'1 agonist to open.

amount of menstrual bleeding. This device is placed inside the uterus by a physician during an office visit and can be left in place for up to 5 years. It does not rely on the patient's memory for effectiveness. The progestin in the IUD is released slowly over time and can decrease the amount and frequency of menses. The IUD does not protect against sexually transmitted infections. Also, this patient has had a DVT which is a contraindication to any form of contraception that contains a combination of estrogen and progestin, like the combination oral contraceptive pill, patch, or ring.

APPROACH TO
Contraception

DEFINITIONS

INTRAUTERINE CONTRACEPTIVE DEVICES (IUD): Small T-shaped device, usually plastic with or without copper or a progestin, placed in the endometrial cavity as a method of long-term contraception.

TYPICAL USE EFFECTIVENESS: Overall efficacy in actual use, when forgetfulness and improper use occur.

PERFECT USE EFFECTIVENESS: Efficacy of a method when always used correctly, consistent and reliable use occur.

BARRIER CONTRACEPTIVE: Prevents sperm from entering upper female reproductive tract.

STEROID HORMONE CONTRACEPTION: Synthetic estrogen and/or progestin to provide contraception in various methods, including oral contraceptive pills, contraceptive patch, contraceptive ring, contraceptive injection, and implant.

YUZPE REGIMEN: Use of specific oral contraceptive regimen first reported by Dr Yuzpe, consisting of two tablets of Ovral oral contraceptives (total of 0.1 mg ethinyl estradiol and 0.5 mg levonorgestrel) at time zero and two tablets after 12 hours.

PLAN B (PROGESTIN ONLY): Levonorgestrel 0.75 mg taken orally at time zero and the same dose after 12 hours.

CLINICAL APPROACH

Contraceptive agents have different effectiveness, which are characterized as theoretical (or perfect) and with typical use (see Table 33–1). The various agents each have particular advantages and disadvantages and unique factors that may make one method better suited for a particular patient. Thus, the history and physical examination should focus on a patient's preference of

Table 33–1 CONTRACEPTIVE FAILURE RATES COMPARING TYPICAL USE AND PERFECT USE

METHOD	% FAILURE WITHIN FIRST YEAR OF USE	
	PERFECT USE	TYPICAL USE
No method	85	85
Periodic abstinence (calendar)	9	25
Diaphragm	6	16
Male condom	2	15
OC (combined and minipill)	0.3	8
Patch	0.3	8
Ring	0.3	6
Depo-Provera	0.3	3
Levonorgestrel implants (Implanon)	0.05	0.05
IUD Mirena (Levonorgestrel) ParaGard (copper-T)	0.1 0.6	0.1 0.8
Female sterilization	0.5	0.5
Male sterilization	0.1	0.15

method, factors such as the ability to remember to take a pill every day, and other medical conditions (see Table 33–2).

Barrier contraceptives prevent sperm from entering the upper female reproductive tract. Various forms include the male condom, female condom, vaginal diaphragm, cervical cap, and spermicides. The *male condom* is made of latex, polyurethane, or animal tissue. It is a sheath placed on an erect penis prior to intercourse and ejaculation. The latex condom is the most effective method of contraception to prevent transmission of sexually transmitted infections. It is the second most commonly used method of reversible contraception in the United States. The *female condom* is a sheath with two polyurethane rings. One ring is placed inside the vagina at the closed end of the sheath and provides an insertion mechanism and anchor. The second ring is at the outer edge of the device and is outside the vagina providing coverage for the labia and the base of the penis. It should offer more protection against transmission of certain infections, like genital herpes. The *vaginal diaphragm*

Table 33-2 CONTRACEPTION AGENTS COMPARED INCLUDING BEST-SUITED PATIENTS

CATEGORY	AGENTS	MECHANISM	BEST SUITED FOR	DISADVANTAGES AND CONTRAINDICATIONS
Barrier	Diaphragm Cervical caps Condoms (male and female)	Mechanical obstruction	Not desiring hormones **Decrease sexually transmitted infections**	Pelvic organ prolapse Patient discomfort with placing devices on genitals **Lack of spontaneity** Allergies to material Diaphragm may be associated with more UTIs
Combined hormonal (estrogen and progestin)	Combined oral contraceptives Contraception patch Vaginal ring	Inhibit ovulation Thickens cervical mucous to inhibit sperm penetration. Alters motility of uterus and fallopian tubes Thins the endometrium	Iron deficiency anemia Dysmenorrhea Ovarian cysts Endometriosis **OCP**—take pill each day **PATCH—less to remember but ? more nausea** **RING**—less to remember, ?vaginal irritation, and discharge	Known thrombogenic mutations Prior thromboembolic event Cerebrovascular or coronary artery disease (current or remote) Cigarette smoking over the age of 35 Uncontrolled hypertension Diabetic retinopathy, nephropathy, peripheral vascular disease Known or suspected breast or endometrial cancer Undiagnosed vaginal bleeding Migraines with aura Benign or malignant liver tumors, active liver disease, liver failure Known or suspected pregnancy

(Continued)

Table 33–2 CONTRACEPTION AGENTS COMPARED (CONTINUED)

CATEGORY	AGENTS	MECHANISM	BEST SUITED FOR	DISADVANTAGES AND CONTRAINDICATIONS
Progestin-only oral	Minipill	Thickens cervical mucous to inhibit sperm penetration Alters motility of uterus and fallopian tubes Thins the endometrium	**Breast-feeding**	Very dependent on taking pill each day at same time Patient needs to remember to take pill
Injectables	Depo-medroxy progesterone acetate	Inhibits ovulation Thins endometrium Alters cervical mucous to inhibit sperm penetration	Breast-feeding Desires long-term contraception Iron deficiency anemia **Sickle cell disease** **Epilepsy** Dysmenorrhea Ovarian cysts Endometriosis	? Depression ? Osteopenia/osteoporosis Weight gain
Implants (subdermal in arm)	Levonorgestrel Implant (Implanon)	Inhibits ovulation Thins endometrium Thickens cervical mucous to inhibit sperm penetration	Breast-feeding Desires long-term contraception (lasts for 3 years) Iron deficiency anemia Dysmenorrhea Ovarian cysts	Current or past history of thrombosis or thromboembolic disorders Hepatic tumors (benign or malignant), active liver disease Undiagnosed abnormal vaginal bleeding Known or suspected carcinoma of the breast or personal history of breast cancer

			Endometriosis	Hypersensitivity to any of the components of Implanon **May lead to irregular vaginal bleeding**
IUD	Levonorgestrel intrauterine device	Thickens cervical mucous Thins endometrium	Desires long-term, reversible contraception Stable, mutually monogamous relationship Menorrhagia Dysmenorrhea (NOTE: decreased bleeding and dysmenorrhea)	**Current STI or recent PID** *(past ok)* Unexplained vaginal bleeding Malignant gestational trophoblastic disease Untreated cervical or endometrial cancer Current breast cancer Anatomical abnormalities distorting the uterine cavity Uterine fibroids distorting endometrial cavity
IUD	Copper-T	Inhibits sperm migration and viability Changes transport speed of ovum Damages ovum	Desires long-term reversible contraception (10 years) Stable, mutually monogamous relationship Contraindication to contraceptive steroids	Current STI Current or PID within the past 2 months Unexplained vaginal bleeding Malignant gestational trophoblastic disease Untreated cervical or endometrial cancer Current breast cancer Anatomical abnormalities distorting the uterine cavity Uterine fibroids distorting endometrial cavity **Wilson disease** */ or Cu allergy* **May cause more bleeding or dysmenorrhea**
Permanent sterilization	Bilateral tubal occlusion	Mechanical obstruction of tubes	Does not desire more children	Contraindications to surgery May want children in the future

must be fit by a physician. It should be placed 1 to 2 hours before intercourse, be used with a spermicide, and be left in place for at least 8 hours after coitus. Drawbacks include higher rate of urinary tract infections and increased risk of ulceration to the vaginal epithelium with prolonged usage. The *cervical cap* is also fit by a physician. Compared to a diaphragm, the cap can be left in place for up to 48 hours and is more comfortable. It is also carries a risk of ulceration and infection of the cervix if left in place for too long. However, the cap is only for use in women with normal cervical cytology due to concern of traumatizing the cervix. Spermicides include gels, foams, suppositories, and jellies placed in the vagina. The active agent is nonoxynol-9 which disrupts the sperm cell membrane and provides a mechanical barrier. The contraceptive *sponge* is made of polyurethane impregnated with 1 mg of nonoxynol-9 and does not have to be inserted into the vagina before each act of intercourse. Its use is associated with lower pregnancy rate in nulliparous women compared to parous women. Advantages of barrier methods include low cost, decreased transmission of certain sexually transmitted diseases, and no requirement for continuous hormonal exposure or ongoing IUD use due to use only at time of coitus. Disadvantages include relatively high failure rate due to required use with each act of intercourse.

Oral contraceptives were initially marketed in the United States in 1960. These quickly became the most-used method of reversible contraception among women. Oral steroid contraceptives come in combination pills at a fixed dose or a phased dose, or a progestin-only pill (minipill). The main effect of the progestin is to inhibit ovulation and cause cervical mucus thickening. The main effect of the estrogen is to maintain the endometrium, prevent unscheduled bleeding, and inhibit follicular development. The most common side effects are relatively mild and include nausea, breast tenderness, fluid retention, or weight gain.

The **main risks of combined hormonal contraception** are due to the estrogen component and include **venous thromboembolism, strokes** in patients with migraines with aura, **myocardial infarction** in women smokers age 35 and older, increased risk of **cholelithiasis**, and **benign hepatic tumors**. Use of oral contraceptives decreases the risk of developing ovarian or endometrial cancer, shortens the duration of menses, decreases blood loss during menses, improves pain from dysmenorrhea and endometriosis, decreases dysfunctional uterine bleeding and menorrhagia, and improves acne.

The World Health Organization contraindications to combined hormonal contraceptives include known thrombogenic mutations, prior thromboembolic event, cerebrovascular or coronary artery disease (current or remote), uncontrolled hypertension, migraines with aura, diabetes with peripheral vascular disease, smoking and age 35 years or older, known or suspected breast cancer, history of, or known or suspected, estrogen-dependent neoplasia, undiagnosed abnormal genital bleeding, benign or malignant liver tumors, active liver disease, liver failure, known or suspected pregnancy.

The **contraceptive patch** delivers norelgestromin and ethinyl estradiol transdermally. It is worn on the buttocks, upper outer arm, lower abdomen, or upper torso excluding the breast. It is changed weekly for 3 weeks followed by a week without a patch to allow for withdrawal bleed. In women weighing greater than 90 kg, efficacy may be less. A recent FDA warning indicated the risk of DVT was twice that of OCP. The **contraceptive ring** allows steroids to be absorbed through the vaginal epithelium into circulation. The ring is worn for 21 days and then removed for 7 days to allow for withdrawal bleed. The patch and ring have similar efficacy and side effects to combination oral contraceptives.

Only one **injectable contraceptive** is currently available in the United States, depomedroxyprogesterone acetate (DMPA). It is administered subcutaneously every 3 months. Women receiving the injection have a very low pregnancy rate. There is a significant disruption of the normal menstrual cycle that usually leads to amenorrhea.

A single subdermal **implant**, placed in a woman's upper arm, releases a steady amount of levonorgestrel. The duration of action for this implant, named Implanon, is 3 years. Return to fertility is delayed about 2 weeks after cessation of pills, patches, or rings, and by about 4 weeks after stopping contraceptive injection. Post-pill amenorrhea may persist for up to 6 months.

An **intrauterine contraceptive device (IUD)** is a small device, usually plastic with or without copper or a progestin, placed in the endometrial cavity as a method of contraception. Two IUDs are currently available in the United States: the copper T380A and the levonorgestrel-releasing intrauterine device. The copper T380A has approved use for 10 years and has a 10-year cumulative pregnancy rate comparable to that of sterilization. Many mechanisms of action have been described for the copper-containing IUD, including inhibition of sperm migration and viability, change in transport speed of the ovum, and damage to or destruction of the ovum.

The **levonorgestrel-releasing intrauterine device** releases 20 μg of levonorgestrel daily and is approved for use for 5 years. It works by thickening the cervical mucus and creating an atrophic endometrium. The small amount of steroid causes minimal amounts of systemic side effects, and it also decreases menstrual bleeding due to the local effect on the endometrium. The levonorgestrel-releasing IUD also has noncontraceptive benefits and can be used to treat patients with menorrhagia, dysmenorrhea, and pain due to endometriosis and adenomyosis.

IUDs are most appropriate for women who are in stable, mutually monogamous relationships at low risk for sexually transmitted infections. Both IUDs have the advantage of requiring a single act of motivation for long-term use. The efficacy is 0.5% to 0.1%. They also have rapid return to fertility after removal of the device. Insertion has an infrequent association with uterine perforation (1:1000) and transiently increases the risk of upper genital infection (1:1000) due to endometrial contamination.

WHO contraindications to IUD insertion include current pregnancy, current sexually transmitted infection, current or pelvic inflammatory disease

within the past 3 months, unexplained vaginal bleeding, malignant gestational trophoblastic disease, untreated cervical cancer, untreated endometrial
cancer, uterine fibroids distorting the endometrial cavity, current breast cancer (for levonorgestrel-releasing IUD only), anatomical abnormalities distorting the uterine cavity, known pelvic tuberculosis, and allergy to component
of IUD or Wilson disease (for copper-containing IUD).

Emergency contraception is the therapy for women who have had unprotected sexual intercourse, including victims of sexual assault. It is also known
as the "morning after pill." The two most common regimens are the combination oral contraceptive method, known as the Yuzpe method, and the
progestin-only regimen. The Yuzpe method consists of 0.1 mg of ethinyl estradiol and 0.5 mg of levonorgestrel in two doses, 12 hours apart, beginning
within 72 hours of unprotected intercourse. The progestin-only (plan B)
method consists of 0.75 mg of levonorgestrel in two doses taken 12 hours
apart. The mechanisms of action may include inhibition of ovulation, decreased
tubal motility, and, possibly, interruption of implantation.

The efficacy of the combination method is accepted to be about a 75%
reduction in pregnancy rate, thus decreasing the risk of a midcycle coital pregnancy from 8 per 100 to about 2 per 100. The progestin-only method appears
to have slightly greater efficacy, with a pregnancy risk reduction of about 85%.

The major side effect of emergency contraception is nausea and/or emesis,
which is more prominent with the combination method. An antiemetic is
often prescribed with the Yuzpe regimen. Emergency contraception should
not be used in patients with a suspected or known pregnancy, or those with
abnormal vaginal bleeding. Those women who do not have onset on menses
within 21 days following the emergency contraception should have a pregnancy test.

The IUD can be inserted up to 5 days after unprotected intercourse for
emergency contraception. Women who receive the IUD under emergency
conditions often choose to maintain the IUD for contraception.

Comprehension Questions

33.1   A 17-year-old G0 P0 woman is noted to desire a reversible form of
        contraception. After reviewing the various options, she chooses depot
        medroxyprogesterone acetate. Which of the following tests is most
        likely to be abnormal after 2 years of use?
        A. Dual energy x-ray absorptiometry (DEXA) scan
        B. Serum glucose level
        C. Serum creatinine level
        D. Ultrasound of the gall bladder

33.2   Which of the following patients can safely receive combination oral contraceptive pills?
        A. 35-year-old female with diabetes with peripheral circulatory problems
        B. 37-year-old female who smokes cigarettes
        C. 25-year-old female with persistent tension headaches
        D. 30 year old whose blood pressure is 160/90 mm Hg

33.3   A 28-year-old G1 P1 woman is noted to have been prescribed an oral contraceptive agent. She was counseled about some risks, but also some benefits. Which of the following is a benefit of combination oral contraception?
        A. Decreased risk of breast cancer
        B. Decreased gallstone formation
        C. Decreased deep venous thrombosis risk
        D. Decreased benign breast masses

33.4   A 28-year-old patient experienced an episode of unprotected intercourse. Her last menstrual period was about 2 weeks previously. She receives combination oral contraceptive agent emergency contraception. Which of the following is the most common side effect of the Yuzpe regimen (combination OC)?
        A. Vaginal spotting
        B. Nausea and/or vomiting
        C. Elevation of liver function enzymes
        D. Glucose intolerance
        E. Renal insufficiency

33.5   A 25-year-old nulliparous woman is being evaluated for possible IUD insertion. Which of the following characteristics is most acceptable for IUD use?
        A. Current sexually transmitted disease
        B. Nulliparity
        C. Recent pelvic inflammatory disease
        D. Enlarged uterus with an irregular cavity

33.6   A 29-year-old G1 P1 woman requests emergency contraception for unprotected intercourse. She is given choices between the progestin-only (plan B) regimen versus the Yuzpe (combination OC) regimen. Which of the following is the main effect of the progestin-only regimen as compared with the Yuzpe regimen in EC?
        A. Higher ectopic pregnancy rate
        B. Less effective prevention of pregnancy
        C. Less nausea
        D. More liver dysfunction

ANSWERS

33.1   **A.** Depot medroxyprogesterone acetate is associated with loss of bone mineral density particularly in adolescents. If it is the best type of contraception for the patient, then the loss in bone mineral density should not discourage the use of the agent, but it should be considered in the choice of the contraception agent.

33.2   **C.** Tension headaches are not a contraindication for oral contraceptive agents. Migraines with aura increase the risk of strokes in patient who take combination hormonal contraception. Other contraindications to combination hormonal contraception include diabetes with vascular disease, smoker over the age of 35, and uncontrolled hypertension.

33.3   **D.** Oral contraceptives have many beneficial effects including decreasing the risk of endometrial and ovarian cancer, decreasing the risk of benign breast disease; there may be a slightly increased risk of breast cancer. Gallstones incidence may also be slightly increased.

33.4   **B.** Because of the high dose of estrogens, nausea and vomiting are the most common side effects.

33.5   **B.** Nulliparity is not a contraindication to IUD insertion. Contraindications include pregnancy, current or recent history of pelvic inflammatory disease, current sexually transmitted disease, current or recent puerperal or postabortion sepsis, purulent cervicitis, undiagnosed abnormal vaginal bleeding, malignancy of the genital tract, known uterine anomalies or fibroids distorting the uterine cavity in a way incompatible with IUD insertion, or allergy to any component of the IUD or Wilson disease.

33.6   **C.** As compared to the combination OC regimen, the progestin-only method has better efficacy and fewer side effects (nausea). Thus, it is the preferred method. Patients who are given the combination OC agents usually require an antiemetic agent.

Clinical Pearls

➤ Emergency contraception is effective when initiated within 72 hours of intercourse.

➤ Emergency contraception consists of high-dose combination hormones, high-dose progestin, or insertion of an IUD.

➤ The main side effects of combination hormonal emergency contraception therapy are nausea and vomiting.

➤ An advantage of IUD insertion is that it can be retained for continued long-term contraception.

➤ The levonorgestrel-releasing IUD can be used to improve bleeding profiles in patients with dysfunctional uterine bleeding and menorrhagia.

➤ Nonuser-dependent methods like the IUD, DMPA, and the subdermal implant, have the lowest failure rates.

➤ Oral contraceptives decrease the risk of ovarian and endometrial cancer; there may be a slightly increased risk of breast cancer. It decreases the duration of menses and the amount of blood loss per cycle.

➤ Smoking over the age of 35 years is an absolute contraindication for combination oral contraceptives.

➤ Sickle cell crises and epilepsy occur less often with IMPA.

➤ The contraceptive patch may be associated with a greater risk of DVT.

REFERENCES

American College of Obstetricians and Gynecologists. Emergency contraception. *ACOG Practice Bulletin 69*. Washington, DC: American College of Obstetricians and Gynecologists; 2005.

American College of Obstetricians and Gynecologists. Intrauterine device. ACOG *Practice Bulletin 59*. Washington, DC: American College of Obstetricians and Gynecologists; 2005.

American College of Obstetricians and Gynecologists. Intrauterine device and adolescents. ACOG *Committee Opinion 392*. Washington, DC: 2007.

American College of Obstetricians and Gynecologists. Use of hormonal contraception in women with coexisting medical conditions. ACOG *Practice Bulletin 73*. Washington, DC: 2006.

Mishell DR, Jr. Family planning. In: Katz VL, Lentz GM, Lobo RA, Gershenson DM, eds. *Comprehensive Gynecology*. 5th ed. Philadelphia, PA: Mosby Elsevier; 2007: 275-325.

Nelson AL. Family planning: reversible contraception, sterilization, and abortion. In: Hacker NF, Gambone JC, Hobel CJ, eds. *Essentials of Obstetrics and Gynecology*, 5th ed. Philadelphia, PA: Saunders; 2009:304-314.

Case 34

A 20-year-old G1 P0 woman at 29 weeks' gestation is hospitalized for acute pyelonephritis. She has no history of pyelonephritis in the past. She has been receiving intravenous ampicillin and gentamicin for 48 hours. She complains of acute shortness of breath. On examination, her heart rate (HR) is 100 beats per minute (bpm), respiratory rate (RR) 45 beats per minute and labored, and blood pressure (BP) is 120/70 mm Hg. Right costovertebral angle tenderness is noted. Her abdominal examination reveals no masses or tenderness. The fetal heart tones are in the 140 to 150 bpm range. The urine culture revealed *Escherichia coli* sensitive to ampicillin.

➤ What is the most likely diagnosis?

ANSWER TO CASE 34:
Pyelonephritis, Unresponsive

Summary: A 20-year-old G1 P0 woman at 29 weeks' gestation has received intravenous ampicillin and gentamicin for 48 hours for acute pyelonephritis. She complains of acute shortness of breath. On examination, her HR is 100 bpm, RR 45 breaths per minute, and BP is 120/70. Right costovertebral angle tenderness is noted. The urine culture revealed *E coli* sensitive to ampicillin.

➤ **Most likely diagnosis:** Acute respiratory distress syndrome (ARDS).

ANALYSIS

Objectives

1. Understand the clinical presentation of pyelonephritis.
2. Know that the primary treatment of pyelonephritis is intravenous antibiotic therapy.
3. Understand that endotoxins can cause pulmonary damage, leading to acute respiratory distress syndrome (ARDS).

Considerations

This patient is 20 years old at 29 weeks' gestation. She presented with pyelonephritis. She had been treated with intravenous ampicillin and gentamicin. The diagnosis is confirmed since *E coli* has been cultured from the urine. She is now presenting with dyspnea and tachypnea. The most likely etiology for her respiratory symptoms is ARDS, with pulmonary injury due to the endotoxin release. This typically occurs after antibiotics have begun to lyse the bacteria, leading to endotoxemia. The endotoxins can induce damage to the myocardium, liver, and kidneys, as well as the lungs. The mechanism is leaky capillaries, which allows fluid from the intravascular space to permeate into the alveolar areas. A chest film may show patchy infiltrates; however, if the disease process is early, the chest radiograph may be normal. Treatment would include oxygen supplementation, careful monitoring of fluids (not to overload), and supportive measures. Occasionally, a patient may require intubation, but usually the condition stabilizes and improves.

APPROACH TO
Pyelonephritis in Pregnancy

DEFINITIONS

PYELONEPHRITIS: Kidney parenchymal infection most commonly caused by gram-negative aerobic bacteria, such as *E coli*.

ENDOTOXIN: A lipopolysaccharide that is released upon lysis of the cell wall of bacteria, especially gram-negative bacteria.

ACUTE RESPIRATORY DISTRESS SYNDROME (ARDS): Alveolar and endothelial injury leading to leaky pulmonary capillaries, clinically causing hypoxemia, large alveolar-arterial gradient, and loss of lung volume.

CLINICAL APPROACH

Pyelonephritis in pregnancy can be a very serious medical condition, with an incidence of 1% to 2% of all pregnancies. It is the most common cause of sepsis in pregnant women. The patient generally complains of dysuria, urgency, frequency, costovertebral tenderness, fever and chills, and nausea and vomiting. The urinalysis usually will reveal pyuria and bacteriuria; a urine culture revealing greater than 100,000 colony-forming units/mL of a single uropathogen is diagnostic. The most common organism is *E coli*, seen in about 80% of cases. *Klebsiella pneumoniae*, *Staphylococcus aureus*, and *Proteus mirabilis* may also be isolated.

Pregnant women with acute pyelonephritis should be hospitalized and given intravenous antibiotics. Cephalosporins, such as cefotetan or ceftriaxone, or the combination of ampicillin and gentamicin are usually effective. The patient should be treated until the fever and flank tenderness have substantially improved and then switched to oral antimicrobial therapy, and then suppressive therapy for the remainder of the pregnancy. Up to one-third of pregnant women with pyelonephritis will develop a recurrent UTI if suppressive therapy is not utilized. A repeat urine culture should be obtained to ensure eradication of the infection. **If clinical improvement has not occurred after 48 to 72 hours of appropriate antibiotic therapy, a urinary tract obstruction (ie, ureterolithiasis) or a perinephric abscess should be suspected.**

Approximately 2% to 5% of pregnant women with pyelonephritis will develop acute respiratory distress syndrome (ARDS), which is defined as pulmonary injury due to sepsis, usually endotoxin related. The endotoxins derived from the gram-negative bacterial cell wall enter the blood stream, especially after antibiotic therapy, and may induce transient elevation of the serum creatinine as well as liver enzymes. Also, the endotoxemia may cause uterine contractions and place a patient into preterm labor. Diffuse bilateral or interstitial infiltrates are typically seen on chest radiograph (Figure 34–1).

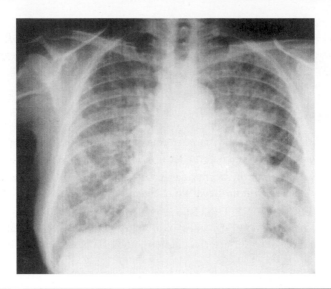

Figure 34–1.   Acute respiratory distress syndrome. Chest radiograph depicts acute respiratory distress syndrome with diffuse pulmonary infiltrates. *Reproduced with permission from Kasper DL, et al.* Harrison's Principles of Internal Medicine. *16th ed. New York, NY: McGraw-Hill; 2005:1593.*

The treatment of ARDS is supportive, with priorities on oxygenation and careful fluid management. In severe cases, mechanical ventilation may be required to maintain adequate oxygen levels.

Comprehension Questions

34.1   A 36-year-old G1 P0 woman at 27 weeks' gestation is noted to have fever, right flank tenderness, and pyuria. She is diagnosed with pyelonephritis. A urine culture is performed. Which of the following is the most commonly isolated etiologic agent causing pyelonephritis in pregnancy?

A. Proteus species
B. Candidal species
C. *Escherichia coli*
D. Klebsiella species

34.2   A 21-year-old G1 P0 woman at 15 weeks' gestation is noted to have
        fever of 101°F (38.3°C), BP of 80/40 mm Hg, and decreased urine out-
        put. She is noted to be in septic shock. Which of the following is the
        most common cause of septic shock in pregnancy?
        A. Pelvic inflammatory disease
        B. Pyelonephritis
        C. Wound infection
        D. Mastitis

34.3   When a pregnant woman with pyelonephritis does not improve on
        adequate antibiotic therapy for 48 hours and experiences continued
        severe flank tenderness and fever, which of the following should be
        next considered?
        A. Obstruction of the urinary tract, such as by nephrolithiasis
        B. Anaerobic organisms
        C. Hemolytic uremic syndrome
        D. Factitious fever

34.4   Asymptomatic bacteriuria is best identified by which of the following?
        A. Careful questioning for dysuria or urinary frequency
        B. Urine culture on the first prenatal visit
        C. Urine culture at 35 weeks' gestation
        D. Urinalysis for any patient with family history of UTI

ANSWERS

34.1   **C.** *Escherichia coli* is the most commonly isolated bacteria in pyelonephri-
        tis. *Proteus* and *Klebsiella* may also be found, but they are not the most
        common. Pregnant women with acute pyelonephritis should be hospital-
        ized and given IV hydration and antibiotics. Cephalosporins, or the com-
        bination of ampicillin and gentamicin, are usually effective. The patient
        should be treated with IV medicines until the fever and flank pain
        resolve, and then switched to oral medication for the remainder of the
        pregnancy. *Candida* species are more often associated with vaginitis and
        not an infection associated with the urinary tract or kidneys.   LPS.

34.2   **B.** Pyelonephritis is the most common cause of septic shock in preg-
        nancy. Endotoxins derived from the gram-negative bacterial cell wall
        enter the bloodstream, especially after antibiotic therapy, and may
        induce transient elevation of serum creatinine as well as liver enzyme
        levels. The endotoxemia may cause uterine contractions and place a
        patient into preterm labor. Another complication that may arise is the
        development of ARDS, pulmonary injury due to sepsis. Mastitis typi-
        cally occurs postpartum and, though rare, if left untreated can lead to
        abscess formation or sepsis. The agent most commonly responsible for
        mastitis is *S aureus*, typically acquired from the back of the baby's
        throat during breast-feeding. An unattended wound infection can lead

to postpartum sepsis as well; especially after cesarean delivery. Pelvic inflammatory disease typically does not lead to sepsis; however, if a tubo-ovarian abscess forms and then ruptures, the patient is likely to go into septic shock. This is a surgical emergency that could be fatal.

34.3   **A.** Urinary obstruction, such as with a stone, should be considered with continued fever and flank tenderness after a 48- to 72-hour course of appropriate antibiotic therapy. Pyelonephritis is typically caused by **aerobic** bacteria such as *E coli, Kebsiella, Proteus, and Staphylococcus aureus.* Hemolytic uremic syndrome (HUS) is a disease characterized by hemolytic anemia, acute renal failure (uremia), and thrombocytopenia, but is not associated with pyelonephritis; however, like pyelonephritis, its etiology is usually due to *E coli* (in HUS, a strain of *E coli* that expresses a Shiga-like toxin). Patients typically present with bloody diarrhea rather than fever and flank pain. Factitious fever is also not associated with pyelonephritis, since the fever associated with this infection is legitimate.

34.4   **B.** Urine culture for every patient at the first prenatal visit helps to identify asymptomatic bacteriuria. Treatment prevents sequelae such as preterm labor and pyelonephritis during pregnancy. Careful questioning would not be of much use since the bacteriuria is asymptomatic. A urine culture at 35 weeks would not be helpful either; by this point, the asymptomatic bacteria may have already led to unfavorable consequences such as preterm labor or pyelonephritis. It is cost-effective and a good practice of preventative medicine for patients to get a urinalysis at every prenatal visit, regardless of family history which does not affect the likelihood of having bacteriuria.

Clinical Pearls

➤ The most common cause of septic shock in pregnancy is pyelonephritis.
➤ When dyspnea occurs in a pregnant woman who is being treated for pyelonephritis, ARDS should be considered.
➤ Endotoxin release from gram-negative bacteria is the cause of acute respiratory distress syndrome associated with pyelonephritis.

REFERENCES

Castro LC, Ognyemi D. Common medical and surgical conditions complicating pregnancy. In: Hacker NF, Gambone JC, Hobel CJ, eds. *Essentials of Obstetrics and Gynecology,* 5th ed. Philadelphia, PA: Saunders; 2009:191-218.
Cunningham FG, Leveno KJ, Bloom SL, Hauth JC, Gilstrap LC III, Wenstrom KD. Renal and urinary tract disorders. In: *Williams Obstetrics.* 22nd ed. New York, NY: McGraw-Hill; 2005:1255-1258.

Case 35

A 31-year-old G1 P0 woman at 24 weeks' gestation complains of a 2-day history of soreness of the right calf. She states that she has been walking slightly more over the past several days. She denies a history of medical illnesses or trauma to her legs. Her family history is unremarkable. On examination, her blood pressure (BP) is 100/60 mm Hg, heart rate (HR) 100 beats per minute (bpm), respiratory rate (RR) 12 breaths per minute, and she is afebrile. The neck is supple. Her heart and lung examinations are normal. The abdomen is nontender and without masses. The fundal height is 23 cm and the fetal heart tones are in the range of 140 to 150 bpm. The right calf is somewhat tender and slightly swollen. No palpable cords are present. The Homans sign is negative.

➤ What is your next step?

ANSWER TO CASE 35:

Deep Venous Thrombosis in Pregnancy

Summary: A 31-year-old G1 P0 woman at 24 weeks' gestation, who has been walking slightly more than usual, complains of a 2-day history of right calf soreness. On examination, her HR is 100 bpm and RR 12 breaths per minute. Her heart and lung examinations are normal. The right calf is somewhat tender and slightly swollen. No palpable cords are present, and the Homans sign is negative.

> ➤ **Next step:** Noninvasive assessment for a deep venous thrombosis of the right leg.

ANALYSIS

Objectives

1. Know that pregnancy is a hypercoagulable state and predisposes to thrombosis.
2. Know that the physical examination is not an accurate method to diagnose deep venous thrombosis.
3. Know the diagnostic and therapeutic measures for deep venous thrombosis.

Considerations

This 31-year-old woman at 24 weeks' gestation has been walking slightly more than usual and complains of calf tenderness. The right calf is mildly tender and swollen. These subtle findings are sufficient to warrant investigations for a deep venous thrombosis. Because of the increased levels of clotting factors (predominantly fibrinogen) and the venous stasis, pregnancy produces a hypercoagulable state. The physical examination is not very sensitive or specific in the assessment of deep venous thrombosis (DVT). The Homans sign, that is, dorsiflexion of the foot to attempt to elicit tenderness in the patient is a poor test, and theoretically may itself cause embolization of clots. For these reasons, many experts advise against the performance of this test. Instead, a noninvasive test, such as Doppler flow studies of the venous system of the affected lower extremity, is an appropriate method to assess for deep venous thrombosis. If the Doppler flow test confirms a thrombosis, anticoagulation with an agent such as heparin should be initiated. In a nonpregnant woman, venography would be an option, that is, injecting radiopaque dye into a vein of the foot and taking radiographic images of the venous system.

APPROACH TO
Deep Venous Thrombosis in Pregnancy

DEFINITIONS

DEEP VENOUS THROMBOSIS: Deposit of a thrombus, platelet, and fibrin in the deep veins usually of the lower extremity or pelvis.

DUPLEX ULTRASOUND FLOW STUDY: Ultrasound technique using both real-time sonography and Doppler flow to assess for deep venous thrombosis.

PULMONARY EMBOLISM: When a fragment of the thrombus is dislodged and migrates into the pulmonary arterial circulation.

CLINICAL APPROACH

Deep venous thrombosis occurs in slightly less than 1% of pregnancies. The pregnant state increases the risk fivefold due to the venous stasis with the large gravid uterus pressing on the vena cava and the hypercoagulable state due to the increase in clotting factors. Cesarean delivery further increases the risk of DVT. Whereas clots involving the superficial venous system pose virtually no danger and may be treated with analgesia, deep venous thrombosis is associated with pulmonary embolism in 40% of untreated cases. The risk of death is increased tenfold when pulmonary embolism is unrecognized and untreated. Therefore, early diagnosis and anticoagulation treatment are crucial.

Signs and symptoms of DVT include "muscle pain," deep linear cords of the calf, and tenderness and swelling of the lower extremity. A 2-cm difference in leg circumferences is also sometimes helpful. Unfortunately, none of these findings are very specific for DVT, and in fact, the examination is normal in half of the cases of DVT. Hence, imaging tests are necessary for confirmation.

In pregnancy, the diagnostic test of choice is Doppler ultrasound imaging, which usually employs a 5 to 7.5 MHz Doppler transducer to measure venous blood flow with and without compression of the deep veins. This modality is nearly as sensitive and specific as the time-honored method of contrast venography.

Management of deep venous thrombosis is primarily anticoagulation with bed rest and extremity elevation. During pregnancy, heparin is usually preferable over Coumadin, since Coumadin may cause congenital abnormalities and is more difficult to reverse. Heparin, which is a potent thrombin inhibitor that blocks conversion of fibrinogen to fibrin, combines with antithrombin III. It stabilizes the clot and inhibits its propagation. After full intravenous anticoagulation therapy for 5 to 7 days, the therapy is generally switched to subcutaneous therapy to maintain the aPTT at 1.5 to 2.5 times control for at least 3 months after the acute event. After 3 months, either full heparinization or "prophylactic heparinization" can be utilized for the remainder of the pregnancy and for 6 weeks postpartum (see Case 22).

Comprehension Questions

35.1   A 27-year-old G1 P1 woman underwent a normal vaginal delivery 10 days previously. She is seen by her physician for right leg pain and calf tenderness. A Doppler flow study indicates a deep venous thrombosis of the right lower extremity. Which of the following is a reason for the hypercoagulable state in pregnancy or the postpartum stage?

       A. Venous stasis
       B. Deceased clotting factors levels
       C. Elevated platelet count
       D. Endothelial damage

35.2   A 38-year-old G2 P1 woman had been diagnosed with a deep venous thrombosis of the right leg when she was at 8 weeks' gestational age. She has been on subcutaneous heparin therapy for 6 months. Which of the following is the most likely result of long-term heparin therapy?

       A. Osteoporosis
       B. Thrombophilia
       C. Fetal intracranial hemorrhage
       D. Diabetes mellitus

35.3   A 28-year-old woman underwent a total abdominal hysterectomy for uterine fibroids. She is diagnosed with a deep venous thrombosis. Which of the following is the most common location of a deep venous thrombosis?

       A. Inferior vena cava
       B. Lower extremities
       C. Ovarian vein
       D. Superior vena cava
       E. Subclavian vein

35.4   A 30-year-old G1 P0 woman at 20 weeks' gestation is diagnosed with a deep venous thrombosis. Which of the following agents is most likely to be contraindicated?

       A. Medroxyprogesterone acetate depot (Depo-Provera) contraception
       B. Intrauterine contraceptive device (IUD)
       C. Combination oral contraceptive
       D. Levonorgestrel silastic implants (Norplant)
       E. Prostaglandin compounds

ANSWERS

35.1   **A.** Venous stasis is one of the main factors contributing to the hyper-coagulable state in pregnancy. Venous stasis is present due to the uterus compressing the vena cava. Usually, the platelet count is slightly lower in the pregnant state. The lower limit of normal is 150,000/mm³ in the nonpregnant patient and 120,000/mm³ in the pregnant woman. There is an increased level of clotting factors in pregnancy, and this along with venous stasis are the two factors that increase the risk of DVT in a pregnant woman fivefold. Endothelial damage is associated with the development of hypertension and not a hypercoagulable state in pregnancy.

35.2   **A.** Heparin is a large, charged glycoprotein that does not cross the placenta very well; therefore, it is safer to use during pregnancy instead of Coumadin, which may lead to congenital abnormalities and is more difficult to reverse. Osteoporosis (anticoagulants have a propensity to inhibit vitamin K, which is involved in bone metabolism) and throm-bocytopenia (not thrombophilia) are long-term complications of heparin use. Heparin is not known to cause diabetes mellitus.

35.3   **B.** The most common locations of DVT associated with gynecologic surgery are the lower extremities and the pelvic veins. The **Virchow triad** (ie, stasis, hypercoagulability, intimal injury) is a model used to explain the increased risk of developing a DVT during the periopera-tive period. The patient is usually left in a supine position during this period; this, along with the vasodilating effects of the anesthesia con-tributes to the **"stasis"** component of the triad. Because the body rec-ognizes blood loss during a surgery, patients typically tend to become **hypercoagulable** as well since an increased number of clotting factors are produced in an attempt to stop the bleeding from surgery. **Vascular wall injury** can occur from the excessive vasodilation caused by the anesthesia, and any injury to blood vessels leads to an accumulation of clotting factors at the site of injury. Also, the longer the surgery, the higher the risk of developing a DVT. The lower extremities and pelvic veins are at an increased susceptibility to DVTs due to the increased diameter of the veins and more "sluggish" flow of blood in this region.

35.4   **C.** The estrogen in the combination oral contraceptive is slightly thrombogenic and may be contraindicated in a woman with a prior DVT. All of the other answer choices are progestin-only methods of contraception, and progesterone is not considered thrombogenic. Progestin-only contraception is contraindicated in women with unex-plained uterine bleeding. Reason being, progestin-only methods are associated with irregular uterine bleeding which consists of amenor-rhea, breakthrough bleeding, irregular spotting, and prolonged periods of amenorrhea or menorrhagia. This would make a pathological diag-nosis more obscure.

Clinical Pearls

➤ The physical examination is not very useful in assessing for deep venous thrombosis.

➤ Venous duplex Doppler sonography is an accurate method to diagnose deep venous thrombosis.

➤ After a deep venous thrombosis or pulmonary embolus is diagnosed, anticoagulation is indicated.

➤ The most common locations for deep venous thrombosis after gynecologic surgery are the lower extremities and the pelvic veins.

REFERENCES

American College of Obstetricians and Gynecologists. Thromboembolism in pregnancy. *Practice Bulletin No. 19*. August 2000.

Castro LC, Ognyemi D. Common medical and surgical conditions complicating pregnancy. In: Hacker NF, Gambone JC, Hobel CJ, eds. *Essentials of Obstetrics and Gynecology*, 5th ed. Philadelphia, PA: Saunders; 2009:191-218.

Cunningham FG, Leveno KJ, Bloom SL, Hauth JC, Gilstrap LC III, Wenstrom KD. Pulmonary disorders. In: *Williams Obstetrics*. 22nd ed. New York, NY: McGraw-Hill; 2005:1055-1070.

Case 36

A 50-year-old G4 P4 woman comes in for a well-woman examination. She had used the contraceptive diaphragm for birth control until she went into menopause 1 year ago. Her family history is unremarkable for cancer. Her surgical history includes a myomectomy for symptomatic uterine fibroids 10 years ago. On examination, her blood pressure (BP) is 120/74 mm Hg, heart rate (HR) 80 beats per minute (bpm), and she is afebrile. Her thyroid is normal on palpation. Her heart and lung examinations are normal. The breast examination shows a 1.5-cm, mobile, nontender mass of the upper outer quadrant of the right breast. No adenopathy or skin changes are appreciated. Mammography and ultrasound examinations of the breasts are normal.

➤ What is your next step?

Choice of Bx type.

ANSWER TO CASE 36:
Dominant Breast Mass

Summary: A 50-year-old postmenopausal woman comes in for a well-woman examination. The breast examination shows a 1.5-cm, mobile, nontender mass of the upper outer quadrant of the right breast. No adenopathy or skin changes are appreciated. Mammography and ultrasound examinations of the breasts are normal.

➤ **Next step:** Excisional biopsy of the breast mass, or stereotactic core needle biopsy.

ANALYSIS

Objectives

1. Understand that any three-dimensional dominant breast mass requires tissue for histologic analysis.
2. Understand that the age of the patient is usually the biggest risk factor for breast cancer.
3. Understand that normal imaging of a palpable breast mass does not rule out cancer.

Considerations

This 50-year-old woman came in for a well-woman examination. The physical examination is aimed at screening for common and/or serious conditions, such as hypertension, thyroid disease, cervical cancer (Pap smear), colon cancer (stool for occult blood), and breast cancer. A single 1.5-cm breast mass is palpated, but there are no associated skin changes, such as nipple retraction or dimpling of the skin. There is no associated adenopathy. Furthermore, the imaging tests (mammography and ultrasonography) are normal. Despite the normal imaging, there is a possibility that the breast mass is malignant. Therefore, biopsy of the mass is indicated. Because of the patient's age, removal of the entire mass (excisional biopsy) is preferable over fine needle aspiration. Fine needle aspiration may miss a malignancy, and at this patient's age, leaving a mass in the breast would make future examinations more difficult.

dominant 3d mass ⇒ excisional Bx.
> 35 yo

< 35 ⇒ FNA,
core Bx

APPROACH TO
Breast Masses

DEFINITIONS

DOMINANT BREAST MASS: A three-dimensional mass that, on palpation, is felt to be separate from the remainder of the breast tissue.

EXCISIONAL BIOPSY: Surgical procedure removing the entire mass.

SKIN DIMPLING: Retraction of the skin, which is suspicious for an underlying malignancy, due to the cancer being fixed to the skin.

BRCA GENE MUTATIONS: BRCA1 gene is located on chromosome 17 and BRCA2 gene is located on chromosome 13. These are tumor suppressor genes, such that a mutation in the gene confers a markedly increased risk of breast cancer and ovarian cancer.

CLINICAL APPROACH

Breast cancer is the most common cancer in women. It is the second leading cause of female cancer deaths, exceeded only by lung cancer. The prevalence of breast cancer is age specific and **age is the most important risk factor.** One in 2500 women will develop breast cancer at the age of 20 years; whereas 1 in 30 women will develop breast cancer at the age of 60 years, giving an overall lifetime risk of 1 in 8. Other risk factors include a family history of mammary cancer, especially of premenopausal onset.

Early diagnosis improves survival. The most common way that breast cancer is first discovered is a mass palpated by the patient. Unfortunately, this frequently occurs at an advanced stage. Routine screening is preferable. Monthly self-breast examination and clinical breast examination every 3 years should be performed for women from ages 20 to 39 years. Women over the age of 40 years should perform a monthly self-breast examination, and have a yearly clinical breast examination; some experts advocate mammography every 2 years between the ages of 40 to 49 years. Annual mammography should be initiated at age 50 years, but may be performed sooner if risk factors warrant the need.

Mammograms carry a false-negative rate of up to 10%. Thus, **any palpable dominant mass, regardless of mammographic findings, requires histologic diagnosis.** The type of biopsy will vary depending on the risk of cancer. For example, a young woman with a clinical examination consistent with a fibroadenoma may have a fine needle aspiration; in contrast, a woman aged 50 years, at greater risk for malignancy due to age, will usually have an excisional biopsy. The greater the risk for cancer, the more the tissue that should be sampled.

If a mammogram detects a suspicious lesion, a biopsy is usually performed. For nonpalpable lesions, the biopsy requires needle-localization excisional biopsy or stereotactic core needle biopsy.

A patient who has two first-degree relatives with breast cancer is a candidate for genetic testing, such as BRCA1 and BRCA2 testing. Patients of Ashkenazi Jewish ancestry are specially of increased risk. A mutation of the BRCA1 gene is associated with a 50% to 70% risk of breast cancer, and a 30% risk of ovarian cancer. The risks with BRCA2 are slightly lower. Identification of these risks also allow for risk reduction medications and possibly surgery such as bilateral mastectomy or prophylactic oophorectomy after child-bearing.

Comprehension Questions

36.1   A 36-year-old woman is noted to have a 2-cm palpable breast mass noted on physical examination. A mammogram is performed suggestive of a cyst. Ultrasound confirms a cystic mass. A fine needle aspiration is performed with 8 cc of blood-colored fluid obtained. The mass is no longer palpable. Which of the following is the next best step for this patient?

   A. Expectant management as the prognosis is excellent
   B. Send the fluid for cytology
   C. Lumpectomy and lymph node dissection
   D. Tamoxifen therapy

36.2   A 26-year-old woman is referred to genetic counseling for her mother who died from breast cancer, and her sister with breast cancer. The patient is noted to have a BRCA1 mutation. Which of the following best describes the genetic transmission of this disorder?

   A. Autosomal dominant
   B. Autosomal recessive
   C. X-linked dominant
   D. X-linked recessive

36.3   A 49-year-old woman is noted to have a 1.5 cm mass of the right breast. It is nontender and there are no skin changes or adenopathy. The mammogram is negative, and the ultrasound likewise is normal. An excisional biopsy reveals an infiltrating intraductal carcinoma. Which of the following would most significantly impact on the patient's prognosis?

   A. Hormone receptor status
   B. Lymph node status
   C. Size of the primary cancer
   D. Presence of skin changes

[handwritten at top of page: aspirate fluid → straw colored → discard; → Bloody Dark → cytology]

ANSWERS

36.1 **B.** When the fluid obtained from a breast cyst is straw-colored and the mass disappears, then the fluid can be discarded and no further therapy is needed. However, when the fluid is a different color such as bloody, then the fluid should be sent for cytology. Lumpectomy and lymph node dissection is performed for proven breast cancer for staging. Tamoxifen therapy is used for postmenopausal women with breast cancer after surgical staging.

36.2 **A.** A mutation to one BRCA gene is associated with an increased risk of breast and ovarian cancer. Thus, this is an autosomal dominant disorder. Half the offsprings would be affected, and both sexes would be equally affected.

36.3 **B.** The patient's lymph node status is the most significant impact on the patient's prognosis. Hormone receptor status does play some role but not as significantly as the lymph node condition. Infiltrating intraductal carcinoma is the most common histological subtype of breast cancer. The size of the primary tumor likewise does play a role. Optimally, the smaller the tumor, the better the survival.

Clinical Pearls

➤ A three-dimensional dominant breast mass must be biopsied, regardless of the imaging results.

➤ Early detection of breast cancer leads to better survival.

➤ In general, the biggest risk factor for the development of breast cancer is age.

➤ Two first-degree family members with breast cancer suggest a familial syndrome, such as mediated by the BRCA1 or BRCA2 gene.

➤ Women at the age of 35 years or greater with a family history of breast cancer should have annual mammography.

➤ The most common cause of unilateral serosanguineous nipple discharge from a single duct is intraductal papilloma.

➤ Infiltrating intraductal carcinoma is the most common histological type of breast cancer.

➤ A breast cyst in which the fluid is straw-colored or clear and the breast mass upon aspiration disappears may be observed.

➤ Upon aspiration of a breast cyst, fluid that is other than straw-colored should be sent for cytology, and a mass that persists after aspiration should be biopsied.

REFERENCES

American College of Obstetricians and Gynecologists. Breast cancer screening. *ACOG Practice Bulletin 42*. April 2003.

American College of Obstetricians and Gynecologists. Elective and risk-reducing salpingo-oophorectomy. *ACOG Practice Bulletin 89*. Washington, DC: 2008.

Balea FA, Katz VL. Breast diseases. In: Katz VL, Lentz GM, Lobo RA, Gersenson DM, eds. *Comprehensive Gynecology*. 5th ed. St. Louis, MO: Mosby-Year Book; 2007:327-355.

Hacker NF, Friedlander ML. Breast disease: a gynecologic perspective. In: Hacker NF, Gambone JC, Hobel CJ, eds. *Essentials of Obstetrics and Gynecology*, 5th ed. Philadelphia, PA: Saunders; 2009:332-344.

Case 37

A 22-year-old parous woman complains of a 3-month history of weight loss, nervousness, palpitations, and sweating. She denies a history of thyroid disease, and is not taking any weight loss medications. She denies abdominal pain, nausea or vomiting, fever, or prior irradiation. On examination, her blood pressure (BP) is 110/60 mm Hg, heart rate (HR) is 110 beats per minute (bpm), and she is afebrile. Her thyroid gland is normal to palpation. She does not have proptosis or lid lag. Her abdomen is nontender and with normal bowel sounds. She is noted to have a fine tremor. Her uterus is normal in size. A mobile, nontender, 9-cm mass is palpated on the right side of the pelvis, which on sonography has the appearance of an adnexal mass with solid and cystic components.

➤ What is the most likely diagnosis?

➤ What is your management of this patient?

ANSWERS TO CASE 37:
Ovarian Tumor (Struma Ovarii)

Summary: A 22-year-old parous woman without a history of thyroid disease complains of a 3-month history of weight loss, nervousness, palpitations, and sweating. She has tachycardia, but her thyroid gland is normal to palpation. She does not have proptosis or lid lag. She is noted to have a mobile, non-tender, 9-cm mass, which on sonography has solid and cystic components.

➤ **Most likely diagnosis:** Hyperthyroidism caused by a benign cystic teratoma containing thyroid tissue (struma ovarii).

➤ **Management of this patient:** Exploratory laparotomy with ovarian cystectomy.

ANALYSIS

Objectives

1. Know that benign cystic teratomas (dermoid cysts) are the most common ovarian tumors in women younger than 30 years.
2. Understand that dermoid cysts sometimes contain thyroid tissue and cause hyperthyroidism.
3. Know that surgical therapy is the treatment of choice for ovarian tumors.
4. Understand how to evaluate and manage adnexal masses in the various age groups.

Considerations

This 22-year-old woman has symptoms of hyperthyroidism with weight loss, palpitations, and nervousness. The most common cause of hyperthyroidism in the United States is Graves disease, but the patient has no history of thyroid disease and her thyroid is normal to palpation. A patient with Graves disease usually will have a nontender goiter, and many times eye-related symptoms (proptosis or lid lag). She has an ovarian mass, which on sonography is noted to be complex, that is, to have both solid and cystic components. There is no mention of ascites in the maternal abdomen; the presence of ascites would be consistent with ovarian cancer. In a young woman (<30 years of age) with a unilateral complex ovarian mass, the most likely diagnosis is a cystic teratoma, or dermoid cyst. These tumors sometimes contain thyroid tissue and may cause hyperthyroidism. The treatment of choice for ovarian neoplasms is exploratory laparotomy with ovarian cystectomy, if benign, or more extensive surgery if malignant. At the time of surgery, the excised cyst is sent for frozen section to determine if it is benign (no further surgery needed) or malignant (surgical staging needed).

APPROACH TO
Adnexal Masses

DEFINITIONS

CYSTIC TERATOMA: A benign germ cell tumor that may contain all three germ cell layers.

STRUMA OVARII: Benign cystic teratoma containing thyroid tissue, which can cause symptoms of hyperthyroidism.

OVARIAN NEOPLASM: An abnormal growth (either benign or malignant) of the ovary; most will not regress.

EPITHELIAL OVARIAN TUMOR: Neoplasm arising from the outer layer of the ovary, which can imitate the other epithelium of the gynecologic or urologic system. This is the most common type of ovarian malignancy, usually occurring in older women.

FUNCTIONAL OVARIAN CYST: Physiologic cysts of the ovary, which occur in reproductive-aged women, of follicular, corpus luteal, or theca lutein in origin.

CLINICAL APPROACH

Germ Cell Tumors

Germ cell tumors (Table 37–1) represent about one-quarter of all ovarian tumors, and are the second most frequent type of ovarian neoplasms. They are found mainly in young women, usually in the second and third decade of life. The most common tumor is the benign cystic teratoma (dermoid). A germ cell malignancy usually presents as a pelvic mass and causes pain due to its rapidly enlarging size. Because of these symptoms, 60% to 70% of patients present at stage I, limited to one or both ovaries.

Mnemonic : DEEP-CT
⟶ (1/4 of ovarian neoplasms)

Table 37–1 GERM CELL CLASSIFICATION

Dysgerminoma
Endodermal sinus tumor
Embryonal carcinoma
Polyembryoma
Choriocarcinoma
Teratoma

Teratomas

Mature benign cystic teratomas (dermoid cysts) constitute over 95% of all ovarian teratomas. They make up 15% to 25% of all ovarian tumors, especially in the second and third decades of life. The most common elements are ectodermal derivatives such as skin, hair follicles, and sebaceous or sweat glands. However, they can also contain tissues of the three embryonic layers, including mesoderm and endoderm. They are usually multicystic and contain hair intermixed with foul-smelling, sticky, keratinaceous and sebaceous debris. Although most are unilateral, they can appear bilaterally 10% to 15% of the time. Ultrasound features of dermoid cysts include a hypoechoic area or echoic band-like strand in a hypoechoic medium or the appearance of a cystic structure with a fat fluid level. Ultrasound is generally very accurate in the diagnosis of dermoid cysts. Torsion is the most frequent complication, with severe acute abdominal pain as the typical initial symptom. This is more commonly seen during pregnancy and the puerperium. Torsion is also more common in children and younger patients. Rupture is an uncommon complication and presents as shock or hemorrhage. A chemical peritonitis can be caused by the spill of the contents of the tumor into the peritoneal cavity. The treatment is usually a cystectomy or unilateral oophorectomy with inspection of the contralateral ovary.

Immature teratomas contain all three germ layers, as well as immature or embryonal structures. They are uncommon and comprise less than 1% of ovarian cancers. They occur primarily in the first and second decades of life and are basically unknown after menopause. Malignant teratomas contain immature neural elements and that quantity alone determines the grade. They are almost always unilateral. The prognosis is directly related to the stage and the cellular immaturity. The treatment is a unilateral salpingo-oophorectomy with wide sampling of peritoneal implants. If the primary tumor is grade 1 and all peritoneal implants are grade 0, no further treatment is warranted. However, if the primary tumor is grade 2 or 3 and if there are implants or recurrences, combination chemotherapy is usually effective.

Struma Ovarii

Struma ovarii is a teratoma in which thyroid tissue has overgrown the other elements. They are usually unilateral, occurring more frequently in the right adnexa, and generally measure less than 10 cm in diameter. Preoperative clinical or radiologic diagnosis is very difficult. Only rarely will patients develop thyrotoxicosis. On MRI, these tumors appear as complex multilobulated masses with thick septa, thought to represent multiple large thyroid follicles. Most of these tumors are benign, but about 10% can have malignant changes. They will rarely produce sufficient thyroid hormone to induce hyperthyroidism. The treatment is usually cystectomy or salpingo-oophorectomy.

Table 37–2 EPITHELIAL OVARIAN TUMORS
Serous
Mucinous
Endometriod
Brenner
Clear cell

Epithelial Tumors

The most common ovarian tumors in women over the age of 30 years are of epithelial origin (Table 37–2).

The **serous subtype** is most common and more often bilateral. **Mucinous** tumors are characterized by their large size, and if ruptured may lead to pseudomyxoma peritonei, in which the mucinous material spills out into the intra-abdominal cavity. Endometrioid tumors of the ovary may coexist with a primary endometrial carcinoma of the uterus. The treatment of epithelial tumors is surgical, and if malignancy is confirmed, cancer staging is indicated. Treatment of epithelial ovarian cancer involves combination chemotherapy following surgical staging. Malignant ascites is common with cancer, as is spread to the small bowel and omentum. Lymphatic extension may also be seen. The tumor marker cancer antigen (CA)-125 is elevated in most epithelial ovarian tumors, and is more specific in postmenopausal women, since a variety of diseases during the reproductive years can elevate the CA-125 level.

Adnexal Masses

The evaluation of adnexal masses is guided by the suspicion of neoplasm (benign or malignant). At the extremes of ages, there are few functional ovarian cysts and the management is straightforward (Table 37–3).

During the reproductive years, functional ovarian cysts, such as follicular and corpus luteal cysts, sometimes make the evaluation difficult. In general, any adnexal mass greater than 8 cm in size is likely to be a tumor and should be explored. Any adnexal mass less than 5 cm in size suggests a functional cyst. Between 5 and 8 cm, the sonographic features may help to distinguish functional versus neoplasm. Septations, solid components, or excrescences (growth on surface or inner lining) are consistent with a neoplastic process, whereas a simple cyst is more suggestive of a functional cyst. Sometimes, a practitioner will choose to observe an adnexal mass that is between 5 and 8 cm in size for 1 month and operate if it is persistent.

Table 37–3 EVALUATION OF ADNEXAL MASSES BASED ON AGE		
AGE GROUP	**OVARIAN SIZE (CM)**	**PLAN**
Prepubertal	>2	Operate
Reproductive age	<5	Observe
	5-8	Sonogram; if septations, solid components or excrescences, then operate; otherwise observe for 1 month
	>8	Operate
Menopausal	>4-5	Operate

Comprehension Questions

37.1 A 5-year-old female is noted to have breast enlargement, vaginal bleeding, and an 8-cm pelvic mass. Which of the following is the most likely etiology?

A. Benign cystic teratoma (dermoid)
B. Endodermal sinus tumor
C. Brenner tumor
D. Choriocarcinoma
E. Granulosa-theca cell tumor

37.2 A 25-year-old woman is noted to have a 4 cm simple cyst of the right ovary. She denies any abdominal pain, nausea or vomiting. Which of the following is the next best step?

A. Expectant management
B. Laparoscopy
C. Exploratory laparotomy
D. Chemotherapy

37.3 Which of the following is the best treatment for a suspected dermoid cyst found in an 18-year-old nulliparous woman?

A. Total abdominal hysterectomy
B. Unilateral salpingo-oophrectomy
C. Ovarian cystectomy
D. Observation

Which of the following sonographic findings (A-D) matches the ovarian tumor type (37.4-37.6)?
  A. Completely solid
  B. Simple cyst
  C. Complex
  D. Ascites is commonly seen

37.4   Granulosa cell tumor

37.5   Benign cystic teratoma (dermoid cyst)

37.6   Follicular cyst

37.7   A 44-year-old woman is noted to have a 30 cm tumor of the ovary. Which of the following is the most likely cell type?
  A. Dermoid cyst
  B. Granulosa cell tumor
  C. Serous tumor
  D. Mucinous tumor

ANSWERS

→ generally sex cord stromal can be at any age.

37.1   **E.** This is a young child with precocious puberty, which suggests an estrogen-secreting tumor. This is most likely a granulosa-theca cell tumor, best treated by surgery. These are stromal sex cord tumors.

37.2   **A.** When the ovarian cyst in the reproductive-aged female is less than 5 cm in diameter, the most likely cause is a physiologic cyst such as a follicular cyst or corpus luteum. Expectant management and reassessment in 1 to 2 months is the best next step.

37.3   **C.** Ovarian cystectomy is the best treatment for benign cystic teratomas. ✓

37.4   **A.** Granulosa cell tumors and Sertoli-Leydig cell tumors are usually solid on ultrasound, and may secrete sex hormones. Typically, granulosa-theca cell tumors produce estrogens, whereas Sertoli-Leydig cell tumors make androgens.

37.5   **C.** Benign cystic teratomas (dermoid cysts) are complex cysts since they usually have both solid and cystic components. The best treatment of a dermoid in a young woman is ovarian cystectomy. Ovarian torsion is the most frequent complication. Immature teratomas contain all three germ layers, as well as immature or embryonal structures. Malignant teratomas contain immature neural elements, and the grade of the tumor is determined by the amount of neural tissue involved.

37.6   **B.** Follicular cysts are generally simple cysts without septations or solid parts. They are among the physiologic cysts of the ovary, which occur in reproductive-aged women. Other physiologic, or functional, cysts include corpus luteal or theca lutein cysts.

37.7   **D.** Mucinous tumors of the ovary can grow to be very large. If they rupture intra-abdominally, they may cause pseudomyxoma peritonei, which leads to repeated bouts of bowel obstruction. They are of epithelial origin. The most common type of epithelial ovarian tumor is the serous type, which unlike the mucinous tumors, occurs bilaterally. The tumor marker CA-125 is elevated in most epithelial ovarian tumors and is more specific in postmenopausal women because a variety of diseases that occur during the reproductive years can show an elevated CA-125 level.

Clinical Pearls

➤ The most common ovarian tumor in a woman younger than 30 years is a benign cystic teratoma (dermoid cyst). The best treatment of a dermoid in a young woman is ovarian cystectomy.

➤ The most common ovarian tumor in a woman older than 30 years is epithelial in origin, most commonly serous cystadenoma.

➤ An ovarian mass larger than 5 cm in a postmenopausal woman most likely represents an ovarian tumor and should generally be removed. An ovarian mass that is larger than 2 to 3 cm in a prepubertal girl likewise should be investigated and many times requires removal.

➤ During the reproductive years, functional ovarian cysts are common and are usually smaller than 5 cm in diameter. Any ovarian cyst larger than 8 cm in a reproductive-aged woman is probably a neoplasm and should be excised.

➤ The tumor marker CA-125 is most specific for ovarian cancer in postmenopausal women.

➤ Mucinous tumors of the ovary can grow to be very large. If they rupture intra-abdominally, they may cause pseudomyxoma peritonei, which leads to repeated bouts of bowel obstruction.

➤ Ascites is a common sign of ovarian malignancy.

➤ Ovarian cancer staging consists of total abdominal hysterectomy, bilateral salpingo-oophorectomy, omentectomy, peritoneal biopsies, peritoneal washings or sampling of ascitic fluid, and lymphadenectomy.

REFERENCES

American College of Obstetricians and Gynecologists. Management of adnexal masses. ACOG *Practice Bulletin 83*. Washington, DC: 2007.

Coleman RL, Gershenson DM. Neoplastic diseases of the ovary. In: Katz VL, Lentz GM, Lobo RA, Gersenson DM, eds. *Comprehensive Gynecology*. 5th ed. St. Louis, MO: Mosby-Year Book; 2007:839-882.

Nelson AL, Gambone JC. Congenital anomalies and benign conditions of the ovaries and fallopian tubes. In: Hacker NF, Gambone JC, Hobel CJ, eds. *Essentials of Obstetrics and Gynecology*, 5th ed. Philadelphia, PA: Saunders; 2009:248-255.

Case 38

A 45-year-old woman complains of profuse serosanguineous drainage from her abdominal incision site that has persisted over 4 hours and has soaked several large towels. The patient states that the incision had been somewhat red and tender for several days. She had staging surgery for ovarian cancer 7 days previously. She denies the passage of blood clots or foul smelling lochia. She states that her vaginal bleeding was scant. Her past medical history is significant for type 2 diabetes mellitus, and her surgical history is unremarkable. On examination, her weight is 270 lb, blood pressure (BP) is 100/70 mm Hg, heart rate (HR) 80 beats per minute, respiratory rate (RR) 12 breaths per minute, and she is afebrile. The thyroid is normal to palpation. The heart and lung examinations are normal. The remainder of the physical examination is unremarkable except for the abdominal incision.

➤ What is the most likely diagnosis?

➤ What is the most appropriate therapy?

ANSWERS TO CASE 38:
Fascial Disruption

Summary: A 45-year-old obese woman complains of a 4-hour history of profuse serosanguineous drainage from her abdominal incision site. She had undergone staging surgery for ovarian cancer 7 days previously.

➤ **Most likely diagnosis:** Surgical site infection (deep incisional) with fascial disruption.

➤ **Most appropriate therapy:** Immediate surgical closure and broad-spectrum antibiotic therapy.

ANALYSIS

Objectives

1. Know the classic presentation of surgical site infection (SSI) with fascial disruption.
2. Understand that both fascial disruption and fascial evisceration are surgical emergencies.
3. Know the risk factors for wound disruptions.

Considerations

This 45-year-old diabetic woman underwent ovarian cancer staging surgery 7 days previously. She now complains of 4 hours of profuse and continuous serosanguineous drainage from her abdominal incision. This is the typical presentation for fascial disruption. Because the rectus fascia is interrupted, the peritoneal fluid escapes through the wound. If this were only a superficial fascial separation, caused by a seroma or other small fluid collection in the subcutaneous fat tissue, then the patient would have only complained of a limited amount of drainage. The patient does not have intestinal contents penetrating through the incision; thus, an evisceration is not suspected. Nevertheless, deep SSI with fascial disruptions is a surgical emergency requiring immediate surgical repair. Broad-spectrum antibiotic therapy is usually administered. This patient has numerous risk factors for fascial dehiscence including obesity, diabetes, cancer, and a probable vertical incision. The time frame from the surgery is fairly typical, which is usually 7 to 10 days following surgery.

APPROACH TO
Wound Complications

DEFINITIONS

WOUND DEHISCENCE: A separation of part of the surgical incision, but with an intact peritoneum.

FASCIAL DISRUPTION: Separation of the fascial layer, usually leading to a communication of the peritoneal cavity with the skin.

SEROSANGUINEOUS: Blood-tinged drainage.

EVISCERATION: A disruption of all layers of the incision with omentum or bowel protruding through the incision.

SURGICAL SITE INFECTION (SSI): Infection related to the operative procedure that occurs at or near the surgical incision within 30 days of an operation. **Deep incision** must involve the deep soft tissue such as fascia or muscle.

CLINICAL APPROACH

Wound Disorders

Wound complications include superficial separation, dehiscence, and evisceration. Separations of the subcutaneous tissue anterior to the fascia are usually associated with infection or hematoma. They affect about 3% to 5% of abdominal hysterectomy incisions. The affected patient usually presents with a red, tender, indurated incision and fever 4 to 10 days postoperatively. The treatment is opening the wound and draining the purulence. A broad-spectrum antimicrobial agent is recommended, with wet-to-dry dressing changes. The wound may be allowed to close secondarily, or be approximated after several days.

Fascial disruption, separation of the fascia but not the peritoneum, occurs in about 1% of all abdominal surgeries, and about 0.5% of abdominal incisions. It is more common with vertical incisions, obesity, intra-abdominal distension, diabetes, exposure to radiation, corticosteroid use, infection, coughing, and malnutrition. This condition often presents as profuse drainage from the incision 5 to 14 days after surgery. SSI with fascial disruption requires repair as soon as possible with the initiation of broad-spectrum antibiotics.

Evisceration is defined as protrusion of bowel or omentum through the incision, which connotes complete separation of all layers of the wound. This condition carries a significant mortality due to sepsis, and is considered a surgical emergency. When encountered, a sterile sponge wet with saline should be placed over the bowel, and the patient taken to the operating room. Antibiotics should be immediately started. The presentation is similar to that of wound dehiscence.

Comprehension Questions

38.1 Which of the following is a risk for wound dehiscence?
A. Diabetes mellitus
B. Use of monofilament suture
C. Horizontal incision
D. Addison disease

38.2 Which of the following is the most common reason for fascial disruption?
A. Suture becomes untied
B. Suture breakage
C. Suture tears through fascia
D. Defective suture material
E. Suture hydrolytic process

38.3 A 59-year-old woman who had staging surgery for ovarian cancer is noted to have clear serous drainage from her incision. The surgeon is concerned that it may represent lymphatic drainage versus a fistula from the urinary tract. Which of the following studies of the fluid would most likely help to differentiate between these two entities?
A. Creatinine level
B. Leukocyte count
C. pH
D. Hemoglobin level
E. CA-125 level

38.4 A 38-year-old woman had an abdominal hysterectomy for symptomatic uterine fibroids, namely menorrhagia that had failed to respond to medical therapy. One week later, she complains of low-grade fever and lower abdominal pain. On examination, she is noted to have a temperature of 100.8°F (38.22°C) and the Pfannenstiel (low transverse) incision is red, indurated, and tender. Which of the following is the best therapy for this condition?
A. Oral antibiotic therapy
B. Observation
C. Opening the incision and draining the infection
D. Antibiotic ointment to the affected area
E. Interferon therapy

ANSWERS

38.1   **A.** Diabetes is associated with an increased risk for fascial separation because it is more difficult for wounds to heal in patients with this disease. The integrity of blood vessels is disrupted in a wound; this, along with the fact that diabetics typically have poor blood circulation, makes it more difficult to adequately profuse the wounded area (blood contains the necessary clotting factors and immunoglobulins required to heal a wound and prevent infection). As a result, diabetics are also at a greater risk for a serious infection. A vertical incision as opposed to a transverse incision is associated with a greater risk of fascial disruption. Addison disease is a state of hypocortisolism, whereas Cushing disease is a state of hypercortisolism. Since increased cortisol levels are associated with immunosuppression, wound dehiscence would be more likely to occur in Cushing disease, not Addison disease.

38.2   **C.** Fascial breakdown (disruption) is not usually due to suture breakage or knot slippage, but rather due to the suture tearing through the fascia. It is more common with vertical incisions, obesity, intra-abdominal distension, diabetes, exposure to radiation, corticosteroid use, infection, coughing, and malnutrition. This condition requires immediate repair and broad-spectrum antibiotics. Fascial disruption and evisceration typically occur between 5 and 14 days postoperatively.

38.3   **A.** A creatinine level may distinguish between urine and lymphatic fluid. The creatinine level would be significantly more elevated in urine.

38.4   **C.** This patient has a superficial wound infection. The best treatment is to open the wound and drain the purulence. A broad-spectrum antimicrobial agent is recommended, with wet-to-dry dressing changes. The wound can be allowed to close secondarily or be approximated after several days. Observation in the face of infection would not be the best management and may lead to septicemia. Ointments and oral antibiotic therapy are not sufficient treatment options until the drainage is removed.

Clinical Pearls

➤ Fascial disruption is a concern when copious amounts of sero-sanguinous fluid are draining from an abdominal incision.

➤ An SSI with fascial disruption or evisceration should be immediately repaired.

➤ The most common time period in which fascial disruption or evisceration occurs is 5 to 14 days postoperatively.

➤ A superficial wound separation usually occurs due to infection or hematoma, and is treated by opening the wound and using wet-to-dry dressing changes.

➤ Obesity, malnutrition, and chronic cough are risk factors for fascial disruption.

REFERENCES

Centers for Disease Control and Prevention. Definitions of nosocomial infections. Appendix A-1. www.cdc.gov. Accessed 1/6/2009.

Droegemuller W. Preoperative counseling and management. In: Stenchever MA, Droegemueller W, Herbst AL, Mishell DR, eds. *Comprehensive Gynecology*. 5th ed. St. Louis, MO: Mosby-Year Book; 2007:771-825.

Gallup DG. Incisions for gynecologic surgery. In: Rock JA, Thomson JD, eds. *Telinde's Operative Gynecology*. 8th ed. Philadelphia, PA: Lippincott-Raven; 1997:308-311.

Case 39

A 25-year-old woman at 10 weeks' gestation complains of severe abdominal pain and feeling faint for the last hour. She had moderately heavy vaginal bleeding that began yesterday morning, and noted that some tissue possibly passed vaginally. The tissue brought into the office floats when placed in saline with a "frond" pattern. Currently, she denies vaginal bleeding but feels lightheaded. On examination, her blood pressure (BP) is 90/60 mm Hg, heart rate (HR) 120 beats per minute (bpm), and temperature 99°F (37.2°C). Her abdomen is diffusely tender, distended, with rebound tenderness, and a fluid wave is present. The cervix is closed.

➤ What is the most likely diagnosis?

➤ What is your next step in the management?

ANSWERS TO CASE 39:

Abdominal Pain in Pregnancy (Ruptured Corpus Luteum)

Summary: A 25-year-old woman at 10 weeks' gestation complains of severe abdominal pain and lightheadedness. Yesterday, she had moderately heavy vaginal bleeding and passed some tissue, which floats with a "frond" pattern. Her BP is 90/60 mm Hg, HR 120 bpm, and temperature 99°F (37.2°C). Her abdomen is diffusely tender, distended, with rebound tenderness, and a fluid wave is present. The cervix is closed.

➤ **Most likely diagnosis:** Ruptured corpus luteum cyst with hemoperitoneum.

➤ **Next step in the management:** Admission to the hospital with surgical intervention (laparoscopy or laparotomy).

ANALYSIS

Objectives

1. Know the symptoms and signs of hypovolemic shock.
2. Know that a hemoperitoneum in pregnancy is usually caused by a ruptured ectopic pregnancy and, less commonly, by a ruptured corpus luteum.
3. Understand that endometrial tissue that floats with a "frond pattern" is almost always diagnostic for an intrauterine pregnancy.

Considerations

This 25-year-old woman is at 10 weeks' gestation and complains of symptoms of hypovolemia. She feels faint, is hypotensive, and has tachycardia. This symptom complex is consistent with hemorrhagic shock. Furthermore, she has severe abdominal pain, abdominal distension, rebound tenderness, and a positive fluid wave. The most likely cause is a hemoperitoneum. The blood in the abdomen causes irritation of the peritoneal lining, causing the rebound tenderness. In nine out of ten cases, a pregnant woman with a hemoperitoneum has an ectopic pregnancy. However, in this case, the patient passed some tissue, which floated in a "frond pattern" when placed in saline. This is very good evidence of products of conception; in fact, the float test is more than 95% accurate for the presence of chorionic villi. An ectopic pregnancy coexisting with an intrauterine pregnancy is exceedingly rare (1 in 10,000). Thus, the hemoperitoneum is likely caused by a ruptured corpus luteum. Another less common possibility includes splenic injury or rupture.

APPROACH TO
Hypovolemia in Pregnancy

DEFINITIONS

CORPUS LUTEUM: A physiologic ovarian cyst formed from mature graafian follicles following ovulation, which secretes progesterone.

HEMORRHAGIC CORPUS LUTEUM: Bleeding occurring in a corpus luteum, which may cause a hemoperitoneum or cyst enlargement.

HEMOPERITONEUM: A collection of blood in the peritoneal cavity. The blood initially clots and then lyses, so that there may be a combination of clots and hemorrhagic fluid that will not clot.

CLINICAL APPROACH

Corpus luteum cysts develop from mature Graafian follicles and are associated with normal endocrine function or prolonged secretion of progesterone. They are usually less than 3 cm in diameter. There can be intrafollicular bleeding because of thin-walled capillaries that invade the granulosa cells from the theca interna. **When the hemorrhage is excessive, the cyst can enlarge and there is an increased risk of rupture.** Cysts tend to rupture more during pregnancy, probably due to the increased incidence and friability of corpus lutea in pregnancy. Anticoagulation therapy also predisposes to cyst rupture, and these women should receive medication to prevent ovulation. Patients with hemorrhagic corpus lutea usually present with the sudden onset of severe lower abdominal pain. This presentation is especially common in women with a hemoperitoneum. Some women will complain of unilateral cramping and lower abdominal pain for 1 to 2 weeks before overt rupture. Corpus luteum cysts rupture more commonly between days 20 and 26 of the menstrual cycle.

The differential diagnosis of a suspected hemorrhagic corpus luteum should include ectopic pregnancy, ruptured endometrioma, adnexal torsion, appendicitis, and splenic injury or rupture. Ultrasound examination may show free intraperitoneal fluid, and perhaps fluid around an ovary. The diagnosis is confirmed by laparoscopy. The first step in the treatment of a ruptured corpus luteal cyst is to secure hemostasis. Once the bleeding stops, no further therapy is required; if the bleeding continues, however, a cystectomy should be performed with preservation of the remaining normal portion of ovary.

Progesterone is largely produced by the corpus luteum until about 10 weeks' gestation. Until approximately the seventh week, the pregnancy is dependent on the progesterone secreted by the corpus luteum. Human chorionic gonadotropin serves to maintain the luteal function until placental steroidogenesis is established. There is shared function between the placenta and corpus luteum from the seventh to tenth week; after 10 weeks, the placenta emerges as the major source of progesterone. Therefore, if the corpus luteum is removed surgically prior to 10 to 12 weeks' gestation, exogenous progesterone is needed to sustain the pregnancy. If the corpus luteum is excised after 10 to 12 weeks' gestation, no supplemental progesterone is required.

Comprehension Questions

39.1   A 19-year-old G1 P0 woman at 28 weeks' gestation arrives to the obstetric (OB) triage area complaining of a 12-hour history of abdominal pain. She denies trauma, vaginal bleeding, or fever. On examination, her temperature is 99°F (37.2°C), HR 100 bpm, BP 100/70 mm Hg. Her abdominal examination reveals hypoactive bowel sounds, diffuse abdominal pain with guarding. Which of the following statements regarding the abdominal pain is most accurate?

A. The absence of vaginal bleeding rules out abruption as an etiology.
B. Ovarian torsion is typically characterized by constant pain.
C. The gallbladder typically moves superior and laterally with pregnancy.
D. Degenerating leiomyoma typically presents with localized tenderness over the fibroid.

39.2   A 25-year-old woman G1 P0 is noted to have vaginal spotting and β-hCG levels have plateaued in the 1800 mIU/mL range. A uterine curettage is performed and no chorionic villi are seen on histologic examination. Which of the following describes the most likely diagnosis for this patient?

A. Complete molar pregnancy
B. Intrauterine pregnancy
C. Incomplete molar pregnancy
D. Ectopic pregnancy
E. Spontaneous abortion

39.3   A 20-year-old G1 P0 woman at 12 weeks' gestation is noted to have a suspected ruptured ectopic pregnancy. On sonography there is a moderate amount of free fluid in the abdominal cavity. The medical student assigned to evaluate the patient is amazed by the apparent stability of the patient. Which of the following is the earliest indicator of hypovolemia?

A. Tachycardia
B. Hypotension
C. Positive tilt
D. Lethargy and confusion
E. Decreased urine output

39.4   A 20-year-old woman is brought into the emergency room with a
        blood pressure of 70/40 mm Hg and heart rate of 130 bpm, and a his-
        tory of heavy vaginal bleeding. Which of the following describes the
        first step in treatment?
        A. Intravenous isotonic fluids
        B. Aggressive oral fluids
        C. Immediate blood transfusion
        D. Immediate uterine curettage
        E. Intravenous dobutamine therapy

ANSWERS

39.1   **D.** Fibroids of the uterus can be associated with red or carneous
        degeneration during pregnancy due to the estrogen levels leading to
        rapid growth of the fibroid. The fibroid outgrows its blood supply
        leading to ischemia and pan. Typically, the pain of a degenerating
        fibroid is localized over the leiomyoma. Abruption can be concealed
        with bleeding behind the placenta. The gallbladder usually does not
        move during pregnancy, whereas the appendix will move superiorly
        and laterally. Ovarian torsion is associated with colicky abdominal
        pain and comes and goes.

39.2   **D.** With no chorionic villi on uterine curettage (therefore, unlikely
        to be an intrauterine pregnancy or spontaneous abortion) and a
        human chorionic gonadotropin level of 1800 mIU/mL, the most
        likely diagnosis is an ectopic pregnancy. Molar pregnancies are asso-
        ciated with a rapid rise in the human chorionic gonadotropin level,
        and will reveal hydropic villi on dilation and curettage (D and C).
        Spontaneous abortion if completed prior to the D and C is a possi-
        bility; however, the patient does not complain of bleeding or passage
        of tissue.

39.3   **E.** Renal blood flow is decreased with early hypovolemia as reflected
        by decreased urine output. This is a compensatory mechanism to
        make blood volume available to the body. Typically before tachycar-
        dia or hypotension occurs, a positive tilt test is noted. By the time
        hypotension is noted at rest in a young, healthy patient, 30% of
        blood volume is lost.

39.4   **A.** The priorities in treating any patient are the ABCs. Since the
        patient's airway and breathing are normal, then attention should be
        paid to circulatory status. Stabilizing the patient with isotonic intra-
        venous fluid infusion is the first step to resuscitation of the patient
        with hypovolemia. Aggressive oral fluids are not absorbed fast
        enough, plus the patient may not be coherent enough to intake fluids.
        For a blood transfusion, it would take too long to retrieve the

patient's blood type and get the appropriate blood products, plus it takes longer to infuse a patient with blood than it does to infuse with IV fluids. A uterine curettage would not be indicated because the source of the bleed has not been identified and it still would not make up for the volume that has already been lost.

Clinical Pearls

➤ The most common cause of hemoperitoneum in early pregnancy is ectopic pregnancy.

➤ A ruptured corpus luteum can mimic an ectopic pregnancy.

➤ Hemorrhagic corpus lutea can occur more commonly in patients with bleeding tendencies either congenital (von Willebrand) or iatrogenic (Coumadin induced).

➤ Nonclotted blood obtained from culdocentesis is consistent with intraabdominal hemorrhage.

➤ When the corpus luteum is excised in a pregnancy of less than 10 to 12 weeks gestation, progesterone should be supplemented.

➤ The first sign of hypovolemia is oliguria (decreased urine output).

➤ By the time hypotension at rest is noted in a young, healthy patient, 30% to 40% of the patient's blood volume is lost.

REFERENCES

Katz VL. Benign gynecologic lesions. In: Katz VL, Lentz GM, Lobo RA, Gersenson DM, eds. *Comprehensive Gynecology*. 5th ed. St. Louis, MO: Mosby-Year Book; 2007: 419-470.

Nelson AL, Gambone JC. Congenital anomalies and benign conditions of the ovaries and fallopian tubes. In: Hacker NF, Gambone JC, Hobel CJ, eds. *Essentials of Obstetrics and Gynecology*, 5th ed. Philadelphia, PA: Saunders; 2009:248-255.

Case 40

A 33-year-old woman complains of 7 months of amenorrhea following a spontaneous abortion. She had a dilation and curettage (D and C) at that time. Her past medical and surgical histories are unremarkable. She experienced menarche at age 11 years and notes that her menses have been every 28 to 31 days until recently. Her general physical examination is unremarkable. The thyroid is normal to palpation, and breasts are without discharge. The abdomen is nontender. The pelvic examination shows a normal uterus, closed and normal-appearing cervix, and no adnexal masses. A pregnancy test is negative.

➤ What is the most likely diagnosis?

➤ What is the next test to confirm the diagnosis?

ANSWERS TO CASE 40:
Amenorrhea (Intrauterine Adhesions)

Summary: A 33-year-old woman complains of 7 months of amenorrhea after she had a D and C for a spontaneous abortion. Her menstrual history was normal previously. The thyroid, pelvic, and breast examinations are normal. The pregnancy test is negative.

➤ **Most likely diagnosis:** Intrauterine adhesions (Asherman syndrome).

➤ **Next diagnostic test:** Hysterosalpingogram (or hysteroscopy).

ANALYSIS

Objectives

1. Know the definition of secondary amenorrhea.
2. Understand how uterine curettage can cause endometrial adhesions and amenorrhea.
3. Know how to diagnose intrauterine adhesive disease (Asherman syndrome).

Considerations

This 33-year-old woman has had 7 months of amenorrhea since experiencing a miscarriage. She had undergone a uterine dilation and curettage at that time. Her menstrual history was unremarkable previously; hence, she meets the definition of secondary amenorrhea (6 months of no menses in a woman with previously normal menses). Pregnancy should be the first condition to be ruled out. Secondary amenorrhea may be caused by hypothalamic etiologies (such as hypothyroidism or hyperprolactinemia), pituitary conditions (such as Sheehan syndrome), or ovarian causes (such as premature ovarian failure). The patient does not have symptoms of hypothyroidism or galactorrhea, postpartum hemorrhage, or hot flushes. Additionally, her history suggests a proximate relationship to the miscarriage. Hence, the most likely diagnosis is intrauterine adhesions, arising from the curettage of the uterus. With this condition, the hypothalamus, pituitary, and ovary are working normally, but the endometrial tissue is not responsive to the hormonal changes. A hysterosalpingogram, a radiologic study where radiopaque dye is injected into the uterine cavity via a transcervical catheter, showing obliteration of the endometrial cavity would establish the diagnosis.

APPROACH TO
Suspected Intrauterine Adhesions

DEFINITIONS

SECONDARY AMENORRHEA: Absence of menses for a period of 6 months or more in a woman who has had spontaneous menses.

INTRAUTERINE ADHESIONS (IUA): Condition when scar tissue or synechiae form to obliterate the endometrial cavity, usually occurring because of uterine curettage following a pregnancy.

HYSTEROSALPINGOGRAM: A radiologic study in which radiopaque dye is injected into the endometrial cavity via a transcervical catheter, used to evaluate the endometrial cavity and/or the patency of the fallopian tubes.

HYSTEROSCOPY: Procedure of direct visualization of the endometrial cavity with an endoscope, a light source, and a distension media.

UTERINE SOUNDING: Assessing the depth and direction of the cervical and uterine cavity with a thin blunt probe.

CLINICAL APPROACH

Intrauterine Adhesions (Asherman Syndrome)

Intrauterine scarring leading to an unresponsive endometrium is most commonly due to injury to the pregnant or recently pregnant uterus. However, any mechanical, infectious, or radiation factor can produce endometrial sclerosis and adhesion formation. The sine qua non for the development of intrauterine adhesions is endometrial trauma, especially to the basalis layer. The adhesions are usually strands of avascular fibrous tissue, but they may also consist of inactive endometrium or myometrium. Myometrial adhesions are usually dense and vascular carrying a poor prognosis. Women with atrophic and sclerotic endometrium without adhesions carry the worst prognosis. This is usually found after radiation or tuberculous endometritis and is not amenable to any therapy. Postpartum curettage performed between the second and fourth weeks after delivery, along with hypoestrogenic states such as breast-feeding or hypogonadotropic hypogonadism, is associated with extensive intrauterine scar formation. Uterine curettage performed after a missed abortion is associated with a higher incidence of intrauterine synechiae than curettage performed after an incomplete abortion or a molar pregnancy. Adhesions may also form after a diagnostic D and C. In general, the routine use of uterine curettage at the time of a diagnostic laparoscopy is unwarranted and may damage the endometrium.

Intrauterine adhesions should be suspected if a woman presents with secondary amenorrhea, a negative pregnancy test, and does not have progestin-induced withdrawal bleeding. There is no consistent correlation between the menstrual bleeding patterns and the extent of intrauterine adhesions. The diagnosis of IUA should be suspected on every patient with infertility, recurrent abortions, uterine trauma, and menstrual abnormalities. **The most common method of diagnosing IUA is by hysterosalpingogram.** In cases of severe intrauterine adhesions, the cavity cannot be sounded, making the procedure very difficult to perform. Vaginal ultrasound can be used in the diagnosis of IUA; however, it lacks specificity. Sonohysterography is an excellent complement to the vaginal ultrasound and can allow for the evaluation of the uterine cavity. Magnetic resonance imaging (MRI) is expensive and does not offer a greater advantage over the other diagnostic modalities. Hysteroscopy allows for direct visualization of the uterine cavity and is considered the "gold standard" for the establishment of the diagnosis and extent of the IUA.

Operative hysteroscopy is the ideal treatment for IUA. The postoperative management may include the insertion of an IUD or a pediatric Foley catheter to prevent the recently lysed adhesions from reforming. In addition, the administration of conjugated estrogens and progesterone (medroxyprogesterone acetate) should be considered. The uterine cavity should be reevaluated prior to attempting conception.

Comprehension Questions

40.1   A 34-year-old woman states that she has had no menses since she had a uterine curettage and cone biopsy of the cervix 1 year previously. Since those surgeries, she complains of severe, crampy lower abdominal pain "similar to labor pain" for 5 days of each month. Her basal body temperature chart is biphasic, rising 1°F for 2 weeks of every month. Which of the following is the most likely etiology of secondary amenorrhea?

A. Hypothalamic etiology
B. Pituitary etiology
C. Uterine etiology
D. Cervical condition

40.2   A 29-year-old woman G2 P0 underwent an evaluation for amenorrhea of
        10 months duration. Her menses had been regular previously. A pregnancy
        test, TSH, prolactin level, FSH, and LH levels were normal. The patient
        had sequential estrogen and progestin therapy without vaginal bleeding.
        Her presumptive diagnosis was intrauterine adhesions, which was con-
        firmed with imaging. Which of the following statements is most accurate?

        A. Her condition usually occurs after uterine curettage for a pregnancy-
           related process.
        B. She would best be diagnosed by laparoscopy.
        C. The patient likely has cramping pain every month.
        D. Her treatment includes endometrial ablation.

40.3   A 32-year-old G1 P1 woman presents with an 8-month history of
        amenorrhea. A pregnancy test is negative. TSH and prolactin levels
        are normal. The FSH level is elevated at 40 IU/L. Which of the fol-
        lowing is the most likely complication for this patient?

        A. She is at significant risk for endometrial cancer.
        B. She is at increased risk for ovarian cancer.
        C. She is at increased risk for osteoporosis.
        D. She is at increased risk for multiple gestations.

40.4   A 41-year-old woman is suspected of having intrauterine adhesions
        because she has had irregular menses since a spontaneous abortion
        18 months previously. Which of the following historical or laboratory
        pieces of information would support this diagnosis?

        A. Presence of hot flushes
        B. FSH level too low to be measurable
        C. Normal estradiol levels for a reproductive-aged woman
        D. Monophasic basal body temperature chart

ANSWERS

40.1   **D.** This patient has two potential causes for amenorrhea: IUA
        caused by the uterine curettage and cervical stenosis due to the cer-
        vical conization. The biphasic basal body temperature chart suggests
        normal functioning of the hypothalamus-pituitary-ovarian axis. The
        crampy abdominal pain most likely is due to retrograde menstrua-
        tion; thus, this is most likely due to a cervical process, cervical
        stenosis. If untreated, this patient would likely develop severe
        endometriosis.

40.2   **A.** Uterine curettage for a pregnancy-related process predisposes to
        IUA. This is best diagnosed with **hysteroscopy** (direct visualization
        of endometrial cavity) and not laparoscopy (visualized intraperitoneal
        cavity). **Cervical stenosis,** and not IUA, is associated with cramping
        pain every month. Ideal treatment for Asherman is **operative**

hysteroscopy. The patient has a work-up for secondary amenorrhea, which is fairly standard consisting of pregnancy test, prolactin and TSH levels which would alter GnRH pulsations, and FSH and LH assessing ovarian failure. Sequential estrogen and progestin without bleeding indicates a uterine/cervical etiology.

40.3   **C.** This patient has secondary amenorrhea. Her pregnancy test is negative. The TSH and prolactin levels are normal. Her serum FSH level is elevated, indicating that she has premature ovarian failure. Due to the low estrogen levels, she is at risk for osteoporosis. She is not at risk for endometrial cancer. Patients with PCOS would be at risk for endometrial cancer due to unopposed estrogen.

40.4   **C.** With IUA, the hormonal status of the woman should be normal. This would exclude the possibility of ovarian failure (hot flushes), low FSH levels, and a monophasic basal body temperature chart since these are all indications of an *abnormal* hormonal status.

Clinical Pearls

> ➤ The most common cause of secondary amenorrhea after uterine curettage is intrauterine adhesions.
> ➤ Intrauterine adhesions are diagnosed by hysterosalpingogram and confirmed by hysteroscopy.
> ➤ Hysteroscopic resection is the best treatment of intrauterine adhesions.
> ➤ Uterine curettage, especially associated with pregnancy, is a risk factor for intrauterine adhesions.
> ➤ The evaluation of secondary amenorrhea includes a pregnancy test, prolactin level, TSH level, and assessment of gonadotropin levels.

REFERENCES

Alexander CJ, Mathur R, Laufer LR, Aziz R. Amenorrhea, oligomenorrhea, and hyperandrogenic disorders. In: Hacker NF, Gambone JC, Hobel CJ, eds. *Essentials of Obstetrics and Gynecology*, 5th ed. Philadelphia, PA: Saunders; 2009:355-367.
Lentz GM. Primary and secondary amenorrhea and precocious puberty. In: Katz VL, Lentz GM, Lobo RA, Gersenson DM, eds. *Comprehensive Gynecology*. 5th ed. St. Louis, MO: Mosby-Year Book; 2007:933-960.

Case 41

A 59-year-old woman comes into the doctor's office for a health maintenance examination. Her past medical history is remarkable for mild
hypertension controlled with an oral thiazide diuretic agent. Her surgical history is unremarkable. On examination, her blood pressure (BP) is
140/84 mm Hg, heart rate (HR) 70 beats per minute (bpm), and she is
afebrile. The thyroid is normal to palpation. The breasts are nontender
and without masses. The pelvic examination is unremarkable.
Mammography revealed a small cluster of calcifications around a small
mass.

➤ What is your next step?

ANSWER TO CASE 41:

Breast, Abnormal Mammogram

Summary: A 59-year-old woman comes into the doctor's office for a health maintenance examination. The breasts are nontender and without masses. Mammography revealed a small cluster of calcifications around a small mass.

> ➤ **Next step:** Stereotactic biopsy or needle-localization excisional biopsy of the breast.

ANALYSIS

Objectives

1. Understand the role of mammography in screening for breast cancer.
2. Know that mammography is not perfect in identifying breast cancer.
3. Know the typical mammographic findings that are suspicious for cancer.

Considerations

This 59-year-old woman is going to her doctor for routine health maintenance. She is taking a thiazide diuretic for mild hypertension. Her blood pressure is mildly elevated. The mammogram reveals a small cluster of calcifications around a small mass, which is one of the classic findings of breast cancer. With this mammographic finding, it is of paramount importance to obtain tissue for histologic diagnosis. Because of the high risk of malignancy, a stereotactic-directed core biopsy, or surgical excisional biopsy, is preferable to a fine needle aspiration. For needle localization, mammographic guidance is employed so that the end of the needle is placed in the center of the suspicious area. The surgeon may then perform a breast biopsy using the needle as a guide. Because the mass is not palpable, a needle-localized approach is needed. The other option is a stereotactic core biopsy guided by computer-assisted imaging techniques.

APPROACH TO

The Abnormal Mammogram

DEFINITIONS

SUSPICIOUS MAMMOGRAPHIC FINDINGS: A small cluster of calcifications, or masses with ill-defined borders.

NEEDLE LOCALIZATION: Procedure in which a sterile needle is placed via mammographic guidance such that the end of the needle is placed in the center of the suspicious area. The surgeon uses this guide to assist in excising breast tissue.

STEREOTACTIC CORE BIOPSY: Procedure in which the patient is prone on the mammographic table and biopsies are taken as directed with computer-assisted techniques.

CLINICAL APPROACH

Although a clinical history and proper clinical breast examinations are important in detecting breast cancer, mammography remains the best method of detecting breast cancer at an early stage.

A mammogram is an x-ray of the breast tissue. Current radiation levels from mammography have been shown to be safe and cause no increased risk in developing breast cancer. The radiation exposure is less than 10 rads per lifetime if annual mammograms begin at age 40 years and continue up to age 90. Both false positives and false negatives of up to 10% have been noted. **Hence, a palpable breast mass in the face of a normal mammogram still requires a biopsy.** Breast implants can diminish the accuracy of a mammogram, particularly if the implants are in front of the chest muscles. Magnetic resonance imaging has recently been shown to be effective in screening for breast cancer, particularly in younger patients and those at risk for breast cancer such as due to BRCA mutation. MRI may identify early breast cancers missed by mammography.

Mammographic findings strongly suggestive of breast cancer include a mass, often with speculated and invasive borders, or an architectural distortion, or an asymmetric increased tissue density when compared with prior studies or a corresponding area in the opposite breast (Figure 41–1).

An isolated cluster of tiny, irregular calcifications, especially if linear and wispy, is an important sign of breast cancer. Skin thickening is also an important prognostic indicator.

If a breast cancer is suspected, biopsy is warranted. A stereotactic biopsy may be used to localize and sample the lesion. This method employs a computerized, digital, three-dimensional view of the breast and allows the physician to direct the needle to the biopsy site. The procedure carries a 2% to 4% "miss rate." Needle-localization biopsies employ multiple mammographic views of the breast and allow the surgeon to localize the lesion for evaluation. The latter procedure is more time consuming, carries a comparable 3% to 5% miss rate, but excises more tissue, which is helpful in "borderline" histologic conditions, such as ductal carcinoma-in-situ.

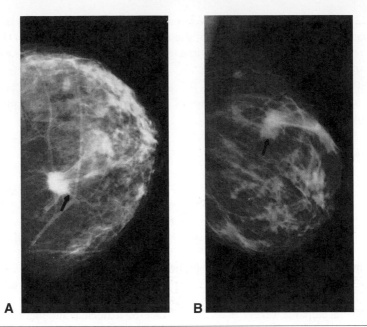

Figure 41–1.   Mammogram showing spiculated mass. Early intraductal carcinoma of the right breast. Craniocaudal (**A**) and oblique mediolateral (**B**) views of the right breast show a spiculated mass in the upper outer quadrant. *Reproduced with permission from Schwartz SI, Shires GT, Spencer FL, et al, eds. Principles of Surgery, 7th ed,. New York: McGraw-Hill, 1999, 545.*

Comprehension Questions

41.1   A 40-year-old woman undergoes a screening mammogram which reveals a lesion of the right breast, showing an ill-defined mass with a cluster of calcifications. She recalls bumping her right breast against a door knob leading to a bruise approximately 1 year previously. Which of the following is the most likely diagnosis?

A. Ductal carcinoma-in-situ

B. Infiltrating intraductal carcinoma

C. Fat necrosis

D. Lobular carcinoma

41.2   A 39-year-old woman physicist is referred by her physician for a screening mammogram. She asks about the amount of radiation exposure, and the cumulative risk of cancers due to the radiation. Which of the following describes the radiation risk with modern mammography given once annually?

A. Increased risk for thyroid cancer
B. No increased risks
C. Increased risk for lung cancer
D. Increased risk of skin cancer in the chest area

41.3   A 55-year-old woman has several coarse calcifications found on mammography that are suspicious for breast cancer. She has no family history of breast cancer and no mass is palpable. Which of the following is the most accurate statement?

A. The best diagnostic method for this patient is fine-needle aspiration.
B. The next best step is MRI of the lesion.
C. Since there is no palpable mass on physical examination, the patient may be observed for changes on mammography in 3 months.
D. One option for this patient is a core tissue biopsy by stereotactic means.

ANSWERS

41.1   **C.** Fat necrosis resulting from trauma to the breast often leads to mammographic findings that are identical to breast cancer. This patient recalls trauma to the breast in the location of the mammographic abnormality. To further evaluate the patient and confirm the diagnosis, a biopsy should be performed. Cancer is still a concern, and infiltrating intraductal carcinoma is the most common histological subtype.

41.2   **B.** Modern mammography has very low radiation and no increased risk of cancer.

41.3   **D.** Mammographic findings that are suspicious for cancer must be addressed. Two viable methods include core biopsy via stereotactic guidance and needle-localization excision. Fine-needle aspiration is not sensitive enough, and no mass is palpable to be able to serve for localizing. MRI does not add to an already suspicious lesion.

Clinical Pearls

➤ Mammographic findings suggestive of cancer include a small cluster of calcifications around a mass, or a mass with irregular borders.

➤ Stereotactic core biopsy or needle-localization excisional biopsy are two accepted methods of assessing suspicious, mammographic, nonpalpable masses.

➤ The amount of radiation from mammography is negligible and has no significant sequelae.

➤ Trauma to the breast may lead to fat necrosis and produce mammographic findings similar to that seen in breast cancer. These lesions should be excised to confirm the diagnosis.

REFERENCES

American College of Obstetrician and Gynecologists. Breast cancer screening. ACOG *Practice Bulletin 42*. April 2003.

Hacker NF, Friedlander ML. Breast disease: a gynecologic perspective. In: Hacker NF, Gambone JC, Hobel CJ, eds. *Essentials of Obstetrics and Gynecology*, 5th ed. Philadelphia, PA: Saunders; 2009:332-344.

Valea FA, Katz VL. Breast diseases. In: Katz VL, Lentz GM, Lobo RA, Gersenson DM, eds. *Comprehensive Gynecology*. 5th ed. St. Louis, MP: Mosby-Year Book; 2007:327-357.

Case 42

A 17-year-old nulliparous adolescent female complains that she has not yet started menstruating. She denies weight loss or excessive exercise. Each of her sisters achieved menarche by 13 years of age. The patient's mother recalls a doctor mentioning that her daughter had a missing right kidney on an abdominal x-ray film. On examination, she is 5 ft 6 in tall and weighs 140 lb. Her blood pressure is 110/60 mm Hg. Her thyroid gland is normal on palpation. She has Tanner stage IV breast development and female external genitalia. She has Tanner stage IV axillary and pubic hair. There are no skin lesions.

➤ What is the most likely diagnosis?

➤ What is the next step in diagnosis?

ANSWERS TO CASE 42:
Amenorrhea (Primary), Müllerian Agenesis

Summary: A 17-year-old nulliparous adolescent female, who may have only one kidney, presents with primary amenorrhea. She denies weight loss or excessive exercise. On examination, she is 5 ft 6 in tall and weighs 140 lb. Her blood pressure is 110/60 mm Hg. Her thyroid gland is normal. She has appropriate Tanner stage IV breast development, axillary and pubic hair, and female external genitalia.

➤ **Most likely diagnosis:** Müllerian (or vaginal) agenesis.

➤ **Next step in diagnosis:** Serum testosterone, or karyotype.

ANALYSIS

Objectives

1. Know the definition of primary amenorrhea, that is, no menses by age 16 years.
2. Know that the two most common causes of primary amenorrhea when there is normal breast development are müllerian agenesis and androgen insensitivity.
3. Understand that a serum testosterone level or karyotype would differentiate the two conditions.

Considerations

This 17-year-old adolescent female has never had a menstrual period; therefore, she has primary amenorrhea. She has **normal Tanner stage IV breast development**, as well as **normal axillary and pubic hair**. Breast development connotes the presence of estrogen, and axillary and pubic hair suggests the presence of androgens. She also has a history of only one kidney. The most likely diagnosis is müllerian agenesis, because a significant fraction of these patients will have a urinary tract abnormality. Also, with androgen insensitivity, there is typically scant axillary and pubic hair since there is a defective androgen receptor. The diagnosis can be confirmed with a serum testosterone, which would be normal in müllerian agenesis, and elevated (in the normal male range) in androgen insensitivity. A karyotype would also help to distinguish the two conditions. Notably, **absence of breast development** would point to a hypoestrogenic state such as **gonadal dysgenesis (Turner syndrome).**

APPROACH TO
Primary Amenorrhea

DEFINITIONS

PRIMARY AMENORRHEA: No menarche by the age of 16 years.

ANDROGEN INSENSITIVITY: An androgen receptor defect in which 46,XY individuals are phenotypically female with normal breast development.

MÜLLERIAN AGENESIS: Congenital absence of development of the uterus, cervix, and fallopian tubes in a 46,XX female, leading to primary amenorrhea.

CLINICAL APPROACH

When a young woman presents with primary amenorrhea, the differential diagnosis can be narrowed based on whether or not normal breast tissue is present, and whether a uterus is present or absent. After pregnancy is excluded, the two most common etiologies that cause primary amenorrhea associated with normal breast development and an absent uterus are androgen insensitivity syndrome and müllerian agenesis (Table 42–1).

An individual with androgen insensitivity syndrome, also known as testicular feminization, has a 46,XY karyotype with normally functioning male gonads that produce normal male levels of testosterone. However, due to a defect of the androgen receptor synthesis or action, there is no formation of

Table 42–1 MÜLLERIAN AGENESIS VERSUS ANDROGEN INSENSITIVITY		
	MÜLLERIAN AGENESIS	**ANDROGEN INSENSITIVITY**
Breast tissue	Normal breast development	Normal breast development
Axillary and pubic hair	Normal	Scant or absent
Uterus and vagina	Absent uterus and blind vagina	Absent uterus and blind vagina
Testosterone level	Normal testosterone	High testosterone (male range)
Karyotype	46,XX	46,XY
Complications	Renal anomalies	Need gonadectomy

male internal or external genitalia. The external genitalia remain female, as occurs in the absence of sex steroids. There are no internal female reproductive organs and the vagina is short or absent. Without androgenic opposition to the small circulating levels of estrogen secreted by the gonads and adrenals and produced by peripheral conversion of androstenedione, breast development is normal or enhanced. **Pubic and axillary hair is absent or scant due to defective androgen receptors.** Therefore, these individuals are genotypically male (46,XY karyotype) but phenotypically female (look like a woman). The abnormal intra-abdominal gonads are at increased risk for malignancy, but this rarely occurs before puberty. Thus, gonadectomy is not performed until after puberty is completed to allow full breast development and linear growth to occur. After these events take place, usually around age 16 to 18 years, the gonads should be removed. The diagnosis of **androgen insensitivity syndrome** should be suspected when a patient has **primary amenorrhea,** an **absent uterus, normal breast development,** and **scant or absent pubic and axillary hair.** The diagnosis can be confirmed with a karyotype evaluation and/or elevated testosterone levels (male normal range).

Women with müllerian agenesis have a 46,XX karyotype, have no uterus or fallopian tubes, and have a short or absent vagina. Externally, they resemble individuals with androgen insensitivity. They do, however, have normally functioning ovaries since the ovaries are not müllerian structures, and have normal breast development. They also have **normal pubic and axillary hair** growth because there is no defect in their androgen receptors. Congenital renal abnormalities occur in about one-third of these individuals. These women are genotypically male (46,XX) and phenotypically female. The diagnosis of müllerian agenesis should be suspected when a patient has primary amenorrhea, an absent uterus, normal breast development, and normal pubic and axillary hair. The presence of normal pubic and axillary hair is what differentiates them from individuals with androgen insensitivity syndrome, and laboratory confirmation can be accomplished with a karyotype examination and/or testosterone level.

Comprehension Questions

42.1   An 18-year-old nulliparous adolescent female complains of not having started her menses. Her breast development is Tanner stage V. She has a blind vaginal pouch and no cervix. Which of the following describes the most likely diagnosis?

A. Müllerian agenesis

B. Kallman syndrome

C. Gonadal dysgenesis

D. Polycystic ovarian syndrome

42.2 A 20-year-old G0 P0 woman is told by her doctor that there is a strong probability that her gonads will turn malignant. She has not had a menses yet. She has Tanner stage I breast development. Which of the following describes the most likely diagnosis?

A. Müllerian agenesis
B. Androgen insensitivity
C. Gonadal dysgenesis
D. Polycystic ovarian syndrome

42.3 A 19-year-old girl has primary amenorrhea, Tanner stage IV breast development, and a pelvic kidney. Which of the following describes the most likely diagnosis?

A. Müllerian agenesis
B. Androgen insensitivity
C. Gonadal dysgenesis
D. Polycystic ovarian syndrome

42.4 Which of the following is the best explanation for breast development in a patient with androgen insensitivity?

A. Gonadal production of estrogens
B. Adrenal production of estrogen
C. Breast tissue sensitivity to progesterone
D. Peripheral conversion of androgens
E. Autonomous production of breast-specific estrogen

42.5 A 15-year-old adolescent female is brought into the pediatrician due to absence of breast development and short stature. A karyotype is performed which reveals 46 XY. Which of the following is the most likely diagnosis?

A. Androgen insensitivity
C. Gonadal dysgenesis
B. Kallmann syndrome
C. Testicular atrophy syndrome

ANSWERS

42.1 **A.** Normal breast development, no cervix, and a blind vaginal pouch may be caused by either müllerian agenesis or androgen insensitivity. Kallman syndrome is associated with delayed puberty (Tanner stage I breasts).

42.2 **C.** The Y-chromosome gonad may become malignant. This patient likely has gonadal dysgenesis since she has Tanner stage I breast development. Although usually 45X is associated with gonadal dysgenesis, the karyotype can also be 46,XX or 46,XY. In other words, this patient has delayed puberty. This is XY gonodal dysgenesis.

42.3   **A.** A **pelvic kidney** most likely is associated with a **müllerian abnormality**. These women have no uterus or fallopian tubes, and have a short or absent vagina. They do, however, have **normally functioning ovaries** because the ovaries are not müllerian structures, and as a result they have normal breast development.

42.4   **D.** Individuals with androgen insensitivity usually have full breast development due to the **peripheral conversion of androgens to estrogens**. Also, because of the defective androgen receptor, the high endogenous androgens do not inhibit breast development as in a normal male, but **pubic and axillary hair is scant or absent.** The gonads and adrenals also produce a small circulating amount of estrogen, but do not contribute as much as the peripheral androgen conversion. Progesterone sensitivity does not influence breast development, nor does a breast-specific estrogen.

42.5   **C.** The most common cause of delayed puberty (**absent breast tissue** after age 14 years), is **gonadal dysgenesis**, which can also occur with a 46,XY karyotype (along with androgen insensitivity). The most common karyotype of gonadal dysgenesis, however, is **45,XO in Turner syndrome**. In androgen insensitivity, normal breast development occurs. **Kallmann syndrome** is an example of a hypogonadotropic hypogonadism, or hypothalamic hypogonadism, disorder caused by a deficiency in the gonadotropin-releasing hormone (GnRH) secreted by the hypothalamus (and therefore, decreased LH and FSH production). Gonadal dysgenesis, on the other hand, is a state of hypergonadotropic hypogonadism. Patients with Kallmann syndrome also typically have a **deficiency or inability to smell**. Females present with delayed puberty and lack of breast development, but have a normal karyotype (46,XX). Treatment is hormone replacement.

Clinical Pearls

➤ A pregnancy test should be the first test for any female with primary or secondary amenorrhea.
➤ The two most common causes of primary amenorrhea in a woman with normal breast development are androgen insensitivity and müllerian agenesis.
➤ Scant axillary and pubic hair suggest androgen insensitivity.
➤ A karyotype and testosterone level help to differentiate between müllerian agenesis and androgen insensitivity.
➤ Renal anomalies are common with müllerian abnormalities.

REFERENCES

Lobo RA. Primary and secondary amenorrhea and precocious puberty. In: Katz VL, Lentz GM, Lobo RA, Gersenson DM, eds. *Comprehensive Gynecology*. 5th ed. St. Louis, MO: Mosby-Year Book; 2007:933-960.

Pisarska MD, Alexander CJ, Azziz R, Buyalos RP. Puberty and disorders of pubertal development. In: Hacker NF, Gambone JC, Hobel CJ, eds. *Essentials of Obstetrics and Gynecology*, 5th ed. Philadelphia, PA: Saunders; 2009:345-354.

Case 43

A 23-year-old woman underwent a dilation and curettage (D and C) for an incomplete abortion 3 days previously. She complains of continued vaginal bleeding and lower abdominal cramping. Over the last 24 hours, she notes significant fever and chills. On examination, her temperature is 102.5°F (39.16°C), blood pressure (BP) 90/40 mm Hg, and heart rate (HR) 120 bpm. The cardiac examination reveals tachycardia and the lungs are clear. There is moderately severe lower abdominal tenderness. The pelvic examination shows the cervical os to be open to 1.5 cm, and there is uterine tenderness. The leukocyte count is 20,000/mm^3 and the hemoglobin level is 12 g/dL. The urinalysis shows 2 wbc/hpf.

➤ What is the most likely diagnosis?

➤ What is the next step in management?

ANSWERS TO CASE 43:

Abortion, Septic

Summary: A 23-year-old woman, who had undergone a D and C procedure 3 days ago for an incomplete abortion, complains of continued vaginal bleeding, lower abdominal cramping, and fever and chills. Her temperature is 102.5°F (39.16°C), BP 90/40 mm Hg, and HR 120 bpm. The lungs are clear. There is moderately severe lower abdominal tenderness. The cervix is open, and there is uterine tenderness. The laboratory studies are significant for leukocytosis and a normal urinalysis.

➤ **Most likely diagnosis:** Septic abortion (with retained products of conception).

➤ **Next step in management:** Broad-spectrum antibiotics followed by dilatation and curettage of the uterus.

ANALYSIS

Objectives

1. Understand the clinical presentation of septic abortion.
2. Know that the treatment of septic abortion involves both antibiotic therapy and uterine curettage.

Considerations

This 23-year-old woman underwent a D and C procedure for an incomplete abortion 3 days previously and now presents with lower abdominal cramping, vaginal bleeding, fever, and chills. The open cervical os, lower abdominal cramping, and vaginal bleeding suggest retained products of conception (POC). The retained POC may lead to ongoing bleeding or infection. In this case, the fever, chills, and leukocytosis point toward infection. The retained tissue serves as a nidus for infection. The most common source of the bacteria is the vagina, via an ascending infection. The best treatment is broad-spectrum antibiotics with anaerobic coverage and a uterine curettage. Usually, surgery is delayed until antimicrobial agents are infused for 4 hours to allow for tissue levels to increase. Hemorrhage may occur with the curettage procedure. Also, the patient should be monitored for septic shock.

APPROACH TO
Septic Abortion

DEFINITIONS

SEPTIC ABORTION: Any type of abortion associated with a uterine infection.

SEPTIC SHOCK: The septic portion refers to the presence of an infection (usually bacterial), and the shock describes a process whereby the patient's cells, organs, and/or tissues are not being sufficiently supplied with nutrients and/or oxygen.

CLINICAL APPROACH

Septic abortion occurs in less than 1% of all spontaneous abortions and about 0.5% of induced abortions. This risk is increased if an abortion is performed with nonsterile instrumentation. This condition is potentially fatal in 0.4 to 0.6/100,000 spontaneous abortions.

Signs and symptoms of septic abortion are uterine bleeding and/or spotting in the first trimester with clinical signs of infection. The mechanism is ascending infection from the vagina or cervix to the endometrium to myometrium to parametrium, and, eventually, the peritoneum. Affected women generally will have fever and leukocyte counts of greater than 10,500 cells/uL. There is usually lower abdominal tenderness, cervical motion tenderness, and a foul-smelling vaginal discharge. The infection is almost always polymicrobial, involving anaerobic streptococci, Bacteroides species, *Escherichia coli* and other gram-negative rods, and group B β-hemolytic streptococci. Rarely, *Clostridium perfringens*, *Hemophilus influenzae*, and *Campylobacter jejuni* may be isolated.

When patients present with signs and symptoms of septic abortion, a CBC with differential, urinalysis, and blood chemistries including electrolytes should be obtained. A specimen of cervical discharge should be sent for Gram stain, as well as for culture and sensitivity. If the patient appears seriously ill or is hypotensive, blood cultures, a chest x-ray, and blood coagulability studies should be done. The blood pressure, oxygen saturation, heart rate, and urine output should be monitored.

The **treatment** has four general parts: (1) **maintain the blood pressure;** (2) **monitor** the blood pressure, oxygenation, and urine output, (3) start **antibiotic therapy;** and (4) perform a **uterine curettage.** Immediate therapeutic steps include intravenous isotonic fluid replacement, especially in the face of hypotension. Concurrently, intravenous broad-spectrum antibiotics with particular attention to anaerobic coverage should be infused. The combination of gentamicin and clindamycin has a favorable response 95% of the time. Alternatives include β-lactam antimicrobials (cephalosporins and extended-spectrum penicillins) or those with β-lactamase inhibitors. Another regimen includes metronidazole plus ampicillin and an aminoglycoside. Because retained POC are common in these situations, becoming a nidus for infection to develop, evacuation of the uterine contents is important. Uterine curettage is usually performed approximately 4 hours after antibiotics are begun, allowing serum levels to be achieved.

Because oliguria is an early sign of septic shock, the urine output should be carefully observed. Also, for women in shock, a central venous pressure catheter may be warranted. Aggressive intravenous fluids are usually effective in maintaining the blood pressure; however, at times, vasopressor agents, such as a dopamine infusion, may be required. Other therapies include oxygen, digitalis, and steroids.

Comprehension Questions

43.1 A 34-year-old woman undergoes an elective termination of pregnancy at 12 weeks' gestation. She develops fever, uterine tenderness, and is diagnosed with a septic abortion. Which of the following is the most likely mechanism of her infection?

A. Instrumental contamination
B. Ascending infection
C. Skin organisms
D. Urinary tract penetration
E. Hematogenous infection

43.2 A 22-year-old woman is diagnosed with a septic abortion after an incomplete abortion, fever, and uterine tenderness. She is treated with triple IV antibiotics and D and C of the uterus. After 48 hours of antibiotic therapy, she still has a fever of 102°F (38.88°C), BP of 80/40 mm Hg, and HR of 105 bpm. A CT scan of the abdomen and pelvis is performed revealing pockets of air within the muscle of the uterus. Which of the following is the best treatment for this patient?

A. Add extended anaerobic coverage to the antibiotic regimen.
B. Add intravenous heparin to the regimen.
C. Continue the present antibiotic therapy.
D. Counsel the patient regarding need for hysterectomy.

43.3 A 32-year-old Hispanic female G1 P0 at 29 weeks' gestation presents to the obstetrical triage unit complaining of fever, chills, and nausea and vomiting of 3 days duration. She also has myalgias. She denies leakage of fluid per vagina and states that she has been in good health. She has not been out of the country for 2 years. Questions about dietary habits reveal that she does not eat raw or uncooked foods, does not eat raw shellfish, but she does eat a fair amount of soft goat cheese. Her temperature is 101°F (38.33°C), BP 100/80 mm Hg, HR 110 bpm. Her abdominal examination reveals tenderness of the uterine fundus. The fetal heart rate is 170 bpm. An ultrasound reveals a single gestation that is viable consistent with 29 weeks' gestational age, and a normal amniotic fluid volume. An amniocentesis is performed revealing green-ish dark fluid, and a Gram stain of the amniotic fluid shows gram-positive rods. Which of the following is the most likely diagnosis?

A. Group B streptococcus infection
B. Clostridial infection
C. *Listeria monocytogenes* infection
C. *Pasteurella multiforme* infection
D. Meconium-stained amniotic fluid with bacterial skin contaminant

ANSWERS

43.1 **B. Ascending infection** is the most likely mechanism of septic abortion. The bacteria involved are typically polymicrobial, particularly **anaerobes** that have ascended from the lower genital tract. Signs and symptoms include uterine bleeding and/or spotting in the first trimester with clinical signs of infection. There is usually lower abdominal tenderness, cervical motion tenderness, and a foul-smelling vaginal discharge. Also, careful attention should be given to the patient's **urine output** since oliguria is an early sign of septic shock.

43.2 **D.** This patient has a septic abortion which has been treated conventionally with IV antibiotics and D and C to remove the nidus of the infection. She is still febrile and hypotensive despite antibiotic therapy for 48 hours. Also, due to the pockets of gas noted on CT scan, she likely has a necrotizing metritis, with gas forming bacteria such as *Clostridial* species. Hysterectomy should be performed urgently as she may suffer severe morbidity or mortality if the procedure is delayed.

43.3 **C.** Chorioamnionitis, also called intra-amniotic infection, almost always complicates pregnancies with rupture of membranes. One exception to this rule is the gram-positive rod *Listeria monocytogenes*, which can be acquired through unpasteurized milk products such as soft goat cheese. The bacterial infection in the maternal gastrointestinal tract, which presents as a flu-like illness, then is spread hematogenously to the fetus, through the placenta. The diagnosis is largely from clinical suspicion and confirmed by amniocentesis. Often the amniotic fluid is meconium stained, and gram-positive rods may be seen on Gram stain. The microbiology laboratory should be alerted not to dismiss this finding as skin (bacteroid) contaminants. Treatment is with IV ampicillin. Many times the infection may be treated with antibiotic therapy and avoid delivery (again, an exception to the usual rule of needing to deliver the baby in chorioamnionitis). Listeria can also cause miscarriage and septic abortion.

Clinical Pearls

➤ The bacteria involved in septic abortion are usually polymicrobial, particularly anaerobes that have ascended from the lower genital tract.
➤ Hemorrhage often complicates the curettage for septic abortion.
➤ Treatment of septic abortion consists of maintaining blood pressure; monitoring the blood pressure, oxygenation, and urine output; antibiotics; and uterine evacuation.

REFERENCES

Katz VL. Spontaneous and recurrent abortion. In: Katz VL, Lentz GM, Lobo RA, Gersenson DM, eds. Comprehensive Gynecology. 5th ed. St. Louis, MO: Mosby-Year Book; 2007:359-387.
Lu MC, Williams III, J, Hobel CJ. Antepartum care: preconception and prenatal care, genetic evaluation and teratology, and antenatal fetal assessment. In: Hacker NF, Gambone JC, Hobel CJ, eds. Essentials of Obstetrics and Gynecology, 5th ed. Philadelphia, PA: Saunders; 2009:71-90.
Soper DE. Upper genital tract infections. In: Copeland LJ, Jarrell JF, eds. Textbook of Gynecology. 2nd ed. Philadelphia, PA: Saunders; 2000:795-797.

Case 44

A 29-year-old parous (G5 P4) woman at 39 weeks' gestation with preeclampsia delivers vaginally. Her prenatal course has been uncomplicated except for asymptomatic bacteriuria caused by *Escherichia coli* in the first trimester treated with oral cephalexin. She denies a family history of bleeding diathesis. After the placenta is delivered, there is appreciable vaginal bleeding estimated at 1000 cc.

➤ What is the most likely diagnosis?

➤ What is the next step in therapy?

ANSWERS TO CASE 44:

Postpartum Hemorrhage

Summary: A 29-year-old parous (G5 P4) woman at 39 weeks' gestation with preeclampsia delivers vaginally. She denies a family history of a bleeding diathesis. After the placenta is delivered, there is appreciable vaginal bleeding, estimated at 1000 cc.

➤ **Most likely diagnosis:** Uterine atony.

➤ **Next step in therapy:** Dilute intravenous oxytocin, and if this is ineffective, then intramuscular prostaglandin F_2-alpha or rectal misoprostal.

ANALYSIS

Objectives

1. Know the definition of postpartum hemorrhage.
2. Understand that the most common cause of postpartum hemorrhage is uterine atony.
3. Know the treatment for uterine atony, and the contraindications for the various agents.

Considerations

This 29-year-old woman delivers at 39 weeks' gestation and has an estimated blood loss of 1000 cc after the placenta delivers. This meets the definition of postpartum hemorrhage, which is a loss of 500 mL or more after a vaginal delivery. The most common etiology is uterine atony, in which the myometrium has not contracted to cut off the uterine spiral arteries that are supplying the placental bed. Uterine massage and dilute oxytocin are the first therapies. If these are ineffective, then prostaglandin F_2-alpha or rectal misoprostal is the next agent to be used in this patient. Because she is hypertensive, methylergonovine maleate (Methergine) is contraindicated. It should be noted that if the uterus is palpated and found to be firm and yet bleeding continues, a laceration to the genital tract should be suspected. Her risk factors for uterine atony include preeclampsia, since she is likely to be treated with magnesium sulfate.

APPROACH TO
Postpartum Hemorrhage

DEFINITIONS

POSTPARTUM HEMORRHAGE (PPH): Classically defined as greater than 500 mL blood loss at a vaginal delivery and greater than 1000 mL during a cesarean delivery. Practically speaking, it means significant bleeding that may result in hemodynamic instability if unabated.

UTERINE ATONY: Lack of myometrial contraction, clinically manifested by a boggy uterus.

METHYLERGONOVINE MALEATE (METHERGINE): An ergot alkyloid agent that induces myometrial contraction as a treatment of uterine atony, contraindicated in hypertension.

PROSTAGLANDIN F_2-ALPHA: A prostaglandin compound that causes smooth muscle contraction, contraindicated in asthmatic patients.

CLINICAL APPROACH

Postpartum hemorrhage is defined as early and late, according to whether it occurs within the first 24 hours or after that period. The most common cause of early PPH is uterine atony, with bleeding arising from the placental implantation site. (See Table 44–1 for risk factors.)

The physical examination reveals a boggy uterus. The initial management should be uterine massage, best accomplished by bimanual compression with an abdominal hand as well as vaginal hand. Concurrently, intravenous dilute oxytocin is given. If these maneuvers are ineffective, other pharmacological uterotonic agents may be given. These include intramuscular methylergonovine (Methergine), intramuscular prostaglandin F_2-alpha, and rectal misoprostol.

Table 44–1 RISK FACTORS FOR UTERINE ATONY
Magnesium sulfate
Oxytocin use during labor
Rapid labor and/or delivery
Overdistension of the uterus (macrosomia, multifetal pregnancy, hydramnios)
Intra-amniotic infection (chorioamnionitis)
Prolonged labor
High parity

Ergot alkyloids should not be given in women with hypertensive disease because of the risk of stroke. Prostaglandin F_2-alpha should not be administered in those with asthma due to the potential for bronchoconstriction. Among these three agents, rectal misoprostol has emerged in many centers as the preferred agent due to high efficacy, low cost, and low side effects. If medical therapy is ineffective, then two large-bore intravenous lines should be placed, the blood bank should be notified, and anesthesiologist alerted. Surgical therapy may include exploratory laparotomy, with interruption of the blood vessels to the uterus such as uterine artery ligation or internal iliac artery ligation. More recently, suture methods that attempt to compress the uterus, such as the B-lynch stitch, have been described. If these fail, then hysterectomy may be life-saving.

hypogastric

Other causes of early PPH include **genital tract lacerations,** which should be suspected with a **firm contracted uterus.** The vaginal side walls and cervix should be especially carefully inspected. Repair of the complete extent of the laceration is important. Uterine inversion, whether partial or complete, must also be considered. Placental causes include accreta or retained placenta. If the uterus is firm and there are no lacerations, one must also consider coagulopathy.

Late PPH, defined as occurring after the first 24 hours, may be caused by **subinvolution of the placental site,** usually occurring at 10 to 14 days after delivery. In this disorder, the eschar over the placental bed usually falls off and the lack of myometrial contraction at the site leads to bleeding. Classically, the patient will not have bleeding until about 2 weeks after delivery, and is not significantly anemic. Oral ergot alkyloid and careful follow-up is the standard treatment; other options include intravenous dilute oxytocin or intramuscular prostaglandin F_2-alpha compounds.

Another causative process is retained products of conception. Women with retained POC generally have uterine cramping and bleeding, and may have fever and/or foul-smelling lochia. Ultrasound examination helps to confirm the diagnosis. The treatment includes uterine curettage and broad-spectrum antibiotics.

Comprehension Questions

44.1 A 24-year-old G1 P0 woman at 39 weeks' gestation had induction of labor due to gestational hypertension. She was placed on magnesium sulfate for seizure prophylaxis. She was placed on oxytocin for 15 hours and reached a cervical dilation of 6 cm. After being at 6 cm dilation for 3 hours despite adequate uterine contractions as judged by 240 Montevideo units, she underwent a cesarean delivery. The baby was delivered without difficulty through a low-transverse incision. Upon delivery of the placenta, profuse bleeding was noted from the uterus, reaching 1500 mL. Which of the following is the most likely cause of hemorrhage in this patient?

    A. Uterine atony
    B. Uterine laceration
    C. Coagulopathy
    D. Uterine inversion
    E. Retained placenta

44.2 A 26-year-old G2 P1001 woman underwent a normal vaginal delivery. A viable 7 lb 4 oz male infant was delivered. The placenta delivered spontaneously. The obstetrician noted significant blood loss from the vagina, totaling approximately 700 mL. The uterine fundus appeared to be well contracted. Which of the following is the most common etiology for the bleeding in this patient?

    A. Retained placenta
    B. Genital tract laceration
    C. Uterine atony
    D. Coagulopathy
    E. Endometrial ulceration

44.3 A 32-year-old woman has severe postpartum hemorrhage that does not respond to medical therapy. The obstetrician states that surgical management is the best therapy. The patient desires future child bearing. Which of the following is most appropriate to achieve the therapeutic goals?

    A. Utero-ovarian ligament ligation
    B. Hypogastric artery ligation
    C. Supracervical hysterectomy
    D. Ligation of the external iliac artery
    E. Cervical cerclage

44.4　　A 34-year-old woman is noted to have significant uterine bleeding after a vaginal delivery complicated by placenta abruption. She is noted to be bleeding from multiple venipuncture sites. Which of the following is the best therapy?

A. Immediate hysterectomy
B. Packing of the uterus
C. Hypogastric artery ligation
D. Ligation of utero-ovarian ligaments
E. Correction of coagulopathy

ANSWERS

44.1　　**A.** Uterine atony is the most common cause of PPH, even after cesarean delivery. With a prolonged labor, such as with arrest of active phase, a patient is at risk for uterine atony. The finding of a boggy uterus would be indicative. Certainly, lacerations or injury to uterine vessels is a potential issue, and should be visible on examination. The treatment for uterine atony during cesarean is similar to a patient who underwent vaginal delivery, including intravenous dilute pitocin, prostaglandin compounds (such as intramuscular PG F_2-alpha or rectal misoprostol). If these measures are unsuccessful, then surgical management of uterine atony includes ligation of blood supply to the uterus to decrease the pulse pressure (suture ligation of the ascending branch of the uterine artery, or the utero-ovarian ligament, or internal iliac artery), or the B-lynch stitch to try to compress the uterus with external suture "netting." Sometimes hysterectomy needs to be performed due to unresponsive hemorrhage.

44.2　　**B.** Genital tract laceration is the most common cause of PPH in a well-contracted uterus. This is most likely arising from a cervical laceration, commonly laterally into or adjacent to the arterial supply of the cervix. Upon recognition of PPH, the physician should address the ABCs, assess the patient's blood pressure and HR, and have IV isotonic crystalloid infusing quickly. A second large-bore IV infusion should be started. The most common cause of PPH is uterine atony and so attention should be directed toward fundal massage and infusion of pitocin. If the fundus is firm and the uterus well contracted, the next step should be to assess for a genital tract laceration. Inspection for whether the bleeding is coming supracervical (uterus) versus cervical or lower in the genital tract is critical. Supracervical bleeding speaks for coagulopathy, retained POC, or atypical uterine atony. The cervix and then vagina should be carefully inspected for lacerations. Often, if the patient is in a regular labor and delivery room, moving the patient to the operating room with adequate lighting and anesthesia can be helpful. Blood products should be on hand if bleeding persists. At times a genital tract laceration may extend high into the vaginal fornix; careful assessment of the full extent of the laceration, and judicious surgical repair is warranted.

44.3   **B.** Ligation of the ascending branch of the uterine arteries or the internal iliac (hypogastric) artery are methods for decreasing the pulse pressure to the uterus and can help in PPH. Ligation of the cardinal ligaments leads to interruption of the uterine arteries, which usually means that a hysterectomy is necessary. Ligation of the external iliac artery would lead to lower extremity necrosis. A cervical cerclage is not a treatment option for hemorrhage; instead, it is a procedure performed in order to prevent preterm labor and delivery in a pregnant woman with an incompetent uterus.

44.4   **E.** Bleeding from multiple venipuncture sites together with abruption suggests a coagulopathy. This is a systemic response, so no type of localized treatment will fix the problem. A patient with disseminated intravascular coagulation (DIC) can present with a simultaneously occurring thrombotic and bleeding problem, which makes it difficult to choose a treatment option.

Clinical Pearls

➤ The most common cause of postpartum hemorrhage is uterine atony.
➤ The most common cause of early PPH with a firm, well-contracted uterus is a genital tract laceration.
➤ The most common cause of late postpartum hemorrhage (after the first 24 hours) is subinvolution of the uterus.
➤ Hypertensive disease is a contraindication for ergot alkyloids, and asthma is a contraindication for prostaglandin F_2-alpha.
➤ The evaluation and treatment of PPH should be systematic and efficient and involves two aspects: stabilization of the circulatory status, and addressing the hemorrhage.
➤ Stabilization of the patient begins by addressing the ABCs, assuring a second large-bore IV infusion of isotonic crystalloid, assuring availability of blood products if needed, and constantly monitoring key hemodynamic parameters (mental status, BP, HR, urinary output, bleeding, capillary refill).
➤ The systematic search for the etiology of PPH should begin with uterine atony, then genital tract lacerations with careful inspection to discern whether the bleeding is supracervical, cervical, or lower genital tract.

REFERENCES

American College of Obstetricians and Gynecologists. Postpartum hemorrhage. ACOG *Practice Bulletin 76*. Washington, DC: 2006.

Cunningham FG, Leveno KJ, Bloom SL, Hauth JC, Gilstrap LC III, Wenstrom KD. Obstetrical hemorrhage. In: *Williams Obstetrics*. 21st ed. New York, NY: McGraw-Hill; 2005:619-670.

Kim M, Hyashi RH, Gambone JC. Obstetrical hemorrhage and puerperal sepsis. In: Hacker NF, Gambone JC, Hobel CJ, eds. *Essentials of Obstetrics and Gynecology*, 5th ed. Philadelphia, PA: Saunders; 2009:128-138.

Case 45

A 16-year-old adolescent female is referred for never having menstruated. She is otherwise in good health. She has an older sister who experienced menarche at age 12 years. She denies excessive exercise or having an eating aversion. There is no family history of depression. On examination, she is 50 in tall and weighs 100 lb. The neck is supple and without masses. Her breasts appear to be Tanner stage I, and her pubic hair pattern is also consistent with Tanner stage I. Abdominal examination reveals no masses. The external genitalia are normal for a prepubescent female. A normal-appearing small cervix is seen on speculum examination. On bimanual examination, a small uterus and no adnexal masses are palpated.

➤ What is the most likely diagnosis?

➤ What is the next step in diagnosis?

ANSWERS TO CASE 45:
Pubertal Delay, Gonadal Dysgenesis

Summary: A healthy 16-year-old adolescent female is referred for never having menstruated. She denies excessive exercise or an eating aversion. On examination, she is 50 in tall and weighs 100 lb. The neck is supple and without masses. Her breasts and pubic hair are both Tanner stage I. The abdominal examination reveals no masses. The pelvic examination is consistent with a prepubescent female.

➤ **Most likely diagnosis:** Gonadal dysgenesis (Turner syndrome).

➤ **Next step in diagnosis:** Serum follicle-stimulating hormone (FSH).

ANALYSIS

Objectives

1. Know that absence of secondary sexual characteristics by age 14 years constitutes delayed puberty.
2. Know that the most common cause of sexually infantile delayed puberty, gonadal dysgenesis, is usually associated with a chromosomal abnormality.
3. Understand that the FSH level can help to determine whether the delayed puberty is due to a CNS problem or an ovarian problem.

Considerations

This 16-year-old adolescent female has never menstruated and, therefore, has primary amenorrhea. Furthermore, she has not yet experienced breast development (which should occur by age 14 years) and thus has delayed puberty. The lack of breast development means a lack of estrogen, which may be caused by either a central nervous system problem (low gonadotropin levels) or an ovarian problem (elevated gonadotropins). She is also of short stature, confirming the lack of estrogen. The absent pubic and axillary hair is consistent with delayed puberty. The most likely diagnosis without further information would be gonadal dysgenesis, such as Turner syndrome. An elevated FSH level would be confirmatory.

† Breast growth in androgen insensitivity

APPROACH TO
Pubertal Delay

See also Case 42.

DEFINITIONS

DELAYED PUBERTY: Lack of secondary sexual characteristics by age 14 years.

GONADAL DYSGENESIS: Failure of development of ovaries, usually associated with a karyotypic abnormality (such as 45,X) and often associated with streaked gonads. Less commonly, the karyotype may be 46,XX or 46,XY.

CLINICAL APPROACH

Maturation of the hypothalamic–pituitary–ovarian axis leads to the onset of puberty. There are four stages of pubertal development: (1) thelarche, (2) pubarche/adrenarche, (3) growth spurt, and (4) menarche. The first sign of puberty is the appearance of breast budding (thelarche), which occurs at a mean age of 10.8 years. This is followed by the appearance of pubic and axillary hair (pubarche/adrenarche), usually at 11 years. The growth spurt typically occurs 1 year after thelarche. The onset of menses (menarche) is the final event of puberty, occurring approximately 2.3 years after thelarche, at a mean age of 12.9 years. Normal puberty takes place between the ages of 8 to 14 years, with an average duration of 4.5 years. Delayed puberty is the absence of secondary sexual characteristics by age 14 years.

Thelarche → Adrenarche → Growth spurt → Menarche
Breast bud → Axillary and pubic hair → Menses

Delayed puberty can be subdivided based on two factors: the gonadotropic and the gonadal state. The FSH level defines the gonadotropic state. The ovarian production of estrogen refers to the gonadal state. The FSH level differentiates between brain and ovarian causes of delayed puberty. Central nervous system defects result in low FSH levels secondary to disruption of the hypothalamic–pituitary axis. With ovarian failure, the negative feedback of estrogen on the properly functioning hypothalamic–pituitary axis is not present, resulting in high FSH levels.

Hypergonadotropic hypogonadism (high FSH, low estrogen) is due to gonadal deficiency. The most common cause of this type of delayed puberty is Turner syndrome. These individuals have an abnormality in or absence of one of the X chromosomes leading to gonadal dysgenesis and a 45,X karyotype. They do not have true ovaries, but rather a fibrous band of tissue referred to as gonadal streaks. Thus, they lack ovarian estrogen production and, as a result, secondary sexual characteristics. The internal and external genitalia are that of a normal female, but remain infantile even into adult life. Other characteristic physical findings are short stature, webbed neck, shield chest, and increased carrying angle at the elbow. Turner syndrome should be suspected in an individual who presents with primary amenorrhea, prepubescent secondary sexual characteristics, and sexually infantile external genitalia. The definitive diagnosis can be made with an elevated FSH level and a karyotypic evaluation. Occasionally, the karyotype with gonadal dysgenesis may be 46,XX or 46,XY. When affected with 46,XY, the gonads should be removed surgically to avoid neoplastic changes. Other causes of hypergonadotropic hypogonadism are ovarian damage due to exposure to ionizing radiation, chemotherapy, inflammation, or torsion.

+ Kallman
= low
GnRH

Hypogonadotropic hypogonadism (low FSH, low estrogen) is usually secondary to a central defect. Hypothalamic dysfunction may occur due to poor nutrition or eating disorders (anorexia nervosa, bulimia), extremes in exercise, and chronic illness or stress. Other causes are primary hypothyroidism, Cushing syndrome, pituitary adenomas, and craniopharyngiomas (the most commonly associated neoplasm).

The diagnostic approach to delayed puberty begins with a meticulous history and physical examination. The history should query chronic illnesses, exercise and eating habits, and age at menarche of the patient's sisters and mother. The physical examination should search for signs of chronic illness, such as a goiter, or neurologic deficits, such as visual field defects indicative of cranial neoplasms. Skull imaging should be obtained to look for intracranial lesions. The laboratory evaluation should include serum measurements of FSH, prolactin, TSH, free T_4, and appropriate adrenal and gonadal steroids. A karyotype evaluation should be performed when the FSH level is elevated.

The management goals for those with delayed puberty are to initiate and sustain sexual maturation, prevent osteoporosis from hypoestrogenemia, and promote the full height potential. Hormonal therapy and human growth hormone can be used to achieve these objectives. Combination oral contraceptives provide the small amounts of estrogen needed to promote growth and development and the progestin protects against endometrial cancer.

Comprehension Questions

45.1 A 15-year-old adolescent female is diagnosed with gonadal dysgenesis based on delayed puberty, short stature, and elevated gonadotropin levels. Which of the following is generally present?

   A. Secondary amenorrhea
   B. 69,XXY karyotype
   C. Tanner stage IV breast development
   D. Osteoporosis
   E. Polycystic ovaries

45.2   A 15-year-old adolescent female is brought into the pediatrician's office due to no breast development. The patient's mother notes that both of patient's sisters had onset of breast development at age 10, and also all of her friends have already begun menstruating. Examination reveals Tanner stage I breast and pubic/axillary hair, and is otherwise unremarkable. Which of the following is the most likely diagnosis?
A. Delayed puberty
B. Development is within normal limits and should be observed
C. Primary amenorrhea
D. Likely craniopharyngioma

45.3   A 16-year-old adolescent female is evaluated for lack of pubertal development. She is diagnosed with gonadal dysgenesis. Which of the following laboratory findings is likely to be elevated in this patient?
A. Follicle-stimulating hormone levels
B. Estrogen levels
C. Progesterone levels
D. Prolactin levels
E. Thyroxine levels

45.4   A 20-year-old individual with a 46,XY karyotype is noted to be sexually infantile phenotypic female and diagnosed as having gonadal dysgenesis. Which of the following is the most important treatment for this patient?
A. Progestin therapy to reduce osteoporosis
B. Estrogen and androgen therapy to enhance height
C. Progesterone therapy to prevent endometrial cancer
D. Gonadectomy
E. Estrogen therapy to initiate breast development

ANSWERS

45.1   **D.** Breast tissue usually is infantile (**Tanner stage I**) with gonadal dysgenesis because no estrogen is produced; these patients are at risk for **osteoporosis**. Breast tissue is a reflection of endogenous estrogen. They have **primary amenorrhea**, and usually a **45,X karyotype**. They have **streak ovaries**, and not polycystic ovaries (PCOS). PCOS is a condition in which there is unopposed estrogen, high levels of circulating androgens, and no pubertal delay is typically present. The LH:FSH ratio is usually greater than 1.

45.2   **A. Delayed puberty** is defined as no secondary sexual characteristics by age 14 years. **Primary amenorrhea** is defined as no menarche by age 16 years. Although this patient is still within normal limits, an abbreviated work-up such as TSH, prolactin level, and possibly bone age x-rays may be ordered. The physical examination should be performed and if there are any stigmata of Turner syndrome, then FSH and karyotype should be pursued.

45.3   **A.** With gonadal dysgenesis, the **FSH level is elevated**. This distinguishes ovarian failure from a central nervous system dysfunction (central defect). The FSH level determines the gonadotropic state, and the ovarian estradiol level dictates the gonadal state. **Estrogen levels are low**; the progesterone, prolactin, and thyroxine levels remain unchanged.

45.4   **D.** The **Y chromosome predisposes intra-abdominal gonads to malignancy**. Even a mosaic karyotype, such as 46,XX/46,XY, would predispose to gonadal malignancy. Had the patient had a karyotype similar to that in Turner syndrome (45,X), another gonadal dysgenesis disorder, a gonadectomy on the streak ovaries, would not be indicated.

Clinical Pearls

➤ The most common cause of sexually infantile primary amenorrhea is gonadal dysgenesis.

➤ The most common karyotype associated with gonadal dysgenesis is 45,X, although 46,XX or 46,XY may be seen.

➤ Delayed puberty is defined as no development of secondary sexual characteristics by age 14 years.

➤ The FSH level distinguishes ovarian failure from central nervous system dysfunction.

➤ The FSH level determines the gonadotropic state, and the ovarian estradiol level dictates the gonadal state.

➤ The most important initial test for primary amenorrhea with normal breast development is a pregnancy test.

REFERENCES

DeUgarte CM, Buyalos RP, Laufer LR. Puberty and disorders of pubertal development. In: Hacker NF, Moore JG, Gambone JC, eds. *Essentials of Obstetrics and Gynecology.* 4th ed. Philadelphia, PA: Saunders; 2004:386-397.

Pisarska MD, Alexander CJ, Azziz R, Buyalos RP. Puberty and disorders of pubertal development. In: Hacker NF, Gambone JC, Hobel CJ, eds. *Essentials of Obstetrics and Gynecology,* 5th ed. Philadelphia, PA: Saunders; 2009:345-354.

Case 46

A 20-year-old parous woman complains of right breast pain and fever. She states that 3 weeks previously, she underwent a normal spontaneous vaginal delivery. She had been breast-feeding without difficulty until 2 days ago, when she noted progressive pain, induration, and redness to the right breast. On examination, her temperature is 102°F (38.8°C), blood pressure (BP) 100/70 mm Hg, and heart rate (HR) 110 beats per minute (bpm). Her neck is supple. Her right breast has induration on the upper outer region with redness and tenderness. There is also significant fluctuance noted in the breast tissue. The abdomen is nontender and there is no costovertebral angle tenderness. The pelvic examination is unremarkable.

➤ What is the most likely diagnosis?

➤ What is your next step in therapy?

➤ What is the etiology of the condition?

ANSWERS TO CASE 46:

Breast Abscess and Mastitis

Summary: A 20-year-old breast-feeding woman who is 3 weeks postpartum complains of right breast pain and fever of 2 days duration. She notes progressive pain, induration, and redness in the right breast. Her temperature is 102°F (38.8°C). There is also significant fluctuance noted in the right breast.

➤ **Most likely diagnosis:** Abscess of the right breast.

➤ **Next step in therapy:** Incision and drainage of the abscess and antibiotic therapy.

➤ **Etiology of the condition:** *Staphylococcus aureus*.

ANALYSIS

Objectives

1. Know the clinical presentation of postpartum mastitis.
2. Know that S *aureus* is the most common etiology in postpartum mastitis.
3. Understand that the presence of fluctuance in the breast probably represents an abscess that needs incision and drainage.

Considerations

This woman is 3 weeks postpartum with breast pain and fever. This is a typical presentation of a breast infection, since mastitis usually presents in the third or fourth postpartum week. Induration and redness of the breast accompanied by fever and chills are also consistent. The treatment for this condition is an antistaphylococcal agent, such as dicloxacillin. Provided that the offending agent is not methicillin resistant, improvement should be rapid. Affected women are instructed to continue to breast-feed or drain the breast by pump. This patient has fluctuance of the breast that speaks for an abscess, which usually requires surgical drainage and will not generally improve with antibiotics alone. If there is uncertainty about the diagnosis, ultrasound examination may be helpful in identifying a fluid collection.

APPROACH TO
Breast Infections

DEFINITIONS

MASTITIS: Infection of the breast parenchyma typically caused by S *aureus*.

BREAST ABSCESS: The presence of a collection of purulent material in the breast, which requires drainage.

GALACTOCELE: A noninfected collection of milk due to a blocked mammary duct leading to a palpable mass and symptoms of breast pressure and pain.

CLINICAL APPROACH

Postpartum breast disorders and infections are common. They include cracked nipples, breast engorgement, mastitis, breast abscesses, and galactoceles. Cracked nipples usually arise from dryness, and may be exacerbated by harsh soap or water-soluble lotions. Treatment includes air-drying the nipples, the use of a nipple shield, or the application of an oil-based lotion.

Breast engorgement is usually noted during the first week postpartum and is due to vascular congestion and milk accumulation. The patient will generally complain of breast pain and induration, and may have a low-grade fever. Infant feedings around-the-clock usually help to alleviate this condition. Fever seldom persists for more than 12 to 24 hours. Treatment consists of a breast binder, ice packs, and analgesics.

Postpartum mastitis is an infection of the breast parenchyma, affecting about 2% of lactating women. These infections usually occur between the second and fourth week after delivery. Other signs and symptoms include malaise, fever, chills, tachycardia, and a red, tender, swollen breast. Importantly, there should be no fluctuance of the breast, which would indicate abscess formation. The most commonly isolated organism is S *aureus*, usually arising from the infant's nose and throat. The treatment for mastitis should be prompt to prevent abscess formation, consisting of an antistaphylococcal agent, such as dicloxacillin. Breast-feeding should be continued to prevent the development of abscess.

About 1 in 10 cases of mastitis are complicated by abscess, which should be suspected with persistent fever after 48 hours of antibiotic therapy or the presence of a fluctuant mass. Ultrasound examination may be performed to confirm the diagnosis. The purulent collection is best treated by surgical drainage, or alternatively by ultrasound-guided aspiration; antistaphylococcal antibiotics should also be used.

The galactocele or milk-retention cyst is caused by blockage of a milk duct. The milk accumulates in one or more breast lobes, leading to a nonerythematous fluctuant mass. They usually resolve spontaneously, but may need aspiration.

Comprehension Questions

46.1   A 32-year-old woman has just delivered a 40-week baby vaginally. She desires to breast-feed. Her physician recommends that she not breast feed. Which of the following conditions is most likely to be present?
        A. Ampicillin therapy for cystitis
        B. Maternal dilantin therapy for seizure disorder
        C. Maternal HIV infection
        D. Maternal inverted nipples

46.2   A 22-year-old nulliparous woman is noted to have a tender, red, right breast and enlarged, tender axillary lymph nodes that have persisted despite antibiotics for 3 weeks. She denies manipulation of her breasts and is not lactating. Which of the following is the most appropriate next step?
        A. Course of oral antibiotic therapy
        B. Sonographic examination of the breasts
        C. Mammographic examination of the breasts
        D. Check the serum prolactin level
        E. Biopsy of the breast

46.3   A 28-year-old G1 P1 woman has delivered vaginally 3 weeks ago. She is breast-feeding, and notes that the baby prefers to breast-feed from the right breast. On the left breast, she notes a 3-day history of a tender mass on the upper outer quadrant. On examination, she is afebrile. The left breast has a fluctuant mass of 4 × 8 cm of the upper outer quadrant without redness. It is somewhat tender. Which of the following is the best treatment for this condition?
        A. Oral antibiotic therapy
        B. Oral antifungal therapy
        C. Bromocriptine therapy
        D. Aspiration
        E. Mastectomy

46.4.   A 29-year-old G1 P1 woman desires to breast-feed her infant, which
        is 1 day old. The infant received an injection of vitamin K. You coun-
        sel the patient on positive health consequences of breast-feeding
        including immunological, bonding, neurodevelopmental, and gas-
        trointestinal effects. Which of the following requires supplementation
        in the first 6 months as it is not present in breast milk?
        A. Iron
        B. Vitamin D
        C. Vitamin E
        D. Vitamin K

ANSWERS

46.1   **C. Maternal HIV infection is a contraindication for breast-feeding**
        because the neonate may contract the infection from infected breast
        milk. Dilantin and ampicillin are safe to take during pregnancy.
        Though challenging, women with inverted nipples are still able to
        breast-feed. There are very few contraindications to breast-feeding:
        infants with classic galactosemia (galactose 1-phosphate uridyltrans-
        ferase deficiency); mothers who have active untreated tuberculosis
        disease or HIV infection; mothers who are receiving diagnostic or
        therapeutic radioactive isotopes or have had exposure to radioactive
        materials; mothers who are receiving antimetabolites or chemother-
        apeutic agents or a small number of other medications until they
        clear the milk; mothers who are using drugs of abuse ("street drugs");
        and mothers who have herpes simplex lesions on a breast.

46.2   **E.** This woman has had persistent tenderness and redness of the breast
        despite not lactating and not having trauma to the breast; these symp-
        toms have worsened despite antibiotic therapy. There is a concern
        about inflammatory breast carcinoma, and she should undergo biopsy.
        ↳ more common is younger Pt. → get Bx

46.3   **D.** This patient has a galactocele. It is not an abscess since there is
        no fever or redness, although untreated, this could become an
        abscess. The best treatment of a **galactocele** (milk-retention cyst) is
        aspiration if it does not resolve spontaneously. This is done to pre-
        vent a breast abscess. A galactocele forms when a milk duct is
        blocked and the milk accumulates in one or more breast lobes, lead-
        ing to a nonerythematous fluctuant mass. It is not an infection,
        therefore antibiotics and antifungals are unnecessary; it is also not
        cancerous, so a mastectomy is not indicated. **Bromocriptine** is an
        ergot alkaloid that blocks the release of prolactin from the pituitary
        (typically in the setting of a prolactinoma), mostly as an attempt to
        allow a woman to be able to have normal menstrual cycles.

46.4   **B.** Vitamin D should be supplemented at 2 months of age. The
         American Academy of Pediatrics (AAP) recommends that unless
         contraindicated, each infant be breast-fed exclusively for the first
         6 months of life because of the health benefits to the baby. Breast-fed
         babies have less infections including meningitis, urinary tract infec-
         tions, and sepsis thought to be due to immunoglobulin and leukocytes
         in the breast milk. They have slightly better neurodevelopmental out-
         comes, and there is evidence of less risk of diabetes and childhood obe-
         sity in later life. Breast milk consists of two proteins, whey and casein,
         and has lower casein proportion than formula milk, allowing for easier
         digestion. Lactoferrin (inhibits certain iron-dependent bacteria of the
         GI tract), secretory IgA, and lysozyme (enzyme which protects against
         Escherichia coli and other bacteria) are found in breast milk. Fat and
         carbohydrate (lactose) is also found. All the vitamins are found in
         breast milk provided the mother's nutrition is sufficient, with the
         exception of vitamin D. The AAP recommends supplementation of
         vitamin D drops at 2 months of age for infants exclusively breast-fed.

Fe 6 mo!

Clinical Pearls

➤ The best treatment for postpartum mastitis is an oral antistaphylococcal
  antibiotic, such as dicloxacillin, and continued breast-feeding or pumping.
➤ The presence of fluctuance in a red, tender, indurated breast suggests
  abscess, which needs surgical drainage.
➤ The best treatment of cracked nipples is air-drying and the avoidance of
  using a harsh soap.
➤ Breast engorgement rarely causes high fever persisting more than 24 hours.

Infant: Vitamin Supplement	Breast Feed	Formula
	Vitamin K birth	Vitamin K @ birth
	400 iu/day D	400 iu/day
	Fe by 6 mo.	Fe by 4 mos.

REFERENCES

Cunningham FG, Leveno KJ, Bloom SL, Hauth JC, Gilstrap LC III, Wenstrom KD.
    The puerperium. In: *Williams Obstetrics*. 22nd ed. New York, NY: McGraw-Hill;
    2005:703-704.
Hobel CJ, Zakowski M. Normal labor, delivery, and postpartum care: anatomic con-
    siderations, obstetric and analgesia, and resuscitation of the newborn. In: Hacker
    NF, Gambone JC, Hobel CJ, eds. *Essentials of Obstetrics and Gynecology*, 5th ed.
    Philadelphia, PA: Saunders; 2009:91-118.

Case 47

An 18-year-old G2 P1 at 35 weeks' gestation has a history of Graves disease and is under treatment with oral propylthiouracil (PTU). She states that over the last day, she has been feeling as though her "heart is pounding." She also complains of nervousness, sweating, and diarrhea. On examination, her blood pressure (BP) is 150/110 mm Hg, heart rate (HR) 140 beats per minute (bpm), respiratory rate (RR) 25 breaths per minute, and temperature 100.8°F (38.2°C). The patient appears anxious, disoriented, and somewhat confused. The thyroid gland is mildly tender and enlarged. The cardiac examination reveals tachycardia with III/VI systolic murmur. The fetal heart rate tracing shows a baseline in the 160 bpm range without decelerations. Deep tendon reflexes are 4+ with clonus. Her leukocyte count is 20,000/mm³.

➤ What is the most likely diagnosis?

➤ What is the best management for this condition?

ANSWERS TO CASE 47:

Thyroid Storm in Pregnancy

Summary: An 18-year-old G2 P1 at 35 weeks' gestation is taking PTU for Graves disease. She has a 1-day history of palpitations, nervousness, sweating, and diarrhea. On examination, her blood pressure (BP) is 150/110 mm Hg, heart rate (HR) 140 beats per minute (bpm), respiratory rate (RR) 25 breaths per minute, and temperature 100.8°F (38.2°C). The patient appears anxious, disoriented, and somewhat confused. The thyroid is mildly tender and enlarged. Deep tendon reflexes are 4+ with clonus. She has a leukocytosis.

➤ **Most likely diagnosis:** Thyroid storm.

➤ **Best management for this condition:** A β-blocker (such as propranolol), corticosteroids, and PTU.

ANALYSIS

Objectives

1. Know that the most common cause of hyperthyroidism in the United States is Graves disease.
2. Recognize the clinical presentation and danger of thyroid storm.

Considerations

This 18-year-old woman at 35 weeks' gestation has a history of hyperthyroidism due to Graves disease. In the United States, the majority of hyperthyroidism is due to Graves disease; the clinical presentation is typically that of a painless, uniformly enlarged thyroid gland with occasional proptosis. She is being treated with propylthiouracil, which is the most commonly used medication for hyperthyroidism in pregnancy. For whatever reason, which is not stated, the patient has symptoms of increased thyrotoxicosis of 1-day duration. Some possible reasons include noncompliance with the medication, or a stressor, such as surgery or an illness. This woman not only has the nervousness and palpitations of hyperthyroidism, but also autonomic instability, which is the hallmark of thyroid storm. Her blood pressure is 150/110 mm Hg and her temperature is elevated. She is disoriented and markedly confused. Thyroid storm must be recognized because it carries a significant risk of mortality. The therapy consists of a β-blocking agent, such as propranolol, corticosteroids, and additional propylthiouracil. In the nonpregnant patient or a pregnant patient who is sufficiently ill, a saturated solution of potassium iodide (SSKI) oral drops may also be used; however, this agent may affect the fetal thyroid gland. Notably, the patient has a high white blood cell count.

This fact is important since rarely, PTU can induce a bone marrow aplasia, leading to leukopenia, and sepsis.

APPROACH TO
Thyrotoxicosis in Pregnancy

DEFINITIONS

HYPERTHYROIDISM: A syndrome caused by excess thyroid hormone, leading to nervousness, tachycardia, palpitations, weight loss, diarrhea, and heat intolerance.

THYROID STORM: Extreme thyrotoxicosis leading to central nervous system dysfunction (coma or delirium) and autonomic instability (hyperthermia, hypertension, or hypotension).

GRAVES DISEASE: The most common cause of thyrotoxicosis in the United States, leading to a diffusely enlarged goiter.

FREE THYROXINE (T_4): Unbound or biologically active thyroxine hormone.

THIONAMIDE ANTITHYROID MEDICATIONS: Propylthiouracil and methimazole (MMI) are the two thionamide medications are approved for use in the United States.

CLINICAL APPROACH

Hyperthyroidism is rare in pregnancy, occurring in about 1 in 2000 pregnancies. Symptoms of thyrotoxicosis include tachycardia, heat intolerance, nausea, weight loss or failure to gain weight despite adequate food intake, thyromegaly, thyroid bruit, tremor, exophthalmos, and systolic hypertension. The most common cause of hyperthyroidism in pregnancy is Graves disease, an autoimmune disorder in which antibodies are produced which mimic the function of TSH. These antibodies stimulate the thyroid gland to produce more thyroid hormone, leading to the symptoms responsible for thyrotoxicosis. The diagnosis of hyperthyroidism is confirmed in the presence of an elevated free thyroxine and low serum TSH levels. Treatment during pregnancy may be medical or surgical; however, generally, hyperthyroidism in pregnancy is managed medically. Propylthiouracil is generally accepted as the drug of choice in pregnancy. PTU inhibits the peripheral conversion of T_4 to T_3 but may cross the placenta somewhat. Methimazole is another option. Both PTU and MMI cross the placenta and can lead to some transient neonatal hypothyroidism. Because MMI has been possibly associated with aplasia cutis congenital (skin or scalp defects), PTU is usually the drug of choice in pregnancy. Radioactive iodine is contraindicated in pregnancy due to fetal effects.

should be antibodies

Methimazole => aplasia cutis

Thyroidectomy is reserved for those patients who are noncompliant with or cannot tolerate medical therapy. Risks from surgery include vocal cord paralysis and hypoparathyroidism.

Thyroid storm is a rare but life-threatening complication of hyperthyroidism. Symptoms suggestive of storm include **altered mental status, hyperthermia, hypertension, and diarrhea.** Congestive heart failure can result from the effects of thyroxine on the myocardium. Because the mortality rate associated with thyroid storm is high, accurate early identification is crucial. These patients are best monitored in an intensive care unit. Propylthiouracil is administered by mouth or nasogastric tube. β-Blockers are used to control the symptoms of tachycardia; however, they should be used with caution in those patients with congestive heart failure. Acetaminophen or cooling blankets are used for hyperthermia. Corticosteroids may also be used to prevent the peripheral conversion of T_4 to T_3.

Maternal hyperthyroidism may result in either fetal hyper or hypothyroidism. When identified antenatally, the fetus should be treated either with maternal administration of propylthiouracil or injection of intraamniotic thyroxine (fetal hypothyroidism). Failure to identify fetal thyrotoxicosis can result in nonimmune hydrops and fetal demise.

Recently, subclinical maternal hypothyroidism has gained interest, since this condition may be associated with adverse neurological development and childhood intelligence. There is some evidence that levothyroxine replacement in the first trimester may lead to better outcomes. Currently, there is no consensus on universal screening for maternal hypothyroidism; however those patients at increased risk or with symptoms should certainly undergo screening.

PTU + Synthroid ?

Comprehension Questions

47.1   A 25-year-old third-year medical student G1 P0 had been diagnosed with borderline hypothyroidism 4 years ago and has thyroid studies done annually. Last year, her thyroid panel was within normal limits. She is currently at 15 weeks' gestation, and has had a thyroid panel drawn today. Which of the following changes is likely to have occurred today as compared to last year's result?
A.   Elevation of TSH levels
B.   Elevation of total thyroxine levels
C.   Decrease in thyroid-binding globulin levels
D.   Decrease in free T_4 levels
E.   No effect on TSH or total thyroxine levels

47.2 A 15-year-old woman G1 P0 at 16 weeks' gestation complains of some intermittent palpitations, and feeling warm more often. Which of the following is the best screening test for hyperthyroidism?

A. Serum thyroid-stimulating hormone (TSH) levels
B. Serum thyroid-binding globulin levels
C. Serum antithyroid antibody levels
D. Serum total thyroxine levels
E. Serum transferrin levels

47.3 A 24-year-old woman delivered vaginally at term about 2 months previously. She was in good health until 1 week ago, when she began to complain of nervousness, tremulousness, and feeling warm. The TSH is 0.01 mIU/L (normal 0.5-5). Which of the following is the most likely diagnosis?

A. Graves disease
B. Destructive lymphocytic thyrotoxicosis
C. Multinodular thyrotoxicosis
D. Autonomous thyroid adenoma
E. Pheochromocytoma

47.4 A 23 year old G1 P0 woman at 16 weeks' gestation is suspected of hypothyroidism. Which of the following is most consistent with hypothyroidism in pregnancy?

	TSH	Free Thyroxine	Thyroid-Binding Globulin	Total Thyroxine
A.	Unchanged	Elevated	Decreased	Unchanged
B.	Decreased	Elevated	Unchanged	Decreased
C.	Increased	Decreased	Elevated	Unchanged
D.	Unchanged	Decreased	Decreased	Elevated
E.	Unchanged	Unchanged	Unchanged	Decreased

ANSWERS

47.1 **B.** Pregnancy due to the estrogen hormone causes **increases in the thyroid-binding globulin and total T_4,** but **does not change the active or free T_4 or the TSH.** In general, pregnancy is a euthyroid state.

47.2 **A. A TSH level is considered the best screening test for hyperthyroidism.** A low level suggests hyperthyroidism; an elevated level suggests hypothyroidism. The diagnosis of hyperthyroidism is confirmed by the presence of an elevated free T_4 level. Maternal hyperthyroidism may result in either fetal hyperthyroidism or hypothyroidism. Failure to identify fetal thyrotoxicosis can result in nonimmune hydrops and fetal demise. For this reason, it is important to screen women in their

[Handwritten annotations at top of page:]
Subacute Thyroiditis → Painful → Subacute granulomatous (de quervains) → post viral
→ Painless → often postpartum → lymphocytic

[Handwritten annotation in left margin:]
So in short-term
T4↑, destroy follicle

prenatal screen for TSH levels. If the TSH is borderline or a more definitive diagnosis is sought, then free T_4 is a good follow-up test.

47.3   **B.** Overall, the most common cause of hyperthyroidism in the United States is Graves disease. However, in the postpartum period, women with hyperthyroidism are more likely to have destructive lymphocytic thyroiditis. This is because the high corticosteroid levels in pregnancy suppress the autoimmune antibodies, and a flare occurs postpartum when the corticosteroid levels fall after the placenta delivers. Often, antimicrosomal and anti-peroxidase antibodies are present. Thus, the postpartum patient is unique in that the cause of hyperthyroidism is lymphocytic thyroiditis rather than Graves disease.

47.4   **C.** With **hypothyroidism**, the **TSH level is elevated** and the free T_4 is decreased. With hyperthyroidism, the TSH is decreased and the free T_4 is increased. Normally, with pregnancy, the only physiologic change is increased total T_4. With early or mild hypothyroidism, one may occasionally find the TSH level as normal (upper limits of normal) and free T_4 as low; however, the findings **most** consistent with hypothyroidism would be elevated TSH and low T_4.

Clinical Pearls

➤ Graves disease is the most common cause of hyperthyroidism in pregnancy. Thyroid storm should be considered when central nervous system dysfunction and autonomic instability are present. The treatments for thyroid storm in pregnancy include PTU, steroids, and β-blockers.

➤ Pregnancy (or use of estrogens) causes total thyroxine to be increased, free T_4 to be unchanged, TSH to be unchanged, and thyroid-binding globulin to be increased.

➤ Postpartum thyroiditis often occurs 1 to 4 months postpartum, is associated with antimicrosomal antibodies, and can lead to hypothyroidism.

➤ Maternal hypothyroidism that is untreated can lead to neonatal and childhood neurodevelopmental delays.

REFERENCES

American College of Obstetricians and Gynecologists. Subclinical hypothyroidism in pregnancy. ACOG *Committee Opinion 381*. Washington, DC: 2007.

Castro LC, Ognyemi D. Common medical and surgical conditions complicating pregnancy. In: Hacker NF, Gambone JC, Hobel CJ, eds. *Essentials of Obstetrics and Gynecology*, 5th ed. Philadelphia, PA: Saunders; 2009:191-218.

Cunningham FG, Leveno KJ, Bloom SL, Hauth JC, Gilstrap LC III, Wenstrom KD. Endocrine disorders. In: *Williams Obstetrics*. 22nd ed. New York, NY: McGraw-Hill; 2005:1189-1208.

Case 48

An 18-year-old G1 P0 at 22 weeks' gestation has a positive *Chlamydia* DNA assay of the endocervix. She denies vaginal discharge, lower abdominal pain, or fever. On examination, her blood pressure (BP) is 110/70 mm Hg, heart rate (HR) is 70 beats per minute (bpm), and she is afebrile. Her heart and lung examinations are normal. Her abdomen is nontender and gravid. The fundal height is 20 cm and fetal heart tones are in the 140 bpm range. The gonococcal culture is negative and the Pap smear result is normal. Her HIV test by enzyme-linked immunosorbent assay (ELISA) is also positive.

➤ What is your next step in therapy of the chlamydial test?

➤ What is the next diagnostic step for the positive HIV test?

➤ What is the optimal treatment for a pregnant woman who has an HIV infection?

ANSWERS TO CASE 48:
Chlamydial Cervicitis and HIV in Pregnancy

Summary: An 18-year-old G1 P0 at 22 weeks' gestation has a positive *Chlamydia* DNA assay of the endocervix. She denies lower abdominal pain and is afebrile. Her abdomen is nontender and gravid. The gonococcal culture is negative.

➤ **Next step in therapy:** Oral erythromycin, azithromycin, or amoxicillin. *(not doxycycline)*

➤ **Next diagnostic step for HIV:** Either Western blot confirmation, or PCR confirmation.

➤ **Optimal treatment of HIV infection in pregnancy:** Assessment of stage of HIV infection, initiation of highly active antiretroviral therapy (HAART), offer elective cesarean delivery, oral zidovudine to the neonate.

ANALYSIS

Objectives

1. Understand that *Chlamydia trachomatis* is a common cause of cervicitis.
2. Know that tetracyclines (doxycycline also) are contraindicated in pregnancy.
3. Know that chlamydial infections may lead to neonatal pneumonia or conjunctivitis if untreated.

Considerations

This 18-year-old nulliparous woman at 22 weeks' gestation has a positive DNA test for *Chlamydia*. These types of tests are often utilized because of their high sensitivity and specificity yet lower cost as compared with chlamydial cultures. This patient has a chlamydial infection, which is more common than gonorrheal involvement; accordingly, her gonorrheal culture was negative. Chlamydial endocervical infection has not been proven to cause adverse problems with pregnancy, such as preterm labor or preterm premature rupture of membranes. It has been implicated in neonatal conjunctivitis and pneumonia. Interestingly, the erythromycin eye ointment given at birth does not prevent chlamydial conjunctivitis, although it does protect against gonococcal eye infection. Babies with documented chlamydial ophthalmic infections are given oral erythromycin for 14 days. Because it is mainly neonatal disease that is the issue, an important time to screen for the organism would be the third trimester, close to the time of delivery. Treatment includes erythromycin or amoxicillin for 7 days or azithromycin as a one-time dose.

APPROACH TO
Cervicitis and HIV in Pregnancy

DEFINITIONS

CHLAMYDIAL NEONATE INFECTION: Conjunctivitis or pneumonia acquired by inoculation during the birth process.

TETRACYCLINE EFFECT: Tetracycline compounds, such as doxycycline, taken by pregnant women can lead to staining of the fetal teeth.

CLINICAL APPROACH

deciduous teeth develop at week 24 → dont use at 24 !

Chlamydia and Gonorrhea

Chlamydia trachomatis is an obligate intracellular organism with several serotypes. It is one of the most common sexually transmitted organisms in the United States, causing urethritis, mucopurulent cervicitis, and late postpartum endometritis. Vertical transmission may occur during the labor and delivery process, leading to neonatal conjunctivitis or pneumonia. It is unclear whether chlamydial infection of the cervix is associated with preterm labor or preterm rupture of membranes; thus, the main concern is for the neonate. Eye prophylaxis is effective for preventing gonococcal conjunctivitis but not chlamydial involvement. **Chlamydial conjunctivitis** is now the **most common cause of conjunctivitis** in the **first month of life**. Late postpartum endometritis, occurring 2 to 3 weeks after delivery, is associated with chlamydial disease.

Usually, chlamydial infections are asymptomatic, although they may cause mucopurulent cervicitis or urethritis. Some risk factors include unmarried status, age under 25, multiple sexual partners, and late or no prenatal care. The discharge is often difficult to detect because of the increased cervical mucus in pregnancy. Direct fluorescent antibody tests and DNA detection tests using polymerase chain reaction (PCR) are highly sensitive and specific, and less costly than culture. Treatment includes oral erythromycin, amoxicillin, or azithromycin. Tetracycline is contraindicated in pregnancy because of the possibility of staining of the neonatal teeth. Because reinfection is common, repeat testing is prudent in the third trimester.

Gonococcal infection may complicate pregnancy, especially in teens or those with a history of sexually transmitted disease. Gonococcal cervicitis is *GC - intracellular* associated with abortion, preterm labor, preterm premature rupture of membranes, chorioamnionitis, neonatal sepsis, and postpartum infection. Disseminated gonococcal disease is more common in the pregnant woman (especially the second or third trimesters), presenting as pustular skin lesions, arthralgias, and septic arthritis. Untreated gonococcal ophthalmia can progress to corneal scarring and blindness. *Chlamydia* commonly is present in a patient who is infected with gonorrhea. Thus, the usual treatment for gonococcal cervicitis is ceftriaxone intramuscularly and an additional antibiotic for *C trachomatis*, such as erythromycin.

HIV Infection

Heterosexual spread of HIV has surpassed intravenous drug use as the **most common mode of transmission in women.** This accounts for over half of recently acquired infections, and usually entails engaging in intercourse with high-risk individuals such as IV drug users. HIV infection leads to progressive debilitation of the immune system, rendering infected individuals susceptible to opportunistic infections and neoplasias that rarely afflict patients with intact immune systems. Furthermore, the unborn fetus may become infected either by transplacental passage or during the delivery process. The neonate may also acquire HIV from infected breast milk. Because measures in pregnancy, during delivery, and postpartum can dramatically **decrease the risk of vertical transmission** to the fetus, HIV serostatus should be obtained on every pregnant woman as early as possible in pregnancy and repeated at the time of labor or delivery. In fact, over the past 5 years, vertical transmission has dramatically decreased.

Initially, patients may either be asymptomatic or have symptoms that mimic a mononucleosis-like illness. Antibodies to the HIV virus are usually detectable 1 month after infection and are almost always detectable within 3 months. Studies have been unable to determine, with certainty, the effect of pregnancy on HIV disease progression. There continues to be correlation between maternal disease stage at the time of diagnosis with the viral load and transmission rates. When loads are reduced to undetectable levels, transmission to the fetus becomes uncommon. Viral load and CD4 T-cell testing are ways to monitor a woman's health status. In pregnancy, the viral load should be evaluated monthly until it is no longer detectable. The goal in pregnancy is to maintain a viral load under 1000 RNA copies per milliliter.

Treatment regimens, include polytherapy to decrease resistance and compliance is a must. Patients should have regular monitoring of liver function tests and blood counts to detect toxicity. Combination retroviral therapy decreases the risk of perinatal transmission to less than 2%. There is evidence that shows that route of delivery can further decrease vertical transmission. Scheduled cesarean delivery (prior to labor or rupture of membranes) should be discussed for HIV-positive women. Those HIV-infected women who choose to deliver vaginally should receive intravenous zidovudine (ZDV) during labor. Breast-feeding should be discouraged. The neonate generally also receives oral ZDV syrup.

Recently, the CDC has recommended that labor and delivery units consider the use of rapid HIV testing (results ready within 45 minutes) for those women with unknown HIV status, so that HIV infection can be identified and measures may be taken to reduce the risk of vertical transmission.

Comprehension Questions

48.1 Which of the following is a characteristic of chlamydial infection?
   A. Has a characteristic appearance on Gram stain
   B. Has a propensity for transitional and columnar epithelium
   C. Causes neonatal pneumonia, usually with a high fever and sepsis
   D. Is one of the leading causes of deafness worldwide

48.2 Which of the following statements is true regarding C *trachomatis* infections?
   A. The organism has a fairly rapid replication cycle, about 6 hours.
   B. Is an obligate intracellular organism.
   C. Erythromycin eyedrops are an effective means of preventing chlamydial conjunctivitis.
   D. Is associated with acute early endometritis.
   E. Is a cause of infectious arthritis.

48.3 A 28-year-old parous woman at 16 weeks' gestation is noted to have a positive *Chlamydia* assay of the endocervix. She is asymptomatic. Which of the following is an acceptable treatment?
   A. Intramuscular azithromycin
   B. Intramuscular ceftriaxone
   C. Oral amoxicillin
   D. Oral ciprofloxacin
   E. Oral doxycycline

48.4 A 18-year-old G1 P0 woman at 38 weeks' gestation comes into the obstetrical unit in active labor. She states that she is HIV infected, but had not received any medications or prenatal care. She is 5 cm dilated. Which of the following is the most appropriate step?
   A. Immediate cesarean delivery
   B. Intravenous acyclovir and allow labor
   C. Intravenous zidovudine and allow labor
   D. Rupture of membranes, placement of fetal scalp electrode, and uterine contraction monitor

48.5 A 27-year-old woman has been diagnosed with an HIV infection based on a positive ELISA and confirmed by the Western blot analysis. Which of the following is the most likely method that the patient became infected?

A. Exposure to infected blood via splash contamination
B. Heterosexual intercourse
C. Homosexual intercourse
D. Intravenous drug use
E. Renal dialysis center

ANSWERS

48.1 **B.** *Chlamydia* is not typically seen on Gram stain because it is an intracellular organism. It does have a propensity for columnar and transitional epithelium, and it is a leading cause of preventable blindness worldwide. It can cause neonatal pneumonia or conjunctivitis.

48.2 **B.** *Chlamydia* is an obligate intracellular organism associated with **late postpartum endometritis** and has a long replication cycle. Erythromycin eyedrops are an effective means of preventing gonococcal eye infection. Gonococcal cervicitis is more likely to disseminate during pregnancy, and a patient may present with septic arthritis, arthralgias, and pustular skin lesions.

48.3 **C.** Oral amoxicillin is well tolerated and effective treatment of chlamydial cervicitis in pregnancy. Oral azithromycin can be tolerated as well. Erythromycin estolate can lead to liver dysfunction in pregnancy; thus, the estolate salt is contraindicated in pregnant women. IM ceftriaxone is used to treat gonococcal cervicitis. Doxycycline, or tetracycline, is contraindicated in pregnancy because of the possibility of staining neonatal teeth. Ciprofloxacin is also contraindicated in pregnancy because it may lead to neonatal musculoskeletal problems.

48.4 **C.** Because labor has already begun, elective cesarean delivery will not affect vertical transmission. In other words, the cesarean would need to be performed prior to rupture of membranes or labor to effectively decrease vertical transmission. **Intravenous ZDV** and minimizing trauma to the baby, such as avoiding fetal scalp electrode or intrauterine pressure catheters or forceps or vacuum delivery, is advisable. Acyclovir is used to prevent viral shedding in patients infected with HSV. The neonate generally also receives oral ZDV syrup.

48.5 **B.** The most common method of HIV transmission to women in the United States is currently heterosexual intercourse.

Clinical Pearls

➤ The best treatments for chlamydial cervicitis in pregnancy are erythromycin, azithromycin, and amoxicillin.

➤ *Chlamydia* can cause conjunctivitis or pneumonia in the neonate.

➤ Ophthalmic antibiotics administered to the neonate help to prevent gonococcal disease but not chlamydial conjunctivitis.

REFERENCES

American College of Obstetricians and Gynecologists. Routine human immunodeficiency virus screening. *ACOG Committee Opinion 411*. Washington, DC: 2008.

Castro LC, Ognyemi D. Common medical and surgical conditions complicating pregnancy. In: Hacker NF, Gambone JC, Hobel CJ, eds. *Essentials of Obstetrics and Gynecology,* 5th ed. Philadelphia, PA: Saunders; 2009:191-218.

Cunningham FG, Leveno KJ, Bloom SL, Hauth JC, Gilstrap LC III, Wenstrom KD. Sexually transmitted diseases. In: *Williams Obstetrics.* 22nd ed. New York, NY:McGraw-Hill; 2005:1301-1325.

Gibbs RS, Sweet RI, Duff PW. Maternal and fetal infectious disorders. In: Creasy RK, Resnk R, Iams JD, eds. *Maternal Fetal Medicine.* 5th ed., Philadelphia, PA: Saunders; 2004:741-801.

Minkoff HL. Human immunodeficiency virus. In: Creasy RK, Resnik R, Iam JD, eds. *Maternal–Fetal Medicine.* 5th ed. Philadelphia, PA: Saunders 2004:803-813.

Case 49

A 24-year-old G2 P1 woman at 22 weeks' gestation complains of an episode of myalgias and low-grade fever 1 month ago. Her 2-year-old son had high fever and "red cheeks." On examination, her blood pressure (BP) is 110/60 mm Hg, heart rate (HR) 82 beats per minute (bpm), and she is afebrile. The heart and lung examinations are normal. The fundal height is 28 cm and fetal parts are difficult to palpate.

➤ What is the most likely diagnosis?

➤ What is the most likely mechanism?

ANSWERS TO CASE 49:
Parvovirus Infection in Pregnancy

Summary: A 24-year-old G2 P1 woman at 22 weeks' gestation complains of an episode of myalgias and low-grade fever 1 month ago. Her 2-year-old son had high fever and "red cheeks." The fundal height is 28 cm and fetal parts are difficult to palpate.

➤ **Most likely diagnosis:** Hydramnios, with probable fetal hydrops due to parvovirus B19 infection.

➤ **Most likely mechanism:** Fetal anemia due to neonatal parvovirus infection, which inhibits bone marrow erythrocyte production.

ANALYSIS

Objectives

1. Know the clinical presentation of parvovirus infection in children and adults.
2. Understand the possible effects of parvovirus B19 infection on pregnancy.
3. Know the clinical presentation of hydramnios.

Considerations

This 22-year-old woman presents with a history of myalgias and low-grade fever. Her 2-year-old son had "red cheeks" and a high fever. This illustrates the difference in the clinical presentation of parvovirus B19 infection in an adult versus that of a child. Adults rarely have high fever, but more often have malaise, arthralgias and myalgias, and a reticular (lacy) faint rash that comes and goes. Up to 20% of adults will have no symptoms. In contrast, children often develop the classic "slapped cheek" appearance and high fever, which is the manifestation of "fifth disease." Parvovirus infections in pregnancy may cause a fetal infection, which may lead to suppression of the erythrocyte precursors of the bone marrow. Severe fetal anemia may result, leading to fetal hydrops. One of the earliest signs of fetal hydrops is hydramnios, or excess amniotic fluid.

This patient's uterine size is greater than that predicted by her dates, and fetal parts are difficult to palpate, which are classic findings of hydramnios. An ultrasound examination would confirm the fetal and amniotic fluid effects. The diagnosis of parvovirus B19 infection is made by serology (see Table 49–1).

Mom Parvovirus B19 → Fetal Infection → Marrow Suppression → Fetal Anemia → Hydrops → Hydramnios

Table 49–1 PREGNANT PATIENT EXPOSED TO PARVOVIRUS B19

IgM	IgG	DIAGNOSIS	MANAGEMENT
Negative	Positive	Prior infection, immune	Reassurance
Negative	Negative	If more than incubation time (20 days) from exposure, then susceptible, not infected	Counsel about perhaps staying away from infected setting
Negative	Negative	If less than 20 days from exposure, then possible early infection* versus not infected	Repeat IgG and IgM in 1-2 weeks
Positive	Negative	Probable acute infection* but possible false-positive IgM.	Repeat IgG and IgM in 1-2 weeks, expect both to be positive indicating acute infection

*Once acute infection is diagnosed, then weekly ultrasounds assessing for hydrops.

APPROACH TO

Parvovirus Infection in Pregnancy

DEFINITIONS

FIFTH DISEASE: Illness caused by a single-stranded DNA virus, parvovirus B19, also known as erythema infectiosum.

FETAL HYDROPS: A serious condition of excess fluid in body cavities, such as ascites, skin edema, pericardial effusion, and/or pleural effusion.

HYDRAMNIOS (OR POLYHYDRAMNIOS): Excess amniotic fluid.

SINUSOIDAL HEART RATE PATTERN: A fetal heart rate pattern that resembles a sine wave with cycles of 3 to 5 per minute, indicative of severe fetal anemia or fetal asphyxia.

CLINICAL APPROACH

Parvovirus B19 infection is common, and up to 50% of adults have been infected during childhood or adolescence. It usually causes minimal or no symptoms in the adult, but may lead to devastating consequences for the fetus.

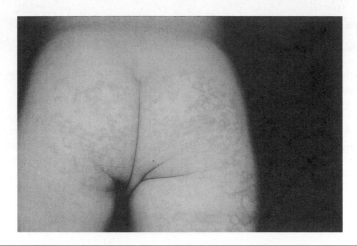

Figure 49-1.   Fifth disease. Lacy reticular rash of erythema infectiosum. *Reproduced, with permission, from Braunwad E et al. eds.* Harrison's Principles of Internal Medicine, *15th ed. New York: McGraw-Hill. 2001: 2416.*

A small, single-stranded DNA virus, parvovirus B19 causes a red "slapped cheek" appearance and fever in children; adults usually are less symptomatic and often have myalgias, and a characteristic lacy reticular rash, which comes and goes (Figure 49–1).

School-aged children are commonly affected, and frequently transmit the virus to adults. Specific IgM antibody confirms the diagnosis. Although there is no universal consensus about how to follow pregnant women who are infected with parvovirus B19, one commonly used strategy includes weekly fetal ultrasounds for 10 weeks assessing for fetal hydrops, and if found then referral for possible intrauterine transfusion. The virus may cause an aplastic anemia by destroying erythroid precursors.

Approximately half of pregnant women will have had parvovirus infection and be immune. IgG and IgM serology are helpful (see Table 49–1). Less than 5% of those susceptible pregnant women who are infected will have fetuses complicated by anemia. There is no vaccine available for parvovirus.

Parvovirus infection may lead to fetal abortion, stillbirth, and hydrops. Hydrops fetalis is defined as excess fluid located in two or more fetal body cavities, and many times is associated with hydramnios (see Table 49–2 for causes of hydramnios); pregnancies less than 20 weeks' gestation are at particular risk. Theories about the mechanism of the hydrops include the observation that the severe anemia may cause heart failure, or induction of the hematopoietic centers in the liver to replace normal liver tissue, leading to low serum protein. The anemia is usually transient. For severely affected fetuses, intrauterine transfusion is one option, while mild cases may sometimes be observed. Other causes of fetal anemia are isoimmunization, such as an Rh-negative woman who is sensitized to develop anti-D antibodies, a large

Table 49–2 CAUSES OF HYDRAMNIOS
Fetal central nervous system anomalies
Fetal gastrointestinal tract malformations
Fetal chromosomal abnormalities
Fetal nonimmune hydrops
Maternal diabetes
Isoimmunization
Multiple gestation
Syphilis

fetal-to-maternal hemorrhage, or thalassemia. An unusual fetal heart rate pattern, called a **sinusoidal pattern,** is associated with severe fetal anemia or asphyxia.

Comprehension Questions

49.1   A 24-year-old G1 P0 woman at 27 weeks' gestation is noted to have fetal size greater than dates. A fetal ultrasound performed reveals fetal hydrops. The fetal heart tones are in the range of 140 bpm. An umbilical venous blood sampling reveals a hemoglobin level of 9 g/dL, consistent with significant anemia. Which of the following is the most likely etiology?

A. Fetal cardiac tachyarrhythmia
B. Immune thrombocytopenia purpura
C. Rh isoimmunization
D. Intrauterine growth restriction
E. Gestational diabetes

49.2   A 32-year-old G2 P1 woman at 32 weeks' gestation is seen in consultation at the maternal fetal medicine center of a hospital. A diagnosis is made of severe fetal anemia, likely from a fetal bone marrow etiology. Which of the following is the most likely cause of the patient's condition?

A. Rh isoimmunization
B. Fifth disease
C. Anti-Duffy antibodies
D. HELLP (hemolysis elevated liver enzymes, low platelets) syndrome
E. Immune thrombocytopenia purpura

49.3   A 22-year-old schoolteacher at 28 weeks' gestation has a history of a
        faint rash and low-grade fever. She states that fifth disease is spreading
        in her school. Serology is obtained for parvovirus B19 revealing that
        the IgM is negative, and the IgG is negative. Which of the following
        statements is most accurate?
        A. This patient is immune to parvovirus B19 and does not need to be
           concerned.
        B. This patient is not infected with parvovirus B19, and is susceptible.
        C. This patient is infected with parvovirus B19 and is at risk for fetal
           hydrops.
        D. There is insufficient information to draw a conclusion about
           whether this patient is infected.

ANSWERS

49.1   **C.** Rh isoimmunization can lead to significant fetal anemia if the
        baby is Rh positive. With the use of Rhogam, this is a rare event
        today. Other causes of isoimmunization, such as anti-Kell disease, are
        still a concern. Fetal cardiac arrhythmias especially supraventricular
        tachycardia is associated with nonimmune hydrops, but does not
        affect the bone marrow. ITP is associated with maternal thrombocy-
        topenia, and rarely fetal thrombocytopenia. IUGR is usually associ-
        ated with polycythemia. Gestational diabetes does not typically
        affect the hemoglobin level.

First
Pregnancy?

49.2   **B.** With fifth disease, the bone marrow is affected leading to anemia
        (typically *aplastic* **anemia** which destroys erythroid precursors). **Rh**
        disease is caused by the mother's (Rh−) antibodies attaching the
        fetus' (Rh+) red blood cells and can cause hemolytic disease of the
        newborn, and in severe cases may lead to hydrops fetalis. Anti-Duffy
        antibodies can also cause hemolytic disease of the newborn in a sim-
        ilar fashion in which the mother's antibodies attack a particular anti-
        gen on the fetus' red blood cells. With **ITP in pregnancy**, antiplatelet
        antibodies may cross the placenta and cause fetal thrombocytopenia
        (can range from minor to severe). **HELLP** syndrome is a serious, pos-
        sibly deadly, complication of pregnancy; the only treatment is deliv-
        ery of the baby.

49.3   **D.** IgM and IgG serology is the most common method to diagnose
        acute fifth disease. Typically, in the acute setting, if the IgG is posi-
        tive and IgM is negative, it indicates that the patient has been
        exposed to parvovirus previously and is immune. When the IgG is
        negative and IgM is positive, then it usually means acute parvovirus
        infection; sometimes a false-positive IgM can occur, so the IgG and
        IgM are repeated in 2 to 3 weeks at which time the IgG should be

positive with a true infection. When the IgG and IgM are both negative, then the patient typically will not be infected and susceptible, provided sufficient time has elapsed past incubation period. In this case, the patient has some symptoms of parvovirus infection in a high-risk setting, so although both IgG and IgM are negative, it would be wise to repeat it in 1 to 2 weeks to ensure that the incubation period (up to 20 days) has elapsed.

Clinical Pearls

➤ Parvovirus infection in pregnancy can cause fetal anemia leading to hydrops fetalis.
➤ Hydramnios is one of the earliest manifestations of fetal hydrops.
➤ A parvovirus infection in the adult commonly leads to subtle findings of myalgias, malaise, and the reticular rash, whereas an infected child often has high fever and a "slapped cheek" appearance.
➤ Some causes of hydramnios include gestational diabetes, isoimmunization, syphilis, fetal cardiac arrhythmias, and fetal intestinal atresias.

REFERENCES

American College of Obstetricians and Gynecologists. Perinatal viral and parasitic infections. ACOG *Practice Bulletin 20*. Washington, DC: 2000.

Castro LC, Ognyemi D. Common medical and surgical conditions complicating pregnancy. In: Hacker NF, Gambone JC, Hobel CJ, eds. *Essentials of Obstetrics and Gynecology*, 5th ed. Philadelphia, PA: Saunders; 2009:191-218.

Cunningham FG, Leveno KJ, Bloom SL, Hauth JC, Gilstrap LC III, Wenstrom KD. Abnormalities of the fetal membranes and amniotic fluid. In: *Williams Obstetrics*. 22nd ed. New York, NY: McGraw-Hill; 2005:817-821.

Case 50

A 24-year-old G1 P1 woman underwent a low-transverse cesarean section 2 days ago for arrest of active phase of labor. She required oxytocin and an internal uterine pressure catheter. She reached and persisted at 6 cm dilation for 3 hours despite adequate uterine contractions as judged by 240 Montevideo units. Her baby weighed 8 lb 9 oz. The past medical and surgical histories were unremarkable. She denies a cough or dysuria. On examination, the temperature is 102°F (38.8°C), heart rate (HR) 80 beats per minute, blood pressure (BP) 120/70 mm Hg, and respiratory rate (RR) 12 breaths per minute. The breasts are nontender. The lungs are clear to auscultation. There is no costovertebral angle tenderness. The abdomen reveals that the skin incision is without erythema. The uterine fundus is firm, at the level of the umbilicus, and somewhat tender. No lower extremity cords are palpated.

➤ What is the most likely diagnosis?

➤ What is the most likely etiology of the condition?

➤ What is the best therapy for the condition?

ANSWERS TO CASE 50:
Postpartum Endomyometritis

Summary: A 24-year-old G1 P1 woman, who underwent a cesarean delivery 2 days previously for arrest of labor, has a fever of 102°F (38.8°C). She denies cough or dysuria. There are no abnormalities of the breasts, lungs, costovertebral region, or skin incision. The uterine fundus is somewhat tender.

➤ **Most likely diagnosis:** Endomyometritis.

➤ **Most likely etiology of the condition:** Ascending infection of vaginal organisms (anaerobic predominance but also gram-negative rods).

➤ **Best therapy for the condition:** Intravenous antibiotics with anaerobic coverage (eg, gentamicin and clindamycin).

ANALYSIS

Objectives

1. Know that the most common cause of fever for a woman who has undergone cesarean delivery is endomyometritis.
2. Know the mechanism of the endomyometritis, that is, ascending infection of "polymicrobial" vaginal organisms.
3. Know that the differential diagnosis of fever in the woman who has undergone cesarean delivery includes mastitis, wound infection, and pyelonephritis.

Considerations

This 24-year-old woman underwent cesarean delivery for arrest of dilation with adequate uterine contractions (see Case 6 for criteria). She presumably had a long labor, an intrauterine pressure catheter, and numerous vaginal examinations. These are all risk factors for the development of postpartum endomyometritis. On examination, she has a fever to 102°F (38.8°C). The scenario reveals that there are no abnormalities of the breasts, which rules out mastitis. The lungs are normal to auscultation, which speaks against atelectasis; in the obstetric patient, atelectasis is an uncommon cause of postoperative fever since the majority of cesarean deliveries are performed under regional anesthesia. This patient's wound appears normal. There is no costovertebral angle tenderness, so the likelihood of pyelonephritis is low. Urinary tract infections involving only the bladder do not usually cause fever. The uterus is only somewhat tender, which does not overtly point to endomyometritis. However, when the remainder of the examination does not reveal a focus, the majority of women who have fever after cesarean delivery have endomyometritis.

APPROACH TO
Fever After Cesarean Delivery

DEFINITIONS

FEBRILE MORBIDITY: Temperature after cesarean delivery equal to or greater than 100.4°F (38°C) taken on two occasions at least 6 hours apart, exclusive of the first 24 hours.

ENDOMYOMETRITIS: Infection of the decidua, myometrium, and, sometimes, the parametrial tissues.

SEPTIC PELVIC THROMBOPHLEBITIS: Bacterial infection of pelvic venous thrombi, usually involving the ovarian vein.

CLINICAL APPROACH

A woman who has febrile morbidity after cesarean delivery most likely has endomyometritis. The mechanism of infection is ascension of bacteria, a mixture of organisms from the normal vaginal flora. In other words, post-cesarean delivery infection is almost always "polymicrobial," with a mix of both aerobic and anaerobic bacteria. The uterine incision site, being devitalized and containing foreign material (ie, suture), is commonly the site for infection. Typically, the fever occurs on postoperative day 2. When intra-amniotic infection occurs during labor, the fever usually continues postpartum. The patient may complain of abdominal tenderness or a foul-smelling lochia. Uterine tenderness is common. **Broad-spectrum antimicrobial therapy** especially with **anaerobic coverage** is important. Intravenous gentamicin and clindamycin is a well-studied regimen and effective in 90% of cases. Other choices include extended penicillins or cephalosporins. In contrast to post-cesarean infection, endometritis after vaginal delivery does not necessarily require anaerobic antimicrobial coverage, and ampicillin and gentamicin are usually sufficient. Regardless of route of delivery, the fever usually improves significantly after 48 hours of antimicrobial therapy. Enterococcal infection may be one reason for nonresponse; ampicillin is the treatment for this organism and often is added if fever persists after 48 hours of therapy. If fever persists despite triple antibiotic therapy for 48 to 72 hours, then a CT scan of the abdomen and pelvis may reveal an abscess or infected hematoma.

Another cause of fever after cesarean delivery is wound infection. Prophylactic antibiotics given during surgery decrease the incidence. When a patient fails to respond to antibiotic therapy, wound infection is the most likely etiology. The fever usually occurs on postoperative day 4. Erythema or drainage may be present in the wound site. The organisms are often the same as those involved with endomyometritis. The treatment includes surgical opening of the wound (and

Table 50–1 APPROACH TO POSTPARTUM FEVER

Evaluate for pulmonary etiology: Cough? atelectasis?
Evaluate for pyelonephritis: Costovertebral angle tenderness? dysuria? pyuria?
Evaluate for breast engorgement: Are breasts engorged, tender, red?
Evaluate for wound infection: Is the wound indurated, erythematous? Is there drainage?
Evaluate for endometritis: Is the uterus tender? Foul-smelling lochia?
If endometritis, begin intravenous gentamicin and clindamycin.
If no response in 48 h, reevaluate and if endometritis is still considered, add
    ampicillin for enterococcus coverage.
If no response after 48 h of triple antibiotics, reevaluate (especially look for wound
    infection). Consider CT imaging to assess for abscess, hematoma, or septic pelvic
    thrombophlebitis.

dressing changes) and antimicrobial agents. The fascia must be inspected for integrity. Necrotizing fasciitis is a serious life-threatening infection that can affect the cesarean wound. Infections in the first 24 hours postoperatively can implicate group A streptococcus, "so called 'flesh eating bacteria." Immediate and extensive surgical debridement is indicated.

Septic pelvic thrombophlebitis (SPT) is a rare bacterial infection affecting thrombosed pelvic veins, usually the ovarian vessels. The bacterial infection at the placental implantation site spreads to the ovarian venous plexuses or to the common iliac veins, sometimes extending to the inferior vena cava. Women with SPT may have a hectic fever and look well, or sometimes have a palpable pelvic mass. The diagnosis may be confirmed by a CT scan or MRI. Treatment includes antimicrobial therapy and some practitioners will also use heparin therapy.

Other considerations in a febrile, postpartum woman should include pyelonephritis (fever, flank tenderness, leukocytes in the urine), pelvic abscess or infected pelvic hematoma, and breast engorgement (Table 50–1).

Comprehension Questions

50.1   A 30-year-old G1 P1 who underwent a cesarean section 3 days previously has a fever of 101°F (38.3°C). The skin incision is indurated, tender, and erythematous. Which of the following is the best management?

A. Initiation of intravenous ampicillin
B. Initiation of intravenous heparin
C. Placement of a warm compress on the wound
D. Opening of the wound

50.2   A 29-year-old woman is diagnosed with postpartum endometritis based on fever, abdominal pain, fundal tenderness, and elimination of other etiologies. Which of the following is the most significant risk factor for postpartum endomyometritis?
A. Numerous vaginal examinations
B. Bacterial vaginosis
C. Cesarean delivery
D. Internal uterine pressure monitors
E. Prolonged rupture of membranes

50.3   A 27-year-old woman G1 P0 at 39 weeks' gestation is noted to be in labor. She underwent artificial rupture of membranes, and experiences fetal bradycardia. Palpation of the vagina reveals a rope-like structure prolapsing through the cervix. She is diagnosed with a cord prolapse and underwent stat cesarean delivery. On postoperative day 2, the patient has a temperature of 102°F (38.8°C), and is diagnosed with endometritis. The patient who works in the microbiology laboratory asks which of the following is the most commonly isolated bacteria in her infection?
A. Bacteroides species
B. *Staphylococcus aureus*
C. Group B streptococcus
D. *Escherichia coli*

50.4   A 22-year-old woman who underwent cesarean delivery has persistent fever of 102°F (38.8°C), despite the use of triple antibiotic therapy (ampicillin, gentamicin, and clindamycin). The urinalysis, wound, breasts, and uterine fundus are normal on examination. A CT scan of the pelvis is suggestive of septic pelvic thrombophlebitis. Which of the following is the best therapy for this condition?
A. Hysterectomy
B. Discontinue antibiotic therapy and initiate intravenous heparin
C. Continue antibiotic therapy and begin intravenous heparin
D. Surgical embolectomy
E. Streptokinase therapy

ANSWERS

50.1   **D.** The best treatment of a wound infection is **opening of the wound**. Prophylactic antibiotics given during surgery decrease the likelihood of becoming infected. In addition to opening the wound, the patient should undergo dressing changes and be started on antimicrobial agents. The fascia must be inspected for integrity. In cesarean wound infections, there are two distinct populations of organisms that may be involved: skin organisms versus vaginal organisms. A Gram stain of the wound may direct toward the correct antibiotic regimen that would be effective for the possible bacteria.

50.2 **C. Cesarean delivery greatly increases the risk of endometritis** due to the fact that the patient most likely had prolonged rupture of membranes, numerous vaginal examinations, and an intrauterine pressure monitor due, for example, to an arrest of labor. Endometritis after vaginal delivery may occur as well, though less frequent, but does not necessarily require anaerobic antimicrobial coverage; therefore, ampicillin and gentamicin are usually sufficient.

50.3 **A. Anaerobic bacteria** are the most commonly isolated organisms in endomyometritis in patients who have undergone cesarean delivery. The most common of these species is *Bacteroides*. The other organisms listed are aerobes.

50.4 **C.** Although there is no universal agreement, the best treatment for septic pelvic thrombophlebitis seems to be the combination of antibiotics and heparin. There are some practitioners who believe that antibiotics alone are sufficient to treat SPT. Heparin alone is not effective. Hysterectomy is not indicated.

Clinical Pearls

➤ The most common cause of fever after cesarean delivery is endomyometritis.
➤ The major organisms responsible for postcesarean endomyometritis are anaerobic bacteria with the most commonly isolated organism bacteroides species.
➤ Atelectasis is rare in obstetric patients due to the large number of women who have regional anesthesia.
➤ When fever in a cesarean patient persists on triple antibiotic therapy, CT imaging should be performed.
➤ Antibiotic therapy and heparin are an accepted treatment for septic pelvic thrombophlebitis.

REFERENCES

Cunningham FG, Leveno KJ, Bloom SL, Hauth JC, Gilstrap LC III, Wenstrom KD. Puerperal infection. In: *Williams Obstetrics*. 22nd ed. New York, NY: McGraw-Hill; 2005:711-724.

Kim M, Hyashi RH, Gambone JC. Obstetrical hemorrhage and puerperal sepsis. In: Hacker NF, Gambone JC, Hobel CJ, eds. *Essentials of Obstetrics and Gynecology*, 5th ed. Philadelphia, PA: Saunders; 2009:128-138.

Case 51

A 31-year-old woman comes in for a well-woman examination. Her last menstrual period was 2 weeks ago. She has no significant past medical or surgical history. She denies having been treated for sexually transmitted diseases. On examination, her blood pressure (BP) is 130/70 mm Hg, heart rate (HR) 70 breaths per minute, and temperature is afebrile. Her thyroid is normal on palpation. Her heart and lung examinations are within normal limits. The abdomen is nontender and without masses. Examination of the external genitalia reveals a nontender, firm, ulcerated lesion approximately 1 cm in diameter, with raised borders and an indurated base located on the right labia majora. Bilateral inguinal lymph nodes are also noted that are nontender. Her pregnancy test is negative.

➤ What is the most likely diagnosis?

➤ What is your next step in diagnosis?

➤ What is the best therapy for this condition?

ANSWERS TO CASE 51:

Syphilitic Chancre

Summary: A 31-year-old woman who comes in for a well-woman examination is noted to have a nontender, firm, 1-cm ulcerated lesion of the vulva; it has raised borders and an indurated base. She also has bilateral, nontender inguinal lymphadenopathy.

➤ **Most likely diagnosis:** Syphilis (primary chancre).

➤ **Next step in diagnosis:** Syphilis serology (RPR or VDRL) and, if negative, darkfield microscopy.

➤ **Best therapy for this condition:** Intramuscular penicillin.

ANALYSIS

Objectives

1. Know the classic appearance and presentation of the chancre lesion of primary syphilis.
2. Know that penicillin is the treatment of choice for syphilis.
3. Understand that the antibody tests (VDRL or RPR) may not yet turn positive with early syphilitic disease and that darkfield microscopy would then be the diagnostic test of choice.

Considerations

This 31-year-old woman came in for a well-woman examination. It was unexpected to find the lesion in the vulvar area. The patient denies any history of sexually transmitted diseases. Nevertheless, she has the classic lesion of primary syphilis, the painless chancre. It is typically a nontender ulcer with clean-appearing edges, often accompanied by painless inguinal adenopathy. In practice, the next step would be serology to assess for a nontreponemal antibody test, such as the RPR or VDRL test. Occasionally, the patient will have a negative nontreponemal test, in which case the next step is scraping of the lesion for darkfield microscopy. Primary syphilis usually manifests itself within 2 to 6 weeks after inoculation. The treatment for syphilis that is less than 1-year duration is one set of injections of long-acting penicillin. If this patient were older, for instance, in her postmenopausal years, squamous cell carcinoma of the vulva would be considered. If the lesion were painful, herpes simplex virus would be the most common diagnosis.

APPROACH TO
Infectious Vulvar Ulcers

DEFINITIONS

NONTREPONEMAL TESTS: Nonspecific antitreponemal antibody test, such as the Venereal Disease Research Laboratory (VDRL) or rapid plasma reagin (RPR) tests. These titers will fall with effective treatment.

SPECIFIC SEROLOGIC TESTS: Antibody tests that are directed against the treponemal organism such as the MHA-TP (micro-hemagglutinin antibody against *Treponema pallidum*) and FTA-ABS (fluorescent-labeled treponemal antibody absorption) tests. These tests will remain **positive for life** after infection.

CLINICAL APPROACH

The **two most common infectious causes of vulvar ulcers** in the United States are **herpes simplex virus and syphilis,** with chancroid much less common. (See Figure 51–1 for an assessment algorithm.)

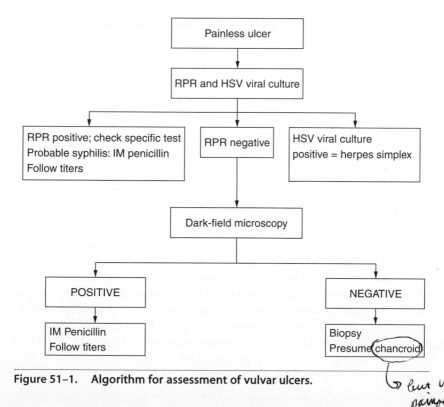

Figure 51–1.   Algorithm for assessment of vulvar ulcers.

⤷ *but usually painful, right?*

Herpes Simplex Virus

Genital herpes is a recurrent sexually transmitted infection (STI) for which there is no cure. It is the most prevalent STI in the United States. This organism is highly contagious, and it is thought that 20% of women in their childbearing years are infected. There are two types of herpes viruses, HSV type 1 and type 2. Type 1 usually causes infections in the oral region, and type 2 in the genital region, however, cross-infection may occur. Recurrence is greater with HSV type 2. The primary episode is usually a systemic as well as local disease, with the woman often complaining of fever or general malaise. Local infection typically induces paresthesias before vesicles erupt on a red base. After the primary episode, the recurrent disease is local, with less severe symptoms. The recurrent herpes ulcers are small and superficial, and do not usually scar. The best diagnostic test is viral culture. Rarely, the infections may be severe enough to warrant hospitalization, such as with encephalopathy or urinary retention. Treatment for immunosuppressed individuals often requires intravenous acyclovir therapy; oral acyclovir is effective in suppressing frequent recurrences.

Syphilis

Syphilis, caused by the bacteria *T pallidum*, may induce a chronic infection. The organism is extremely tightly wound, and too thin to be seen on light microscopy. The typical incubation period is 10 to 90 days. The disease can be divided into **primary, secondary, latent, and tertiary stages. Primary** syphilis classically presents as the **indurated, nontender chancre.** The ulcer usually arises 3 weeks after exposure and disappears spontaneously after 2 to 6 weeks without therapy. Nontreponemal tests (such as the RPR or VDRL) sometimes do not become positive with the appearance of the chancre; if the serology is negative in the face of a painless ulcer, then **darkfield** microscopy is an accepted diagnostic step. Another option is biopsy of the lesion with special stains for syphilis.

Secondary syphilis usually is systemic, occurring about 9 weeks after the primary chancre. The classic macular papular rash may occur anywhere on the body, but usually on the palms and soles of the feet, or the flat moist lesion of condylomata lata on the vulva may be seen (Figure 51–2). These lesions have a high concentration of spirochetes.

Latency of varying duration occurs after secondary disease; latency is subdivided into **early latent** (<1 year in duration), or **late latent** (>1 year). If untreated, about one-third of women may proceed into tertiary syphilis, which may affect the cardiovascular system or central nervous system. Optic atrophy, tabes dorsalis, and aortic aneurysms are some of the manifestations. Penicillin is the treatment of choice for syphilis. Because of the long replication time, prolonged therapy is required. For example, a long-acting penicillin, benzathine penicillin G, is often used. **One injection** of penicillin 2.4 million units intramuscularly is standard treatment for early disease (primary, secondary, and latent up to 1 year of duration). Patients with late-latent syphilis (>1 year) should be treated with a total of 7.2 million units intramuscularly

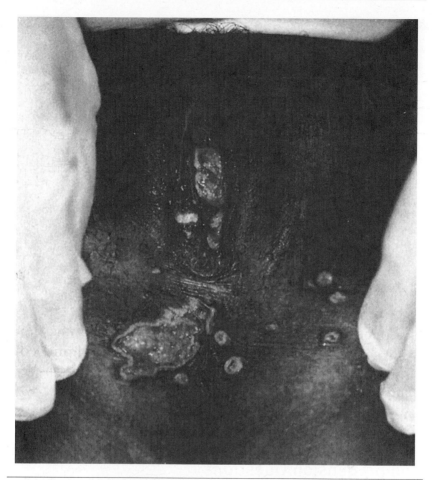

Figure 51–2.   Genital condyloma lata of secondary syphilis. *Reproduced with permission from Cunningham FG, et al. Williams Obstetrics, 21st ed. New York: McGraw-Hill, 2001:1487.*

divided as 2.4 million units every week for a total of three courses. For women allergic to penicillin, oral erythromycin or doxycycline may be used (Table 51–1). In pregnancy, penicillin is the only known effective treatment to prevent congenital syphilis.

Neurosyphilis requires more intensive therapy, usually intravenous penicillin in the hospital.

After therapy, the nontreponemal test is followed quantitatively every 3 months for at least 1 year. An appropriate response is a four-fold fall in titers in 3 months, and a negative titer in 1 year. When the titer does not fall appropriately, one possible etiology is neurosyphilis, which may be diagnosed by lumbar puncture.

Table 51–1 TREATMENT OF SYPHILIS

DURATION	TREATMENT
Primary, secondary, early latent (<1 year)	Penicillin 2.4 million units IM
Late latent (>1 year) or unknown duration	Penicillin 2.4 million units IM every week × 3 doses
Neurosyphilis	IV Penicillin × 4-6 doses

Data from the CDC 2002 Guidelines for treatment of sexually transmitted diseases.

[handwritten notes: "Sex", "Mom → Baby", "early or Late"]

Chancroid

Chancroid is a sexually transmitted disease, usually manifesting a soft, tender ulcer of the vulva. Although common worldwide, it is very rare in the United States. It is more common in males than in females. The typical ulcer is tender, with ragged edges on a necrotic base. Tender lymphadenopathy may also coexist with these infections. The etiologic organism is *Haemophilus ducreyi*, a small gram-negative rod. Gram stain usually reveals the classic "school of fish." After ruling out syphilis and herpes, chancroid should be suspected. Biopsy and/or culture help to establish the diagnosis. Treatment includes oral azithromycin or intramuscular ceftriaxone.

Comprehension Questions

51.1 A 19-year-old woman is noted to have a RPR titer of 1:16, and the confirmatory (MHA-TP) test is positive. She had no history of syphilis. She is treated with benzathine penicillin 2.4 million units intramuscularly. Three months after therapy, she is noted to have an RPR titer of 1:2. The next month (4 months after treatment), the titer is 1:1. Two months later, 6 months after treatment, the repeat RPR is noted be 1:32. Which of the following is the most likely diagnosis?

A. Resistant organism
B. Inadequately treated syphilis
C. Laboratory error
D. Reinfection
E. Systemic lupus erythematosus

51.2   Which of the following statements about *T pallidum* is correct?
    A. It is a protozoan.
    B. Gram stain is a very sensitive method of diagnosis.
    C. It causes neonatal disease mainly by direct inoculation of the baby by the genital lesion.
    D. Alternative treatments include doxycycline and erythromycin.

51.3   An 18-year-old G1 P0 at 14 weeks' gestation is noted to have a positive RPR with a positive confirmatory MHA-TP test. The patient states that she is allergic to penicillin, with hives and swelling of the tongue and throat in the past. Which of the following is the most appropriate next step?
    A. Desensitize and treat with penicillin
    B. Oral erythromycin
    C. Oral doxycycline
    D. Pretreat with prednisone, then administer penicillin
    E. Intramuscular ceftriaxone

51.4   A 29-year-old woman was diagnosed with syphilis. She is noted to have a persistently elevated RPR titer of 1:32, despite treatment with benzathine penicillin 2.4 million units each week for a total of 3 weeks. She complains of slight dizziness and a clumsy gait of 6 months duration. Which of the following is the best test to diagnose neurosyphilis?
    A. Plain x-ray films of the skull
    B. Electroencephalograph (EEG)
    C. CT scan of the head
    D. Lumbar puncture
    E. Psychiatric evaluation

ANSWERS

51.1   **D.** When RPR titers fall abruptly to therapy and then suddenly rise, the most likely scenario is **reinfection**. It is common, however, for individuals with systemic lupus erythematosus to have a positive RPR, but they would not show the fluctuations in the titer as with this scenario. Syphilis has not been noted to become resistant to penicillin.

51.2   **D.** Alternatives to treatment for patients allergic to penicillin include erythromycin and doxycycline. Syphilis is a spirochete and not a protozoan. It is very thin and tightly wound and therefore not visible on light microscopy.

51.3   **A. Penicillin is the best treatment of syphilis in pregnancy.** When a pregnant woman with syphilis is allergic to penicillin, she should undergo desensitization and receive penicillin. Penicillin is the only known effective treatment for preventing congenital syphilis.

Doxycycline use may lead to discoloration of the child's teeth, and erythromycin has not been shown to be an effective treatment in treating an infected fetus.

51.4   **D.** Typically, after a patient undergoes therapy for syphilis their RPR titer does not fall appropriately, one possible etiology is **neurosyphilis**, which may be diagnosed by lumbar puncture. The classic examination of neurosyphilis is unsteady balance and Argyll Robertson pupils. Cerebrospinal fluid for RPR may point toward neurosyphilis, although there is no definitive test. Neurosyphilis requires more intensive therapy such as IV penicillin in the hospital.

Clinical Pearls

> Syphilis of less than 1 years' duration can be treated with a single intramuscular course of penicillin; infection of greater than 1 years' duration is treated by three courses of penicillin at 1-week intervals.
> The nontender ulcer with indurated edges is typical for the chancre lesion of primary syphilis. If serology is negative, then darkfield examination warranted.
> The best treatment for syphilis in pregnancy is penicillin.
> Pregnant women with syphilis and an allergy to penicillin should undergo penicillin desensitization and then receive penicillin.
> The three most common infectious vulvar ulcers in the United States are herpes simplex virus and syphilis, and much less common is chancroid.

REFERENCES

Centers for Disease Control and Prevention. 2006 Guidelines for treatment of sexually transmitted diseases. 2006;55(RR11).

Eckert LO, Lentz GM. Infections of the lower genital tract. In: Katz VL, Lentz GM, Lobo RA, Gersenson DM, eds. *Comprehensive Gynecology*. 5th ed. St. Louis, MO: Mosby-Year Book; 2007:569-606.

McGregor JA, Lench JB. Vulvovaginitis, sexually transmitted infections, and pelvic inflammatory disease. sepsis. In: Hacker NF, Gambone JC, Hobel CJ, eds. *Essentials of Obstetrics and Gynecology*, 5th ed. Philadelphia, PA: Saunders; 2009:265-275.

Case 52

A 24-year-old woman G2 P1 at 30 weeks' gestation was admitted to the hospital 2 days ago for premature rupture of membranes. Her antenatal history has been unremarkable. Today, she states that her baby is moving normally and she denies any fever or chills. Her past medical and surgical histories are unremarkable. On examination, her temperature is 100.8°F (38.2°C), blood pressure (BP) 100/60 mm Hg, and heart rate (HR) 90 beats per minute. Her lungs are clear to auscultation. No costovertebral angle tenderness is found. The uterine fundal height is 30 cm and the uterus is slightly tender. No lower extremity cords are palpated. The fetal heart tones are persistently in the 170 to 175 bpm range without decelerations.

➤ What is the most likely diagnosis?

➤ What is the best management for this patient?

➤ What is the most likely etiology of this condition?

ANSWERS TO CASE 52:
Intra-amniotic Infection

Summary: A 24-year-old G2 P1 woman at 30 weeks' gestation was admitted 2 days ago for premature rupture of membranes. Her temperature is 100.8°F (38.2°C). The uterine fundus is slightly tender. There is persistent fetal tachycardia in the 170 to 175 bpm range.

➤ **Most likely diagnosis:** Intra-amniotic infection (chorioamnionitis).

➤ **Best management for this patient:** Intravenous antibiotics (ampicillin and gentamicin) and induction of labor.

➤ **Etiology of this condition:** Ascending infection from vaginal organisms.

ANALYSIS

Objectives

1. Know that infection and labor are the two most common acute complications of preterm premature rupture of membranes.
2. Know the clinical presentation of intra-amniotic infection, and that fetal tachycardia is an early sign of this infection.
3. Understand that broad-spectrum antibiotic therapy and delivery are the appropriate treatment of intra-amniotic infection.

Considerations

This 24-year-old woman at 30 weeks' gestation has preterm premature rupture of membranes. Upon presentation to the hospital, the practitioner should assess for infection; in the absence of signs of infection, corticosteroid therapy should be administered to reduce the risk of respiratory distress syndrome (RDS). Additionally, broad-spectrum antibiotic therapy is given to help reduce the incidence of intra-amniotic infection. Because the risk of prematurity outweighed the risk of infection, expectant management was chosen for this patient. After 2 days in the hospital, the patient developed a fever, mild uterine tenderness, and fetal tachycardia. These symptoms are consistent with intra-amniotic infection. Upon recognition of this diagnosis, the patient should be given intravenous antibiotic therapy, such as ampicillin and gentamicin. Neonates are most commonly affected by group B streptococci and gram-negative enteric organisms such as *Escherichia coli*. Delivery is also an important aspect of therapy for both neonatal and maternal well-being. A vaginal delivery is acceptable, so induction of labor was chosen in this case.

APPROACH TO
Preterm Prom

DEFINITIONS

PREMATURE RUPTURE OF MEMBRANES: Rupture of membranes prior to the onset of labor.

PRETERM PREMATURE RUPTURE OF MEMBRANES: Rupture of membranes in a gestation less than 37 weeks, prior to onset of labor.

LATENCY PERIOD: The duration of time from rupture of membranes to onset of labor.

CLINICAL APPROACH

Preterm premature rupture of membranes (PPROM) is defined as rupture of membranes prior to the onset of labor and at less than 37 weeks of pregnancy. This complication occurs in about 1% of all pregnancies. Approximately one-third of preterm births are associated with PPROM. Risk factors are noted in Table 52–1.

The history consistent with PPROM is that of a loss or "gush" of fluid per vagina, which is very accurate and should be taken seriously. The diagnosis is confirmed with a speculum examination showing the pooling of amniotic fluid in the posterior vaginal vault, alkaline changes of the vaginal fluid, and a ferning pattern of the fluid when seen on microscopy. Occasionally, the speculum examination may be negative, but clinical suspicion is high; in these cases, an ultrasound examination revealing oligohydramnios is consistent with PPROM.

The outcome is dependent on the gestational age. Approximately half of patients with PPROM will go into labor within 48 hours, and 90% within 1 week. Complications of preterm delivery, such as respiratory distress syndrome,

Table 52–1 RISK FACTORS FOR PPROM
Lower socioeconomic status
Sexually transmitted diseases
Cigarette smoking
Cervical conization
Emergency cerclage
Multiple gestations
Hydramnios
Placental abruption

are common. Other complications include chorioamnionitis, placental abruption, and necrotizing enterocolitis.

Chorioamnionitis affects about 1% of all pregnancies, and 7% to 10% of those with PPROM with prolonged rupture of membranes. Maternal fever, maternal tachycardia, uterine tenderness, and malodorous vaginal discharge are some clinical indicators. An **early sign is fetal tachycardia,** a baseline heart rate of greater than 160 bpm.

The treatment of PPROM is controversial. Prior to 32 weeks' gestation, antenatal steroids may be given to enhance fetal lung maturity in the absence of overt infection. Broad-spectrum antibiotic therapy has been shown to delay delivery and decrease the incidence of chorioamnionitis. Expectant management is undertaken when the risk of infection is thought to be less than the risk of prematurity. After a gestational age of 34 to 35 weeks, the treatment is usually delivery. Some of the risks of expectant management include stillbirth, cord accident, infection, and abruption. When infection is apparent, broad-spectrum antibiotics, such as intravenous ampicillin and gentamicin, should be initiated and labor should be induced. Also, the infant should be delivered when there is evidence of fetal lung maturity, such as by the presence of phosphatidyl glycerol (PG) on the vaginal pool amniotic fluid.

Comprehension Questions

52.1   A 31-year-old G1 P0 at 33 weeks' gestation is admitted for preterm premature rupture of membranes. Which of the following statements is correct?

A.   Intramuscular corticosteroid therapy should be given to enhance fetal lung maturity if there is no evidence of infection.

B.   Broad-spectrum antibiotic therapy is indicated only with maternal fever.

C.   Labor is the most common acute complication to be expected.

D.   Vaginal candidiasis is a risk factor for preterm premature rupture of membranes.

52.2   A 30-year-old G2 P1 woman at 28 weeks' gestation with preterm premature rupture of membranes is suspected of having intra-amniotic infection based on fetal tachycardia. The maternal temperature is normal. Which of the following is the most accurate method to confirm the intra-amniotic infection?

A.   Serum maternal leukocyte count

B.   Speculum examination of the vaginal discharge

C.   Amniotic fluid Gram stain by amniocentesis

D.   Palpation of the maternal uterus

E.   Height of oral temperature

52.3 An 18-year-old Hispanic G1 P0 woman has a clinical presentation of intra-amniotic infection. She denies any leakage of fluid per vagina, and repeated speculum examinations fail to identify rupture of membranes. Which of the following organisms is most likely to be the underlying etiology?

A. Group B streptococci
B. Listeria monocytogenes
C. *Clostridia difficile*
D. *Chlamydia trachomatis*
E. *Escherichia coli*

52.4 A 32-year-old woman at 33 weeks' gestation notes leakage of clear vaginal fluid. She denies uterine contractions. The estimated fetal weight on sonography is 2000 g. Vaginal fluid shows the presence of phosphatidyl glycerol. Which of the following is the next step?

A. Expectant management
B. Intramuscular corticosteroids
C. Induction of labor
D. Ultrasound-guided amniocentesis

ANSWERS

52.1 **C. Labor is the most common complication associated with PROM.** Antibiotics should be given to prolong the pregnancy and decrease the risk of infection. The gestational age is **greater than 32 weeks, so no antenatal steroids** are required. Vaginal candidiasis is not a risk factor for PPROM; however, a lower socioeconomic status, STDs, cigarette smoking, cervical conization, emergency cerclage, multiple gestation, hydramnios, and placental abruption are risk factors.

52.2 **C. Amniocentesis-revealing organisms on Gram stain are diagnostic of infection.** A serum maternal leukocyte count may be at high values suggestive of infections, but it would not be specific for an intra-amniotic infection. Similarly, a speculum examination may reveal an infectious-appearing vaginal discharge; however this would neither confirm that an infection is present or that a specific type of infection is present, especially since increased vaginal discharge is common in pregnancy. Palpation of the maternal uterus and height of an oral temperature would also not be diagnostic.

52.3 **B. *Listeria* may induce chorioamnionitis without rupture of membranes;** the mechanism is transplacental spread. A history of ingesting unpasteurized milk products (eg, some varieties of goat cheese) should raise clinical suspicion of *Listeria*. **Group B streptococci and gram-negative enteric organisms such as *E coli* are the most common organisms to affect neonates.**

52.4   **C.** It is fetal renal anomalies that lead to oligohydramnios, and not vice
          versa. Severe oligohydramnios at an early gestational age can cause pul-
          monary hypoplasia. When **fetal lung maturity** is demonstrated on vagi-
          nal amniotic fluid by the presence of PG, delivery is the best next step
          when there is leakage of fluid. Expectant management and intramus-
          cular corticosteroids place the mother at an increased risk of develop-
          ing an intra-amniotic infection. Corticosteroids suppress the immune
          system, and expectant management prolongs the time frame that an
          ascending infection from the vagina can cause an intra-amniotic infec-
          tion. Expectant management is undertaken when the risk of infection
          is thought to be less than the risk of prematurity, but this is not the case
          for this scenario with a fetus that shows signs of lung maturity. There is
          no indication for an ultrasound-guided amniocentesis.

Clinical Pearls

➤ Pregnancies complicated by premature rupture of membranes after 34- to
   35-weeks gestation are usually managed by induction of labor.
➤ Pregnancies with PPROM less than 32-weeks gestation are usually managed expectantly.
➤ The earliest sign of chorioamnionitis (intra-amniotic infection) is usually
   fetal tachycardia.
➤ Pregnancies complicated by PPROM and chorioamnionitis should be
   treated with broad-spectrum antibiotics (like ampicillin and gentamicin)
   and delivery.
➤ Clinical infection is a contraindication for corticosteroid use.

REFERENCES

American College of Obstetricians and Gynecologists. Premature rupture of mem-
     branes. *ACOG Practice Bulletin 80*. Washington, DC:2007.
Cunningham FG, Leveno KJ, Bloom SL, Hauth JC, Gilstrap LC III, Wenstrom KD.
     Preterm birth. In: *Williams Obstetrics*. 22nd ed. New York, NY: McGraw-Hill;
     2005:855-880.
Hobel CJ. Obstetrical complications: preterm labor, PROM, IUGR, postterm preg-
     nancy, and IUFD. In: Hacker NF, Gambone JC, Hobel CJ, eds. *Essentials of
     Obstetrics and Gynecology*, 5th ed. Philadelphia, PA: Saunders; 2009:146-159.

Case 53

An 18-year-old nulliparous woman complains of a vaginal discharge with a fishy odor over the past 2 weeks. She states that the odor is especially prominent after intercourse. Her last menstrual period was 3 weeks ago. She denies being treated for vaginitis or sexually transmitted diseases. She is in good health and takes no medications other than an oral contraceptive agent. On examination, her blood pressure (BP) is 110/70 mm Hg, heart rate (HR) 80 beats per minute, and temperature is afebrile. The thyroid is normal to palpation. The heart and lung examinations are normal. Her breasts are Tanner stage V as is the pubic and axillary hair. The external genitalia are normal; the speculum examination reveals a homogeneous, white vaginal discharge and a fishy odor. No erythema or lesions of the vagina are noted.

➤ What is the most likely diagnosis?

➤ What is the best treatment for this condition?

ANSWERS TO CASE 53:
Bacterial Vaginosis

Summary: An 18-year-old nulliparous woman complains of a fishy vaginal discharge, which is worse after intercourse. The speculum examination reveals a homogeneous, white vaginal discharge and a fishy odor. No erythema or lesions of the vagina are noted.

➤ **Most likely diagnosis:** Bacterial vaginosis (BV).

➤ **Best treatment for this condition:** Metronidazole orally or vaginally; clindamycin is an alternative.

ANALYSIS

Objectives

1. Know the three common infectious causes of vaginitis or vaginosis, which are BV, Trichomoniasis, and *Candida vulvovaginitis*.
2. Know the diagnostic criteria for bacterial vaginosis.
3. Know the treatments for the corresponding causes of vaginitis and vaginosis.

Considerations

This 18-year-old woman complains of a vaginal discharge that has a fishy odor, which is the most common symptom of bacterial vaginosis. The discharge associated with BV has a typical white, homogenous vaginal coating, described like "spilled milk over the tissue." The pH is not given in this scenario. Also, although a whiff test is not performed with KOH, the worsening of the discharge after intercourse is presumably due to the alkaline semen. The vaginal epithelium is not erythematous or inflamed, which also fits with bacterial vaginosis. Of the three most common causes of infectious vaginal discharge (*Candida*, *Trichomonas*, and BV), bacterial vaginosis is the one etiology that is not inflammatory; there is a predominance of anaerobic bacteria rather than a true infection. Hence, antibiotic therapy aimed at anaerobes, such as metronidazole or clindamycin, is appropriate.

(handwritten top margin: 5/6 350 1724)

APPROACH TO
Vaginal Infections

DEFINITIONS

BACTERIAL VAGINOSIS: Condition of excessive anaerobic bacteria in the vagina, leading to a discharge that is alkaline.

CANDIDA VULVOVAGINITIS: Vaginal and/or vulvar infection caused by *Candida* species, usually with heterogenous discharge and inflammation.

TRICHOMONAS VAGINITIS: Infection of the vagina caused by the protozoa *Trichomonas vaginalis*, usually associated with a frothy green discharge and intense inflammatory response.

CLINICAL APPROACH

The **three most common types of vaginal infections** are **bacterial vaginosis, trichomonal vaginitis,** and **candidal vulvovaginitis** (Table 53–1).

Bacterial vaginosis is not a true infection, but rather an overgrowth of anaerobic bacteria, which replaces the normal lactobacilli of the vagina. Although it may be sexually transmitted, this is not always the case. The most common symptom is a fishy or "musty" odor, often exacerbated by menses or intercourse, since both of these situations introduce an alkaline substance. The vaginal pH is elevated above normal. The addition of 10% potassium hydroxide (KOH) solution leads to the release of amines, causing a fishy odor

(handwritten: → "whiff test")

Table 53–1 CHARACTERISTICS OF VARIOUS VAGINAL INFECTIONS

	BACTERIAL VAGINOSIS	TRICHOMONAL VAGINITIS	CANDIDAL VULVOVAGINITIS
Appearance	Homogeneous, white discharge	Frothy, yellow to green	Curdy, lumpy
Vaginal pH	>4.5	>4.5	<4.5
Whiff test (fishy odor with KOH)	++++	++	None
Microscopy	Clue cells	Trichomonads	Pseudohyphae
Treatment	Metronidazole *(handwritten: or clindamycin)*	Metronidazole	Oral fluconazole or imidazole cream

(handwritten annotations: next to Pseudohyphae "diflucan"; below treatment arrow "terconazole or miconazole")

(whiff test). There is no inflammatory reaction; hence, the patient will not complain of swelling or irritation, and typically, the microscopic examination does not usually reveal leukocytes. Microscopy of the discharge in normal saline (wet mount) typically shows clue cells (Figure 53–1), which are coccoid bacteria adherent to the external surfaces of epithelial cells.

Bacterial vaginosis is associated with genital tract infection, such as endometritis, pelvic inflammatory disease and pregnancy complications, such as preterm delivery and preterm premature rupture of membranes. Treatment includes oral or vaginal metronidazole. Patients should be instructed to avoid alcohol while taking metronidazole to avoid a disulfiram reaction.

Trichomonas vaginalis is a single-cell anaerobic flagellated protozoan that induces an intense inflammatory reaction. It is a common sexually transmitted disease. *Trichomonas vaginalis* can survive for up to 6 hours on a wet surface. Aside from causing infection of the vagina, this organism can also inhabit the urethra or Skene glands. The most common symptom associated with trichomoniasis is a profuse "frothy" yellow-green to gray vaginal discharge or vaginal irritation. Intense inflammation of the vagina or cervix may be noted, with the classic punctate lesions of the cervix (strawberry cervix). A fishy odor is common with this disorder, which is somewhat exacerbated

[handwritten margin notes: BV not inflam. ↓ Trich. inflam. (strawberry cervix)]

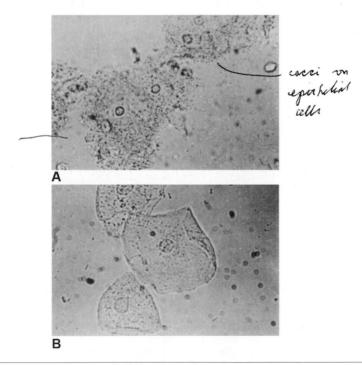

[handwritten annotations: cocci on epithelial cells]

Figure 53–1.   Vaginal epithelial "clue cells." Clue cells (**A**) with a granular appearance in contrast to normal cells (**B**). *Reproduced with permission from Kasper DL, et al. Harrison's Principles of Internal Medicine. 16th ed. New York: McGraw-Hill, 2005:767.*

with KOH. Microscopy in saline will often display mobile, flagellated organisms. If the wet mount is cold or there are excess leukocytes present, the movement of the trichomonads may be inhibited. Optimal treatment consists of a fairly high dose of metronidazole (2 g orally) as a one-time dose, with the partner treated as well. Resistant cases may require the same dose every day for 7 days. A newer anti-protozoal agent, Tinidazole, has a similar dosing, side-effect profile, and contraindication for concurrent alcohol; due to its expense, its main role is for metronidazole-resistant cases.

Candidal vaginitis is usually caused by the fungus, *Candida albicans*, although other species may be causative. The lactobacilli in the vagina inhibit fungal growth; thus, antibiotic therapy may decrease the lactobacilli concentration, leading to *Candida* overgrowth. Diabetes mellitus, which suppresses immune function, may also predispose patients to these infections. Candidiasis is usually not a sexually transmitted disease. The patient usually presents with intense vulvar or vaginal burning, irritation, and swelling. Dyspareunia may also be a prominent complaint. The discharge usually appears curdy or like cottage cheese, in contrast to the homogenous discharge of bacterial vaginosis. Also, unlike the alkaline pH of BV and *Trichomonas* infection, the vaginal pH in candidiasis is typically normal (<4.5). The microscopic diagnosis is confirmed by identification of the hyphae or pseudohyphae after the discharge is mixed with potassium hydroxide. The KOH solution lyses the leukocytes and erythrocytes, making identification of the candidal organisms easier. Treatment includes oral Diflucan or topical imidazoles, such as terconazole (Terazol), or miconazole (Monistat).

Comprehension Questions

53.1 An 18-year-old G0 P0 adolescent female is being seen at the physician's office for vaginal discharge. A presumptive diagnosis of bacterial vaginosis is made. Which of the following is a finding consistent with BV?

A. pH less than 4.5
B. Frothy vaginal discharge
C. Predominance of anaerobes
D. Flagellated organisms

53.2 A 26-year-old woman completed a course of oral antibiotics for cystitis 1 week ago. She complains of a 1-day history of itching, burning, and a yellowish vaginal discharge. Which of the following is the best therapy?

A. Metronidazole
B. Erythromycin
C. Fluconazole
D. Hydrocortisone
E. Clindamycin

53.3 Which of the following organisms may be isolated from a wet surface 6 hours after inoculation?
A. *Candida albicans*
B. *Trichomonas vaginalis*
C. *Gardenerella* species
D. Peptostreptococci

53.4 A 27-year-old woman complains of a fishy odor and a vaginal discharge. The speculum examination reveals an erythematous vagina and punctations of the cervix. Which of the following is the most likely diagnosis?
A. Candidal vaginitis
B. Trichomonal vaginitis
C. Bacterial vaginosis
D. Human papillomavirus
E. Herpes simplex virus

ANSWERS

53.1 **C.** There is a predominance of **anaerobes** in **bacterial vaginosis**. The vaginal pH in BV usually is greater than 4.5, and the discharge is homogenous. The most common symptom is a **fishy or "musty" odor** when introduced to an alkaline substance (ie, 10% KOH, semen, or menses). **Clue cells** are found on microscopy. BV is associated with genital tract infection, such as endometritis, pelvic inflammatory disease, and pregnancy complications, such as preterm delivery and PPROM. Frothy discharge is more typical of trichomoniasis.

53.2 **C.** After **antibiotic therapy, candidal organisms** often **proliferate** and may induce an overt infection. The mechanism is likely that the lactobacilli are eliminated by the antibiotic, allowing overgrowth of yeast. Treatment of candidal vulvovaginitis is oral **fluconazole** or imidazole cream. **Metronidazole** is used to treat BV and *T vaginitis*. Patients should be instructed to avoid alcohol while taking metronidazole to avoid a *disulfiram reaction*. **Erythromycin** may be used in the treatment of syphilis in nonpregnant women allergic to penicillin. **Clindamycin** is typically used in conjunction with gentamicin in the treatment of infections requiring broad-spectrum antibiotics, necessitating anaerobic coverage (ie, postpartum endomyometritis). Hydrocortisone is most commonly indicated for severe allergic reactions.

53.3 **B.** *Trichomonas vaginalis* is a hardy organism and may be isolated from a wet surface up to 6 hours after inoculation. Its difficulty to kill is the reason that therapy is metronidazole 2 gm orally all at once, to be able to obtain sufficiently high tissue levels to be effective. Not uncommonly, a single course is not effective, and a 2- or 3-day course of metronidazole a high dose orally is needed.

53.4   **B.** Erythematous vagina and punctations of the cervix (**strawberry cervix**) are classic findings of the inflammatory effects induced by trichomoniasis. Classic findings in candidal vaginitis include the curdy or cottage cheese appearance of the vaginal discharge with hyphae or pseudohyphae found on microscopy after discharge is mixed with KOH. HPV is associated with findings of cervical dysplasia. Herpes simplex virus is the most common cause of infectious vulvar ulcer disease in the United States.

Clinical Pearls

➤ The three most common types of vaginal infections are trichomoniasis, candidal vaginitis, and bacterial vaginosis.

➤ Both BV and trichomoniasis is associated with alkaline pH and positive whiff test.

➤ Candidal vulvovaginitis is a common infection in women who are pregnant, taking broad-spectrum antibiotics, diabetic, or immunocompromised.

➤ Bacterial vaginosis is associated with preterm delivery, postpartum endometritis, and pelvic inflammatory disease.

➤ Trichomonal vaginitis is associated with an intense inflammatory process and may induce punctations of the cervix known as "strawberry cervix."

REFERENCES

American College of Obstetricians and Gynecologists. Vaginitis. ACOG *Practice Bulletin 72*. Washington, DC: 2006.

Eckert LO, Lentz GM. Infections of the lower genital tract. In: Katz VL, Lentz GM, Lobo RA, Gersenson DM, eds. *Comprehensive Gynecology*. 5th ed. St. Louis, MO: Mosby-Year Book; 2007:569-606.

McGregor JA, Lench JB. Vulvovaginitis, sexually transmitted infections, and pelvic inflammatory disease. sepsis. In: Hacker NF, Gambone JC, Hobel CJ, eds. *Essentials of Obstetrics and Gynecology*, 5th ed. Philadelphia, PA: Saunders; 2009:265-275.

Case 54

A 42-year-old parous woman has noticed increasing hair growth on her face and abdomen over the past 8 months. She denies the use of steroid medications, weight changes, or a family history of hirsutism. Her menses previously had been monthly, and now occur every 35 to 70 days. Her past medical and surgical histories are unremarkable. On examination, her thyroid is normal to palpation. She has excess facial hair and male pattern hair on her abdomen. Acne is also noted on the face. The cardiac and pulmonary examinations are normal. The abdominal examination reveals no masses or tenderness. Examination of the external genitalia reveals possible clitoromegaly. Pelvic examination shows a normal uterus and cervix and an 8-cm, right adnexal mass.

➤ What is the most likely diagnosis?

➤ What is the probable management?

ANSWERS TO CASE 54:
Hirsutism, Sertoli–Leydig Cell Tumor

Summary: A 42-year-old woman with an 8-month history of increasing hirsutism and irregular menses. She denies the use of steroid medications, weight changes, or a family history of hirsutism. Pelvic examination shows an 8-cm, right adnexal mass.

➤ **Most likely diagnosis:** An ovarian tumor, probable Sertoli–Leydig cell tumor.

➤ **Probable management:** Ovarian cancer (surgical) staging.

ANALYSIS

Objectives

1. Understand the differential diagnosis of hirsutism.
2. Know the work-up and approach to a woman with virilism and hirsutism.
3. Know the typical history and physical examination for the various causes of hirsutism.

Considerations

This 42-year-old woman has the onset of excess male-pattern hair over the past 6 months, as well as features of virilism (clitoromegaly). This is evidence of excess androgens. The rapid onset speaks of a tumor. Adrenal or ovarian tumors are possibilities. This woman has a large adnexal mass, and so the diagnosis is straightforward. She has irregular menses because of the androgen effect of inhibiting ovulation. The patient does not have the stigmata of Cushing disease, such as hypertension, buffalo hump, abdominal striae, and central obesity. Likewise, she does not take any medications containing anabolic steroids. Polycystic ovarian syndrome (PCOS) is probably the most common cause of hyperandrogenism, but it does not fit this patient's clinical presentation. PCOS usually presents with a gradual onset of hirsutism and irregular menses since menarche. A Sertoli–Leydig cell tumor of the ovary is a solid stromal type of tumor, the androgen counterpart of granulosa-theca cell tumor. These tumors are usually of low malignant potential and slow growing, but nevertheless may metastasize and often recur. Hence, surgical staging is the treatment of choice.

APPROACH TO
Hirsutism

DEFINTIONS

HIRSUTISM: Excessive male pattern hair in a female.

VIRILISM: Androgen effect other than hair pattern, such as cliteromegaly, male balding, deepening of the voice, and acne.

CLINICAL APPROACH

Hirsutism should be viewed as both an endocrine and cosmetic problem. It is most commonly associated with anovulation; however, other causes of increased androgen levels need to be ruled out, such as adrenal and ovarian diseases. The most sensitive marker of excess androgen production is hirsutism, followed by acne, oily skin, increased libido, and virilization. **Virilization** consists of clitoromegaly, deepening of the voice, balding, increased muscle mass, and male body habitus. Adrenal hyperplasia or androgen-secreting tumors of the adrenal gland or ovary are causes of virilization. The treatment depends on the underlying etiology.

The pattern of hair growth is genetically predetermined. Differences in hair growth between ethnic groups are secondary to variations in hair follicle concentration and 5-α-reductase activity. Hair growth can be divided into three phases: anagen (growing phase), catagen (involution phase), and telogen (quiescent phase). Hair length is determined by the length of the anagen phase, and the stability of hair is determined by the length of the telogen phase. Hair found on the face, axilla, chest, breast, pubic area, and anterior thighs are termed "sex hair" because they respond to sex hormones. Androgens (especially testosterone) initiate growth of and increase the diameter and pigmentation of "sex hair." Androgens may be produced by the ovary, adrenal gland, or by peripheral conversion. Dehydroepiandrosterone sulfate (DHEA-S) is derived almost exclusively from the adrenal gland. Dihydrotestosterone (DHT) is metabolized from testosterone by 5-α-reductase; increased activity of 5-α-reductase leads to an increase in DHT and stimulation of hair growth. The majority of testosterone is bound to sex hormone-binding globulin (SHBG) and it is the unbound portion that is primarily responsible for androgenicity. Hyperandrogenism decreases SHBG, and thus, exacerbates hirsutism.

The appearance and cosmetic changes associated with hirsutism depend on the number of follicles present, ratio of growth to resting phases, asynchrony of growth cycles, and thickness and degree of pigmentation of individual hairs. The history should focus on the onset and duration of symptoms (faster growth is associated with tumors of adrenal and ovary, whereas slow onset since menarche is more likely polycystic ovarian syndrome). The severity of symptoms should be characterized (eg, virilization is rare and is usually associated with androgen-secreting tumors). The regularity of the menses and symptoms of thyroid disease should also be sought. The physical examination should focus on the location of hair growth and its severity, thyromegaly, body shape and habitus, the presence of breast discharge, skin changes (acanthosis or abdominal striae), adnexal or abdominal masses, and the external genitalia. Helpful laboratory tests include assays for serum testosterone, dihydroepiandrostenedione sulfate (DHEA-S), 17-hydroxyprogesterone (which is elevated with congenital adrenal hyperplasia), prolactin, and TSH. A markedly elevated testosterone level suggests an androgen-secreting ovarian tumor, such as a Sertoli–Leydig cell tumor. With a high DHEA-S level, the examiner should be suspicious of an adrenal process, such as adrenal hyperplasia or a tumor.

The differential diagnosis for hirsutism (Table 54–1) includes anovulation, late-onset adrenal hyperplasia, androgen-secreting tumors (adrenal or ovarian in origin), Cushing disease, medications, thyroid disease, and hyperprolactinemia.

A genetic defect in the enzyme 21-hydroxylase causes most of the cases of congenital adrenal hyperplasia (CAH). While classic CAH is the most common cause of ambiguous genitalia in the newborn, late-onset of nonclassical CAH can present in adult females with symptoms of hirsutism and anovulation. An elevated morning fasting 17-hydroxyprogesterone level is highly

Table 54–1   DIFFERENTIAL DIAGNOSIS OF HIRSUTISM

DISEASE	HISTORY	PHYSICAL EXAMINATION	LABORATORY TEST	TREATMENT
Cushing syndrome	Glucose intolerance	Hypertension, buffalo hump, central obesity	Dexamethasone suppression test	Surgical
Adrenal tumor	Rapid-onset virilism	Abdominal mass	DHEA-S	Surgical
Congenital adrenal hyperplasia	Ambiguous genitalia, family history	Hypotension	Elevated 17-hydroxy-progesterone	Replace cortisol and mineralo-corticoid
Polycystic ovarian syndrome	Onset since menarche	Hirsutism, rarely virilization	Elevated LH-FSH ratio	Oral contraceptive pills
Sertoli–Leydig cell tumor	Rapid onset	Hirsutism, virilism, adnexal mass	Elevated testosterone level	Surgical

adrenocarcinoma (handwritten annotation in left margin)

suggestive of CAH. Treatment depends on the etiology; however, in general, the goal is to decrease the amount of DHT available. This can be accomplished by inhibiting adrenal or ovarian androgen secretion, changing SHBG binding, impairing peripheral conversion of androgen to active androgen, and inhibiting activity at target tissues. Treatment options include weight loss, combined oral contraception pills, spironolactone (a diuretic that is an androgen antagonist), progesterone-containing medications, electrolysis, laser vaporization, waxing, and shaving. The patient must be warned that there is a slow response to treatment with medications (an average of 6 months). To help with more immediate results, nonmedical therapies (waxing and shaving) may be used initially until the new medication begins to work effectively.

Comprehension Questions

54.1 A 6-year-old girl is noted to have breast development and vaginal spotting. No abnormal hair growth is noted. A 10-cm ovarian mass is palpated on rectal examination. Which of the following is the most likely diagnosis?
A. Benign cystic tumor (dermoid)
B. Idiopathic precocious puberty
C. Sertoli–Leydig cell tumor
D. Congenital adrenal hyperplasia
E. Granulosa-theca cell tumor

54.2 A 15-year-old G0 P0 complains of increasing hair over her face and chest. She also has a deepening voice and clitoromegaly. There have been two neonatal deaths in the family. Which of the following is the best diagnostic test for the likely diagnosis?
A. Testosterone level
B. Dexamethasone suppression test
C. 17-hydroxyprogesterone level
D. LH and FSH levels
E. Karyotype

54.3 A 22-year-old nulliparous woman with irregular menses of 7 years' duration complains of primary infertility. She has a family history of diabetes. She has mild hirsutism on examination. Which of the following is the most likely therapy?
A. Cortisol and mineralocorticoid replacement
B. Excision of an adrenal tumor
C. Surgical excision of an ovarian tumor
D. Oral clomiphene citrate
E. Intrauterine insemination

54.4   A 24-year-old woman complains of bothersome hirsutism and skipping
        periods. She does not have evidence of voice changes, hair loss, or cli-
        toromegaly. The pelvic examination does not reveal adnexal masses.
        The serum DHEA-S, testosterone, and 17-hydroxyprogesterone levels
        are normal. The LH to FSH ratio is 2:1. Which of the following is the
        most likely diagnosis?
        A. Polycystic ovarian syndrome
        B. Familial hirsutism
        C. Ovarian tumor
        D. Adrenal tumor
        E. Cushing syndrome

ANSWERS

54.1   **E. Isosexual** (no virilization) **precocious puberty** with an **adnexal
        mass** usually is a **granulosa cell tumor** of the ovary. **Dermoid cysts** are
        also found on the ovary. They present as a pelvic mass that causes pain
        due to its rapidly enlarging size, however they do not cause isosexual
        precocious puberty. A **Sertoli–Leydig cell tumor** is the androgen
        counterpart to the granulose-theca cell tumor. With a Sertoli–Leydig
        cell tumor, testosterone levels are markedly elevated and patients typ-
        ically present with hirsutism, virilism, and an adnexal mass.
        Congenital adrenal hyperplasia is the most common cause of ambigu-
        ous genitalia in the newborn; however, late onset can present in adult
        females with symptoms of hirsutism and anovulation.

54.2   **C.** The most common neonatal endocrine cause of death (salt wasting)
        is **congenital adrenal hyperplasia (21-hydroxylase deficiency).**
        An elevated testosterone level would be found with a **Sertoli–Leydig
        cell tumor.** A dexamethasone suppression test is used in the diagno-
        sis of **Cushing syndrome.** An elevated LH-FSH ration is found with
        PCOS. A **karyotype** may be used in finding the etiology behind a
        young girl's presentation of primary amenorrhea or pubertal delay.

54.3   **D.** Most likely polycystic ovarian syndrome **(PCOS)**; the initial
        treatment for **infertility** is **clomiphene citrate.** Since the symptoms
        were not of rapid onset, the etiology is not likely to involve a tumor.
        Intrauterine insemination is usually indicated for the rare cervical
        factor infertility, and not **ovulatory disfunction.**

54.4   **A. Polycystic ovarian syndrome** is the **most common cause of hirsutism
        and irregular menses**. Treatment may be **spironolactone** (androgen antag-
        onist) and **oral contraceptives.** Familial hirsutism usually is not associated
        with oligomenorrhea or an abnormal LH/FSH ratio. Symptoms do not
        correlate with an ovarian tumor (since the patient has abnormal hair
        growth, hirsutism); also, laboratory values indicate normal adrenal func-
        tion, thus ruling out adrenal tumor and Cushing syndrome.

Clinical Pearls

> ➤ The rapid onset of hirsutism or virilization usually indicates the presence of an androgen-secreting tumor.
> ➤ The two most common locations of androgen production and secretion are the ovary and the adrenal gland.
> ➤ The most common cause of hirsutism and irregular menses is polycystic ovarian syndrome.
> ➤ The most common cause of ambiguous genitalia in the newborn is congenital adrenal hyperplasia, usually due to 21-hydroxlase enzyme deficiency.
> ➤ Hyperandrogenism in the face of an adnexal mass usually indicates a Sertoli–Leydig cell tumor of the ovary, and is treated surgically.

REFERENCES

Alexander CJ, Mathur R, Laufer LR, Aziz R. Amenorrhea, oligomenorrhea, and hyperandrogenic disorders. In: Hacker NF, Gambone JC, Hobel CJ, eds. *Essentials of Obstetrics and Gynecology*, 5th ed. Philadelphia, PA: Saunders; 2009:355-367.

Coleman RL, Gershenson DM. Neoplastic diseases of the ovary. In: Katz VL, Lentz GM, Lobo RA, Gersenson DM, eds. *Comprehensive Gynecology*. 5th ed. St. Louis, MO: Mosby-Year Book; 2007:839-880.

Speroff L. Hirsutism. In: Speroff L, Fritz MA. *Clinical Gynecologic Endocrinology and Infertility*. 7th ed. Philadelphia, PA: Linppincott, Williams and Wilkins; 2005:499-530.

Case 55

A 20-year-old G1 P0 woman at 16 weeks' gestation by last menstrual period has received a serum maternal α-fetoprotein test that returned as 2.8 multiples of the median. She is fairly sure of her last menstrual period and has regular menses. She denies a family history of congenital anomalies or chromosomal abnormalities. On examination, her blood pressure (BP) is 100/70 mm Hg, heart rate (HR) 70 beats per minute, and temperature is afebrile. The heart and lung examinations are normal. The fundal height is midway between the symphysis pubis and the umbilicus. Fetal heart tones are in the range of 140 bpm.

➤ What is your next diagnostic step?

ANSWER TO CASE 55:
Serum Screening in Pregnancy

Summary: A 20-year-old G1 P0 woman at 16 weeks' gestation by a fairly certain last menstrual period has received a serum maternal α-fetoprotein test that returned as 2.8 multiples of the median.

➤ **Next diagnostic step:** Basic obstetric ultrasound examination to assess for dates and multiple gestations.

ANALYSIS

Objectives

1. Understand that the most common causes of abnormal serum screening are wrong dates and multiple gestations.
2. Know that an elevated maternal serum α-fetoprotein (msAFP) level may be associated with an open neural tube defect.
3. Know that a low msAFP level may be associated with fetal Down syndrome.

Considerations

This patient is at 16 weeks' gestation by a fairly certain last menstrual period, which is consistent with the clinical examination. The gestational age window of 16 to 20 weeks is the appropriate time to screen with serum testing. The msAFP returned as 2.8 multiples of the median (MOM), which exceeds the usual cut-off of 2.0 or 2.5 MOM. The interpretation of the msAFP depends on gestational age and number of fetuses. The components of a certain last menstrual period are: (1) patient sure of date of last menstrual period (LMP), (2) regular menses, (3) LMP was normal, (4) patient has had no spotting or bleeding after LMP. The uterine size correlates with the dates. At 16 weeks' gestation, the fundus is usually midway between the symphysis pubis and the umbilicus. At 20 weeks' gestation, the fundal height is generally at the level of the umbilicus. Although this patient has a sure LMP and size and date consistency, there is still a significant risk of a dating abnormality or a multifetal gestation. Hence, the next appropriate step is the basic ultrasound examination. If there is a dating error, the msAFP result would be recalculated based on the corrected gestational age. If the msAFP is still abnormally elevated, then at an early gestational age such as 16 weeks, repeating the serum test is an option. For women with abnormally elevated msAFP at a later gestational age, such as 20 weeks, genetic counseling and referral for amniocentesis may be considered.

APPROACH TO
Abnormal Serum Screening in Pregnancy

DEFINITIONS

ALPHA-FETOPROTEIN: A glycoprotein made by the fetal liver, analogous to the adult albumin.

FIRST-TRIMESTER SCREENING: Use of biochemical markers and/or transvaginal sonography measuring the aspect in the posterior neck region called the "nuchal translucency" giving a risk of Down syndrome and trisomy 18.

NEURAL TUBE DEFECT: Failure of closure of the embryonic neural folds leading to an absent cranium and cerebral hemispheres (anencephaly) or nonclosure of the vertebral arches (spina bifida).

OPEN NEURAL TUBE DEFECT: A neural tube defect that is not covered by skin.

MATERNAL SERUM α-FETOPROTEIN: α-Fetoprotein level drawn from maternal blood; this may be elevated due to increased amniotic fluid α-fetoprotein.

TRISOMY SCREEN: Three or four serum markers that may indicate an increased risk of chromosomal abnormalities. A common combination includes maternal serum α-fetoprotein, human chorionic gonadotropin, inhibin-A, and unconjugated estriol. ⤷ Quad Screen

CLINICAL APPROACH

The triple (or trisomy) screen is used in pregnant women between 15 and 21 weeks' gestation to identify those pregnancies that may be complicated by neural tube defects, Down syndrome, or trisomy 18. It is a multiple marker test, and the term "triple" is often used to denote that it analyzes three chemicals in the maternal serum to determine the risk for neural tube defects or fetal aneuploidy: α-fetoprotein (AFP), human chorionic gonadotropin (hCG), and unconjugated estriol. Although the triple screen may be offered to women over the age of 35 years, or advanced maternal age, genetic amniocentesis provides more diagnostic information.

α-Fetoprotein is a glycoprotein synthesized initially by the fetal yolk sac and then later by the fetal gastrointestinal tract and liver. It passes into the maternal circulation by diffusion through the chorioamniotic membranes. When there is an opening in the fetus not covered by skin, levels of AFP increase in the amniotic fluid and maternal serum. Maternal serum AFP is measured in multiples of the median (MOM). Different laboratories have different cut-off levels for abnormal AFP; in general, levels greater than 2.0 to 2.5 MOM are suspicious for neural tube defects and warrant further evaluation.

Table 55–1 CAUSES OF ELEVATED MSAFP
Underestimation of gestational age
Multiple gestations
Neural tube defects ✖
Abdominal wall defects
Cystic hygroma
Fetal skin defects
Sacrococcygeal teratoma
Decreased maternal weight
Oligohydramnios

However, an abnormally elevated serum AFP level does not necessarily coincide with fetal neural tube defects. Other causes of elevated maternal serum AFP are listed in Table 55–1.

In contrast to neural tube defects, which have an abnormally elevated maternal serum AFP, those pregnancies complicated by Down syndrome have a low maternal serum AFP. Again, other causes of abnormally decreased levels of AFP have been identified and are listed in Table 55–2.

Unconjugated estriol is also decreased in fetuses with Down syndrome. Human chorionic gonadotropin, however, is elevated in these fetuses. By combining these serum chemicals into a multiple marker screening test, approximately 60% of all Down syndrome pregnancies can be identified. With trisomy 18, all of the serum markers are abnormally low. Different variations of the multiple marker test exist, such as one that adds inhibin A as a fourth analyte to further improve detection rates.

Recently, first-trimester Down syndrome screening has become available to women. This allows prediction of abnormal pregnancies at an earlier gestational age. First-trimester screening combines two serum analytes: pregnancy-associated plasma protein (PAPP-A) and free β-hCG with sonographic measurement of nuchal translucency. The nuchal translucency is an echolucent area seen at the back of the fetal neck. In abnormal pregnancies, the levels of PAPP-A and free β-hCG tend to be decreased, whereas the nuchal translucency is thickened. When performed between 10- to 13 weeks' gestation, 85% of Down syndrome may be identified, and 90% of trisomy 18 may be identified. Furthermore, first-trimester screening may be combined with second-trimester screening to improve the detection rate of Down syndrome to 90%.

The first step in the management of an abnormal triple screen is a basic ultrasound to determine the correct gestational age, to identify the possibility of multiple gestation, and to exclude fetal demise. The most common cause of abnormal serum screening is wrong dating. If the risk of trisomy or neural tube defects is still increased after a basic sonogram, amniocentesis or targeted ultrasound is offered. A targeted examination can correctly identify fetuses with neural tube defects by direct visualization of the fetal head and spine.

Table 55–2 CAUSES OF LOW MSAFP

Overestimation of gestational age
Chromosomal trisomies ✸
Molar pregnancy
Fetal death
Increased maternal weight

Furthermore, ultrasound may also detect those fetuses suspicious for having Down syndrome by identification of a thickened nuchal fold, shortened femur length, or echogenic bowel. Other conditions associated with an abnormally high or low maternal serum AFP, such as abdominal wall defects, oligohydramnios, and fetal skin defects, can be identified with ultrasound.

Because high-resolution sonography can detect up to 95% of neural tube defects, some practitioners will not proceed with invasive testing for an elevated msAFP. However, when amniocentesis is chosen for an elevated msAFP, the amniotic fluid is tested for AFP levels. Fetal karyotype is also obtained through amniocentesis, which will identify fetal aneuploidy, such as the trisomies. Fetal loss rate from an amniocentesis is about 0.5%. Other complications include rupture of membranes and chorioamnionitis.

The identification of a fetus affected by a neural tube defect or a chromosomal abnormality can be an ethical and moral dilemma for the parents, whose previous hopes and dreams for having a "normal" child are now extinguished. The parents should not be forced into any decision, but should be provided information in an unbiased fashion.

Comprehension Questions

55.1   A 23-year-old G1 P0 woman at 20 weeks' gestation undergoes an ultrasound examination for size greater than dates. The ultrasound reveals hydramnios with an amniotic fluid index of 30 cm. The fetal abdomen reveals a cystic mass in the right abdominal region, and a cystic mass in the left abdominal area. Which of the following is the most likely associated condition?

A. Gestational diabetes
B. Congenital ovarian tumors
C. Down syndrome
D. Rh isoimmunization

55.2	A 28-year-old woman delivers a baby with a cleft palate and cleft lip. The baby is otherwise healthy. The patient asks about whether there is genetic reason for this anomaly. Which of the following is the best explanation of the genetics of this condition?

A. Autosomal dominant
B. Autosomal recessive
C. X-linked dominant
D. X-linked recessive
E. Multifactorial

55.3	A 22-year-old woman G2 P1 at 25 weeks' gestation with a sure last menstrual period asks for serum screening. The patient's sister has one child with Down syndrome and, otherwise, there is no family history of anomalies or genetic disorders. Which of the following is the most appropriate response?

A. Amniocentesis is the appropriate test.
B. Serum screening should be performed.
C. Explain to the patient that it is too late for serum screening, but that her risk for Down syndrome is not much higher than her age-related risk.
D. The patient being only 22 years of age does not need serum screening.
E. The patient has a 25% chance of her baby having Down syndrome.

55.4	A 28-year-old woman G1 P0 at 16 weeks' gestation is noted to have an elevated msAPF at 2.9 multiples of the median (MOM). She underwent a targeted ultrasound examination which did not reveal a neural tube defect. Her physician also undertakes a diligent search for an etiology for the elevated msAFP without identifying an etiology. Which of the following conditions is this patient at increased risk?

A. Increased incidence of stillbirth
B. Gestational diabetes
C. Placenta previa
D. Molar pregnancy
E. Down syndrome

55.5	A 22-year-old woman is seen for her first prenatal visit at 16 weeks' gestation with a family history of congenital deafness and neonatal renal disease. The patient's hearing is normal. Which of the following is the best next step?

A. Amniocentesis for karyotype
B. Amniocentesis for rubella PCR
C. Genetic counseling
D. Glucose challenge testing

ANSWERS

55.1 **C.** This baby has the "double bubble" of duodenal atresia. The hydramnios results from the inability of the baby to swallow. Duodenal atresia is strongly associated with fetal Down syndrome. Gestational diabetes is associated with hydramnios occasionally; however, duodenal atresia is not related. Rh isoimmunization can also lead to hydramnios and hydrops but not duodenal atresia.

55.2 **E.** The genetics for cleft palate and cleft lip in the absence of other anomalies is multifactorial, and not a clear genetic transmission. The risk of recurrence is generally about 5%. The risk is higher if one of the parents also has a cleft lip/palate. Other disorders that are multifactorial include cardiac malformations and neural tube defects.

55.3 **C.** The window for serum screening is usually between 15 and 21 weeks, so that her gestational age of 25 weeks is too late. The history of her sister having a baby with Down syndrome confers only a very small if any increased risk for her own pregnancy. If the patient herself had a prior baby with Down syndrome, the risk would be substantially increased, and genetic counseling with possible amniocentesis for karyotype would be appropriate.

55.4 **A.** Pregnancies with elevated msAFP, which after evaluation are unexplained, are at increased risk for stillbirth, growth restriction, preeclampsia, and placental abruption. Thus many practitioners will perform serial ultrasound examinations, monitor for these complications, and perform fetal antenatal testing such as biophysical profile testing.

55.5 **C.** Genetic counseling is appropriate with a family history of possible heritable syndromes. A glucose challenge test would not be helpful in evaluating heritable syndromes because it is used as a screen for gestational diabetes. Genetic counseling is recommended before a risky procedure, such as an amniocentesis, is performed because based on the family history it may not be indicated in this situation.

Clinical Pearls

Genetic Testing Pre-Amnio

➤ The most common cause of abnormal triple screening is wrong dates.
➤ The next step in the evaluation of abnormal triple screening is the basic ultrasound.
➤ Up to 95% of neural tube defects are detectable by targeted sonography.
➤ About 60% of Down syndrome cases are detected with the triple screen with an elevated human chorionic gonadotropin level, low msAFP, and low unconjugated estriol.
➤ An elevated msAFP suggests a neural tube defect, but there are many other etiologies.

REFERENCES

American College of Obstetricians and Gynecologists. Screening for fetal chromosomal abnormalities. ACOG *Practice Bulletin 77*. Washington, DC:2007.

Cunningham FG, Leveno KJ, Bloom SL, Hauth JC, Gilstrap LC III, Wenstrom KD. Prenatal diagnosis and fetal therapy. In: *Williams Obstetrics*. 22nd ed. New York, NY: McGraw-Hill; 2005:313-339.

Lu MC, Williams III, J, Hobel CJ. Antepartum care: preconception and prenatal care, genetic evaluation and teratology, and antenatal fetal assessment. In: Hacker NF, Gambone JC, Hobel CJ, eds. *Essentials of Obstetrics and Gynecology*, 5th ed. Philadelphia, PA: Saunders; 2009:71-90.

Case 56

A 23-year-old G0 P0 female presents to the office with complaints of irregular cycles since menarche. Upon further questioning, she also has noticed an increase in facial hair and acne for many years. She denies any history of medical problems and has a strong family medical history of diabetes. On examination, she is noted to have a normal blood pressure (BP), pulse, respiratory rate, and temperature. She is obese with a body mass index (BMI) of 34. She is noted to have some hirsutism and acanthosis nigricans (of neck and inner thighs). Her pelvic examination is limited by her obesity but normal. She does not desire pregnancy at this time. Her pregnancy test is negative.

➤ What is the most likely diagnosis?

➤ What complications is the patient at risk for?

➤ What is your next diagnostic step?

➤ What is your therapeutic plan for this patient?

ANSWERS TO CASE 56:

Polycystic Ovarian Syndrome

Summary: A 23-year-old female with long-standing history of irregular cycles, obesity, hirsutism, and acne.

➤ **Most likely diagnosis**: Polycystic ovarian syndrome.

➤ **Complications**: Diabetes mellitus, endometrial cancer, hyperlipidemia, metabolic syndrome, cardiovascular disease.

➤ **Diagnostic steps**: TSH, prolactin, serum testosterone, dehydroepiandrosterone sulfate (DHEA-S), and 17-hydroxyprogesterone, pelvic ultrasound.
↳ *CAH*

➤ **Therapeutic plan**: Regulate menstrual cycles with combination oral contraceptives and screen for metabolic abnormalities (DM, lipid panel, etc). Encourage diet and exercise.

[handwritten: androblastoma - 3βMSB]
[handwritten: • metformin ?]

ANALYSIS

Objectives

1. Know the clinical presentation and diagnostic criteria of polycystic ovarian syndrome.
2. Understand the workup needed for the diagnosis.
3. Become familiar with basic management strategies.

Considerations

The patient is a 23-year-old G0 P0 female with classic clinical presentation of polycystic ovarian syndrome (PCOS). The diagnostic criteria are oligo-ovulation (oligomenorrhea), hyperandrogenism excluding other etiologies, and some include evidence of small multiple cysts of the ovary on transvaginal ultrasound. LH to FSH ratio, while historically noted as a criteria, is inconsistently demonstrated and is not a consistent finding. She has chronic menstrual cycle irregularities, obesity, and signs of hyperandrogenism (acne, hirsutism). The presence of acanthosis is a sign of insulin resistance. After exclusion of secondary causes of hyperandrogenism (late-onset congenital adrenal hyperplasia, hyperprolactinemia, adrenal/ovarian tumors, Cushing syndrome, thyroid disorders) the diagnosis can be made. Management depends on fertility desires. When the patient does not desire a pregnancy, her menstrual cycles are best regulated with combined oral contraceptive pills. Diet and exercise are important to the patient. She should be assessed for metabolic abnormalities which may predispose her to long-term metabolic diseases such as type 2 diabetes and cardiovascular disease. Ovulation induction may be necessary if the patient desires a pregnancy.

APPROACH TO
Polycystic Ovarian Syndrome

DEFINITIONS

PCOS: A condition of unexplained hyperandrogenic chronic anovulation associated with excessive estrogen.

HIRSUTISM: Excessive terminal hair growth in male pattern of distribution.

BMI: Statistical measurement used to identify obesity taking into account a person's height and weight (weight in kg divided by height in m^2). The normal BMI range is considered to be 18.5 to 24.9.

ACANTHOSIS NIGRICANS: Velvety, mossy, verrucous, hyperpigmented skin usually noted on the back of the neck, in the axilla, and under the breasts, usually a sign of insulin resistance.

CLINICAL APPROACH

One would think by the name PCOS, the development of polycystic ovaries is a central feature for the hyperandrogenic chronic anovulation state. However, the polycystic ovary can occur with any state of anovulation and should be viewed as a sign but not a disease. Consequences of persistent anovulation include: infertility, menstrual irregularities, androgen excess (hirsutism, acne, alopecia), and increased risk of endometrial cancer, cardiovascular disease, and diabetes mellitus. **Hyperandrogenic anovulation is reported to occur in 4% to 6% of women.**

When evaluating patients with suspected PCOS, a thorough history and physical should be performed. Other causes of hyperandrogenic anovulation should be excluded. Important information to obtain from the patient include her menstrual history, onset and duration of androgen excess, medications, family history (especially of diabetes and cardiovascular disease), and lifestyle factors (exercise, smoking, alcohol). When performing the physical examination, careful attention needs to be made to body hair distribution and other signs of androgen excess (acne, temporal balding). The presence of acanthosis should be noted and a pelvic examination should be performed to assess for ovarian enlargement.

Laboratory studies which need to be considered are **TSH, prolactin, lipid profile, glucose-intolerance screening, endometrial biopsy** (in patients with long-standing anovulation and unopposed estrogen exposure), **17-hydroxyprogesterone** (congenital adrenal hyperplasia). **Testosterone and dehydroepiandrosterone (DHEAS)** levels can be assessed when clinical signs of excess androgen stimulation are present or if an androgen-secreting tumor is suspected. The majority of testosterone is produced by the ovary, whereas, DHEAS is almost exclusively secreted by the adrenal gland.

Overall treatment goals are to:

1. Reduce circulating androgen levels
2. Protect the endometrium from unopposed estrogen and reduce risk of endometrial cancer
3. Encourage weight loss and healthy lifestyle changes
4. Induce ovulation when pregnancy is desired
5. Monitor for the development of diabetes and cardiovascular disease and modify risk factors if possible (smoking cessation, lipid-lowering agents, etc)

Combination oral contraceptives have been the primary management of long-standing PCOS. They are effective in regulating dysfunctional bleeding and limiting unopposed estrogen (thus reducing endometrial cancer risk), increasing the sex hormone–binding globulin (decreases free androgen levels), and suppresses ovarian androgen production. Weight loss can reduce both the hyperinsulinemia and hyperandrogenism with as little as 5% weight loss from initial weight. Insulin-lowering agents, such as metformin, can be helpful in reducing the hyperinsulinism and thus limiting the risk of developing cardiovascular disease and diabetes mellitus.

For patients desiring pregnancy, clomiphene citrate is the agent of choice, while metformin is only an adjunct.

Comprehension Questions

56.1   A 32-year-old G0 P0 woman is noted to have irregular menses and hirsutism. Which of the following is consistent with polycystic ovarian syndrome?

A. Elevated 17-hydroxyprogesterone level
B. Finding of a 9-cm right ovarian mass
C. Vaginal bleeding after a 5-day course of progesterone oral therapy
D. DEXA scan showing osteopenia

56.2   A 29-year-old G0 P0 woman with a diagnosis of PCOS is being counseled about the dangers of her condition. In particular, she is cautioned about the possibility of developing metabolic syndrome. Which of the following is the most significant consequence of metabolic syndrome?

A. Hyperthyroidism
B. Cardiovascular disease
C. Breast cancer
D. Renal insufficiency

56.3 A 28-year-old G0 P0 woman has a chronic history of oligomenorrhea and amenorrhea. She undergoes an endometrial biopsy in light of her long history of anovulation, which returns as Grade 1 adenocarcinoma of the endometrium. MRI imaging seems to indicate that the endometrial cancer is isolated to the uterus. The patient desires to have children if possible. Which of the following is the best therapy for this patient?

A. Endometrial ablation
B. Radical hysterectomy
C. Cervical conization
D. High-dose progestin therapy
E. Oral contraceptive agent

ANSWERS

56.1 **C.** PCOS is characterized by obesity, anovulation, hyperandrogenism due to ovarian secretion of testosterone, after excluding other etiologies such as CAH, Sertoli-Leydig cell tumor, and hypothyroidism and hyperprolactinemia. An elevated 17-hydroxyprogesterone level would indicate CAH. A 9-cm ovarian mass would suggest a Sertoli-Leydig cell tumor. With PCOS, the DEXA scan usually shows good bone density due to the excess estrogen environment. Women with PCOS usually will have a positive progestin challenge test; in other words, they have bleeding with a 5- to 10-day course of oral progestin.

56.2 **B.** Metabolic syndrome is characterized by hyperlipidemia, glucose intolerance, hypertension, and central obesity. Patients with metabolic syndrome are at greatly increased risk of cardiovascular disease, particularly when the glucose intolerance is present.

56.3 **D.** Young patients with chronic anovulation due to PCOS are at risk for endometrial cancer. The lesions are almost always Grade 1, and are usually treated with hysterectomy and surgical staging. In selected circumstances, high-dose progestin therapy and repeat of the endometrial sampling in 2 to 3 months is possible for those who desire a pregnancy. Hysterectomy is usually recommended after childbirth. The chronic estrogen exposure without progestin is the reason for development of endometrial cancer.

Clinical Pearls

➤ PCOS is a common cause of chronic hyperadnrogenic anovulation and its diagnosis is made after other secondary causes have been ruled out.
➤ Testosterone is largely secreted by the ovary where as DHEAS is secreted by the adrenal gland.
➤ Patients with PCOS should be screened for glucose intolerance and lipid abnormalities.
➤ Combined oral contraceptive pills are the primary management for irregular cycles and also decrease androgen levels.
➤ An endometrial biopsy should be considered in patients with long-standing anovulation and unopposed estrogen.

REFERENCES

Alexander CJ, Mathur R, Laufer LR, Aziz R. Amenorrhea, oligomenorrhea, and hyperandrogenic disorders. In: Hacker NF, Gambone JC, Hobel CJ, eds. *Essentials of Obstetrics and Gynecology*, 5th ed. Philadelphia, PA: Saunders; 2009:355-367.

American College of Obstetricians and Gynecologist. Polycystic Ovary Syndrome. ACOG *Practice Bulletin 41*. Washington DC: American College of Obstetricians and Gynecologists; 2004.

Lobo RA. Abnormal uterine bleeding. In: Katz VL, Lentz GM, Lobo RA, Gersenson DM, eds. *Comprehensive Gynecology*. 5th ed. St. Louis, MO: Mosby-Year Book; 2007:915-930.

Speroff L, Fritz M. Anovulation and the polycystic ovary. In: *Clinical Gynecologic Endocrinology and Infertility*. 7th ed. New York, NY: Lippincott Williams and Wilkins; 2005: 465-498.

Case 57

A 55-year-old G3 P3 woman complains of a 1-month history of pelvic pressure and feeling as though there is "something falling out of my vagina." She had undergone a total abdominal hysterectomy 10 years previously for symptomatic uterine fibroids. She had three vaginal deliveries. She denies other medical problems. She has no urinary incontinence or dysuria. On examination, her blood pressure (BP) is 120/70 mm Hg, heart rate (HR) 90 bpm, respiratory rate (RR) is 12 breaths per minute, temperature 98°F (36.6°C), and weight 160 lb. Her breasts are nontender and without masses. Her heart and lung examinations are normal. On pelvic examination, her external genitalia are somewhat atropic but without lesions. At the introitus, a mucosal bulging is seen, which increases in size with the patient bearing down. This mass is reducible upon digital pelvic examination. There are no adnexal masses. The physician places a cotton tip applicator into the urethra, but there is no movement of the applicator with Valsalva. On rectal examination, there is normal sphincter tone.

➤ What is the most likely diagnosis?

➤ What is the underlying etiology?

➤ What are the options for therapy?

ANSWERS TO CASE 57:

Pelvic Organ Prolapse

Summary: This 55-year-old G3 P3 woman, who underwent a total abdominal hysterectomy previously, has a 1-month history of pelvic pressure, sensation of "something falling out of her vagina." On examination, there is vulvar atrophy. There is a mucosal bulging through the introitus. The remainder of the pelvic examination including the rectal examination and Q-tip test is normal.

➤ **Most likely diagnosis:** Vaginal vault prolapse.

➤ **Underlying etiology:** Enterocele with small bowel in hernia sac behind the vaginal cuff.

➤ **Options for therapy:** Pessary device or surgical fixation of the vagina to a sturdy structure such as the sacrospinous ligament or sacrum.

ANALYSIS

Objectives

1. Understand the anatomical support of the pelvic organs provided by the pelvic diaphragm and endopelvic fascia.
2. Describe the types of pelvic organ prolapse (POP) based on location: cystocele (anterior), enterocele (central), rectocele (posterior), paravaginal (lateral).
3. Describe the symptoms of the various types of POP defects and treatment options.

Considerations

This 55-year-old patient has a sensation of something falling out of the vagina. She has had three vaginal deliveries, which is a risk factor. She has had a total abdominal hysterectomy in the past. The history does not indicate chronic cough or lifting, which would also be risk factors. On examination, the vaginal cuff is noted at the introitus. Examination of the anterior compartment (bladder) is normal in support, including Q-tip test. If the urethra were not well supported, Valsalva would cause the urethral Q-tip to rotate through a large angle. The posterior compartment is also well supported (rectum). There is no mention of the lateral support. Almost inevitably, an enterocele is present associated with vaginal vault prolapse. It is unlikely that conservative measures, such as pelvic muscle strengthening exercises, will alleviate this patient's symptoms. Therefore the best treatments include either pessary, which is a synthetic device used to act as a "hammock" to suspend the pelvic organs, or surgery. Surgical repair includes dissection and ligation of the hernia sac associated with the enterocele. Then fixation of the vagina is achieved to a sturdy structure such as the sacrospinous ligament (vaginal approach) or abdominal sacrocolpopexy (fixing the vaginal cuff to the sacrum using a synthetic mesh).

APPROACH TO
Pelvic Organ Prolapse

DEFINITIONS

CYSTOCELE: Defect of the pelvic muscular support of the bladder allowing the bladder to fall down into the vagina. Often the urethra is hypermobile. This is an anterior POP defect.

ENTEROCELE: Defect of the pelvic muscular support of the uterus and cervix (if still in situ) or the vaginal cuff (if hysterectomy). The small bowel and/or omentum pushes the organs into the vagina. This is a central POP defect.

RECTOCELE: Defect of the pelvic muscular support of the rectum, allowing the rectum to impinge into the vagina. The patient may have constipation or difficulty evacuating stool. This is a posterior POP defect.

PARAVAGINAL DEFECT: Defect in the levator ani attachment to the lateral pelvic side wall leading to lack of support of the vagina, known as a lateral pelvic defect.

CLINICAL APPROACH

Pelvic organ prolapse may affect up to 50% of parous women to some extent, particularly those over the age of 40 years, and with greater incidence after menopause. The symptoms vary and can include a heaviness or pressure sensation in the pelvis, a bulging mass (central), difficulty voiding or incomplete bladder emptying, urinary incontinence (anterior), constipation or having to use one's fingers to push on the vagina to splint to achieve a bowel movement (posterior), sexual dysfunction or pain with intercourse (see Figure 57–1).

The pelvic diaphragm, a muscular and ligamentous network, which attaches from the pubic bone to the sacrum to the lateral pelvic side walls act to support the pelvic organs. Multiple vaginal births, coughing, lifting, connective tissue disorders, genetic predisposition, lack of estrogen, and obesity are among the risk factors for POP. The **pelvic diaphragm** consists of multiple muscles such as the **pubococcygeus, puborectalis,** and **levator ani.** The bladder sits on the pelvic diaphragm and defects will lead to its falling down from the normal location.

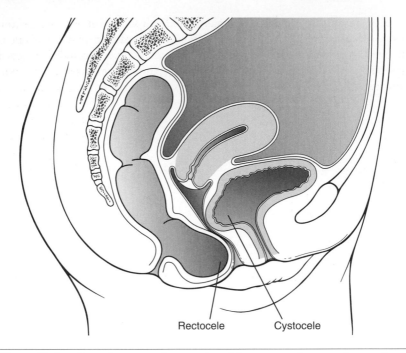

Figure 57–1.   Note the types of anatomic pelvic organ prolapse such as cystocele, and rectocele.

Physical examination can be revealing and indicate what type of defect is present. The examination should be conducted with the patient in the supine as well as standing positions. The bladder should be examined for support, with a cystocele noted if it is bulging into the vagina. When the patient bears down, it should be noted whether the bladder moves further downward. Additionally, a cotton applicator tip may be placed into the urethra and the angle of excursion of the Q-tip should be observed at rest and with Valsalva. A positive Q-tip test of a 60-degree angle of excursion or greater indicates a hypermobile urethra. The rectum should likewise be examined both vaginally and with a rectal examination. The perineal body is often attenuated and weakened with a posterior defect. If the patient has her uterus and cervix, then its position should be noted in relationship to the hymeneal ring. With bearing down, the cervix may descend. Various systems are used to grade the degree of uterine prolapse; one such system is to delineate mild (above the hymen), moderate (at the hymen), complete (beyond the hymen). Sometimes the entire uterus is prolapsed out the patient's introitus, so called procidentia. Women who have had a hysterectomy previously are at risk for vaginal cuff prolapse due to failure to fix the vagina to supporting cardinal or uterosacral ligaments. A paravaginal defect is assessed by palpating the lateral aspects of the vagina for its support and mobility.

Once the extent and type of POP is discerned, the patient can be counseled about therapy. In general, mild POP defects can be treated with pelvic floor strengthening exercises and observation. More significant defects may be treated by pessary devices, which act as a hammock to support the pelvic organ. Different pessary devices are made for different types of defects. Surgical options include resection of redundant tissue, identification of hernia sac and resection if applicable, and then support of the pelvic muscular defect either with suture to a ligamentous support, or using synthetic mesh. Fixation of the vaginal cuff to the sacrospinous ligament for instance is called a sacrospinous ligament fixation procedure. Using a synthetic material to fix the vaginal cuff to the sacral bone is called a sacrocolpopexy. Recently the FDA issued a warning that synthetic meshes in the vagina may lead to erosion and other complications.

Comprehension Questions

57.1   A 48-year-old G3 P3 woman has leakage of urine with coughing and sneezing. She denies dysuria or urinary urgency. Which of the following is likely to be present on physical examination?

A. Hypermobile urethra
B. Rectocele
C. Hypertrophic bladder
D. Paravaginal defect

57.2   A 62-year-old woman complains of constipation and difficulty having bowel movements. She states that she often needs to use her fingers to push vagina backward to achieve a bowel movement. Her history is otherwise unremarkable. Which of the following is the best treatment for this patient?

A. Hysterectomy
B. Anterior colporrhaphy
C. Posterior colporrhaphy
D. Resection and repair of enterocele

57.3   A 35-year-old woman is undergoing a hysterectomy for uterine fibroids that have been symptomatic and failed medical therapy. The surgeon is attempting to ensure that the patient does not have subsequent vaginal vault prolapse. One step that is taken is to use suture to fix the vaginal vault to the uterosacral ligaments. The patient is also noted to have a spacious cul-de-sac area. Which of the following techniques may be used to further decrease the likelihood of vaginal vault prolapse?

A. Obliteration of the vaginal cavity
B. Fixation of the vagina to the anterior abdominal wall
C. Obliteration of the cul-de-sac
D. Prophylactic pessary

ANSWERS

57.1 **A.** This patient has symptoms consistent with pure stress urinary incontinence, typically due to the bladder falling out of its normal intraabdominal position. When she bears down (Valsalva), the pressure to the bladder causes loss of urine. Another component of the urinary incontinence is loss of the vesicourethral angle and hypermobile urethra. The common denominator is probably childbirth, leading to damage of the pelvic support.

57.2 **C.** This woman has symptoms of a rectocele, which is a posterior vaginal defect. Because the support structure to the rectum is defective, the rectum is impinging into the vagina. When the patient bears down to have a bowel movement, the stool gathers in the pouch toward the vagina, instead of out the anal opening. When the patient splints against the rectum with her fingers, she acts as to alleviate the damaged muscular "endopelvic fascia," and simultaneous with Valsalva, stool can be directed toward the anal opening. The surgical repair in this instance is a posterior colporrhaphy consisting of incision of the vaginal mucosa posteriorly, identification of the edges of the endopelvic fascia, and surgical repair of these edges that have separated.

57.3 **C.** One important risk factor for subsequent vaginal vault prolapse is a very spacious and deep cul-de-sac. A surgical technique of obliterating the cul-de-sac region is called culdoplasty. For instance, a circumferential sequence of purse-string sutures can be used to suture the cul-de-sac area closed. This procedure reduces the opportunity for small bowel to push into the vaginal vault and enterocele formation. Caution must be taken to avoid injury to the rectum and the ureter.

Clinical Pearls

➤ Pelvic organ prolapse is very common and is associated with multiparous women over the age of 40 years.
➤ Treatment of POP can entail pessary devices or surgical repair.
➤ Anterior defects lead to cystoceles and possibly urinary incontinence. The treatment is anterior repair (colporrhaphy).
➤ Central defects lead to enteroceles and vaginal vault prolapse or uterine prolapse. The treatment is resection of the enterocele hernia sac and fixation of the vagina to secure ligamentous tissue.
➤ Posterior defects lead to rectoceles and constipation or difficulty having bowel movements. Treatment is posterior repair (colporrhaphy).
➤ Lateral defects lead to lack of lateral vaginal support. Repair is a paravaginal repair, reattachment of the levator ani muscle to its tendinous insertion site of the pelvic side wall.

REFERENCES

American College of Obstetricians and Gynecologists. Pelvic organ prolapse. *ACOG Practice Bulletin 85.* Washington, DC: 2007.

Lentz GM. Anatomical defects of the abdominal wall and pelvic floor. In: Katz VL, Lentz GM, Lobo RA, Gersenson DM, eds. *Comprehensive Gynecology.* 5th ed. St. Louis, MO: Mosby-Year Book; 2007:501-537.

Tarnay CM, Bhatia NN. Genitourinary dysfunction, pelvic organ prolapse, urinary incontinence, and infections. In: Hacker NF, Gambone JC, Hobel CJ, eds. *Essentials of Obstetrics and Gynecology,* 5th ed. Philadelphia, PA: Saunders; 2009:276-289.

Case 58

A 31-year-old G4 P3003 woman at 36 weeks' gestation is admitted to the labor and delivery unit for evaluation of uterine contractions. She has a known twin pregnancy, and throughout the pregnancy, she had significant nausea and vomiting, but otherwise her prenatal course has been unremarkable. Serial ultrasound examinations have been performed showing concordant growth of the twins. She takes prenatal vitamins, an iron supplement, and folic acid. On examination, blood pressure (BP) is 110/70 mm Hg, pulse is 80 beats per minute (bpm), and respiratory rate is 18 breaths per minute. Fundal height is 41 cm. Her cervix is 4 cm dilated and 90% effaced. Ultrasound examination reveals a twin pregnancy with a dividing membrane, and adequate amniotic fluid. The twins are presenting vertex/vertex. After 2 hours of labor, the patient dilates to 6 cm. Artificial rupture of membranes is undertaken to allow for a fetal scalp electrode of twin A. A moderate amount of vaginal bleeding is noted after rupture of membranes. Twin A's fetal heart rate tracing initially was in the 140 bpm baseline, and then increases to 170 bpm, and now has a sinusoidal appearance.

➤ What is the most likely diagnosis?

➤ What is the cause of this condition?

➤ What is the next step in management?

ANSWERS TO CASE 58:
Twin Gestation with Vasa Previa

Summary: A 31-year-old G4 P3 woman at 36 weeks' gestation with a twin pregnancy presents in labor. Upon rupture of membranes, there is moderate vaginal bleeding noted. Twin A has fetal tachycardia and now a sinusoidal heart rate pattern.

➤ **Most likely diagnosis:** Twin gestation with vasa previa.

➤ **Cause of this condition:** The exact pathophysiologic mechanism of vasa previa is not known, but it is associated with a velamentous cord insertion (explained below) and accessory placental lobes.

➤ **Next Step:** Stat cesarean and alert pediatricians for likelihood of anemia in twin A.

ANALYSIS

Objectives

1. Become familiar with the mechanisms responsible for twinning.
2. Understand the implications of twin gestation for a pregnancy (both maternal and fetal effects).
3. Recognize risk factors for and complications of vasa previa.

Considerations

This 31-year-old woman presents with a known twin gestation and ultrasound findings consistent with a vasa previa, where a fetal vessel overlies the internal cervical os. This presents a danger to the fetus when rupture of membranes occurs, as the fetus can rapidly exsanguinate. Prenatal diagnosis of this condition is of the utmost importance, as there is nearly a two-fold increased survival with prenatal diagnosis; unfortunately, it is difficult to diagnose prenatally. The twin gestation has its own set of possible complications that must be considered. These include the increased risk of congenital anomalies, preterm labor, preeclampsia, postpartum hemorrhage, and maternal death.

DEFINITIONS

VELAMENTOUS CORD INSERTION: Umbilical vessels separate before reaching the placenta, protected only by a thin fold of amnion, instead of by the cord or the placenta itself; these vessels are susceptible to tearing after rupture of membranes.

VASA PREVIA: Umbilical vessels that are not protected by cord or membranes, which cross the internal cervical os in front of the fetal presenting part; this most commonly occurs with a velamentous cord insertion or a placenta with one or more accessory lobes.

BILOBED OR SUCCENTURIATE-LOBED PLACENTA: A placenta with either one or more accessory lobes.

MONOZYGOTIC TWINS: Twins formed by the fertilization of one egg by one sperm.

DIZYGOTIC TWINS: Twins formed by the fertilization of two eggs by two sperm.

CHORIONICITY: The number of placentas in a twin or higher order gestation; in monozygotic twins, can either be monochorionic or dichorionic. Dizygotic twins are always dichorionic.

AMNIONICITY: The number of amniotic sacs in a twin or higher order gestation; monozygotic twins may be monoamnionic or diamnionic whereas dizygotic twins are always diamnionic.

CLINICAL APPROACH

The incidence of twin gestation has dramatically increased in the United States over the last two or three decades. This is a result of the increasing use of infertility treatments, including ovulation induction and in vitro fertilization. This dramatic increase has created a new public health concern, as twin pregnancies are associated with a higher rate of preterm delivery and all of the complications associated with it. The other complications of twin gestation include a higher rate of congenital malformations, a two-time increased risk of preeclampsia and postpartum hemorrhage, and twin-twin transfusion (TTT) syndrome.

There are two types of twinning possible: monozygotic and dizygotic. Monozygotic twins are formed when one egg is fertilized by one sperm followed by an error in cleavage; the incidence is not related to race, heredity, or parity. The exact mechanism of monozygotic twinning is not known, but may be caused by a delay in normal events, such as when tubal motility is decreased. Oral contraceptives (OCPs) slow tubal motility, so it is important to know if a mother has used OCPs within 3 months of becoming pregnant. This is associated with an increased incidence of twinning. The chronicity and amnionicity of monozygotic twins is determined by the timing of division of the embryos (see Table 58-1). Relative to dizygotic twins, monozygotic twins are associated with a higher incidence of discordant growth and malformations, with monochorionic twins being associated with a much higher rate of spontaneous abortion.

Dizygotic twins are formed by the fertilization of two eggs by two sperm. The incidence is influenced by race, heredity, maternal age, parity, and fertility drugs. The incidence is 1:100 in white women and 1:80 in black women. The

Table 58–1 CHORIONICITY AND AMNIONICITY OF MONOZYGOTIC TWINS	
TIMING OF DIVISION (AFTER FERTILIZATION)	RESULTING CHRONICITY AND AMNIONICITY
First 72 hours	Dichorionic/diamnionic
Day 4-8	Monochorionic/diamniotic
Day 8	Monochorionic/monoamniotic
After day 8	Conjoined twins

rate of dizygotic twinning increases with maternal age and peaks at 37 years. There is an increased incidence of a twin pregnancy when the mother is a dizygotic twin. Fertility treatments are responsible for many twin gestations. Clomiphene induces ovulation and promotes the maturation of multiple follicles, therefore increasing the number of eggs available for fertilization. In vitro fertilization involves the transfer of two to four embryos to the uterus. If more than one implants, a twin or higher order gestation occurs. All dizygotic twins are dichorionic/diamnionic.

In any kind of twin gestation, it is important to remember that maternal screening and physiology may be different from that in a singleton pregnancy. Increased maternal serum α-fetoprotein (MSAFP) may be misleading, especially in the case of a vanishing twin, where only one fetus is seen on ultrasound. Nausea and vomiting can be increased in a twin gestation. Hemodynamically, blood volume and stroke volume are increased more than in a singleton pregnancy. However, the red cell mass increases proportionately less, so there is greater physiologic anemia. Blood pressure at 20 weeks is usually lower than in a singleton pregnancy, but is higher by delivery. Finally, there is a greater increase in size and weight of the uterus, as might be expected.

Complications more common with multiple gestations include preeclampsia, gestational diabetes, anemia, deep venous thrombosis, postpartum hemorrhage, need for cesarean delivery; fetal or placental complications include preterm delivery, intrauterine growth retardation (IUGR), polyhydramnios, stillbirth, fetal anomalies, placenta previa, abruption, and twin-twin transfusion syndrome. In TTT syndrome, one twin is the donor and the other the recipient such that one twin is larger with more amniotic fluid and the other twin smaller with oligohydramnios. Treatment includes laser ablation of the shared anastomotic vessels at special centers, or serial amniocentesis for decompression. When there is no dividing membrane between the twins, cord entanglement can occur, leading to a 50% perinatal mortality rate. Thus, an important part of the ultrasound evaluation of twin gestations is identification of a dividing membrane.

When multiple gestation is diagnosed, the patient should be followed in a high-risk clinic with serial ultrasound examinations for growth and comparison weight. The patient should be carefully followed for the above complications. Delivery can be vaginal when both twins are presenting as vertex. When the first twin is nonvertex, most of the time cesarean is performed. The first twin is vertex, nonvertex second twin is individualized.

Vasa previa is a serious condition that can cause fetal death rapidly after rupture of membranes. Survival is increased more than two fold by prenatal diagnosis, from 44% to 97%. However, prenatal diagnosis is difficult. It is difficult to identify on vaginal examination, especially before membrane rupture, and ultrasound may give some hint. Currently accepted risk factors are a bilobed, succenturiate-lobed, or low-lying placenta, multifetal pregnancy, and pregnancy resulting from in vitro fertilization. Women with these risk factors or suggestive ultrasound findings should have a color Doppler ultrasound. If vasa previa is identified, a planned cesarean delivery should take place before rupture of membranes, around 35 to 36 weeks of gestation. Digital vaginal examination is contraindicated in cases of vasa previa.

Because fetal blood volume at term is only 250 to 500 cc, it is not hard to imagine that the fetus may exsanguinate within minutes of an umbilical vessel being torn. Fetal heart rate abnormalities such as tachycardia, recurrent decelerations, prolonged bradycardia, and a sinusoidal pattern can indicate serious fetal compromise and should prompt evaluation for its cause. If fetal bleeding is uncertain, the Apt test and Kleihauer-Betke test can be used to differentiate fetal from maternal blood.

Comprehensive Questions

58.1 A 28-year-old G1 P0 woman is diagnosed as having a twin gestation at 15 weeks' gestation. Careful examination of the membranes reveals that there is a very thin membrane between the two fetuses. Which of the following statements is most accurate?

A. It is likely that one fetus is a male and the other a female.
B. It is likely that this is a dizygotic gestation.
C. It is likely that this is a monozygotic gestation.
D. It is likely that there are two separate placentas.

58.2   A 25-year-old G2 P1001 woman at 27 weeks' gestation has been fol-
        lowed for twin gestation. She is undergoing her third ultrasound exam-
        ination today. Her ultrasound findings are as follows:

	Twin A	Twin B
Estimated weight	500 g	1100 g
Amniotic fluid	2 cm	26 cm

Which of the following is the best next step for this patient?
A. Chorionic villus sampling
B. Repeat ultrasound in 3 weeks
C. Laser ablation of vessels
D. Revision of dates for twin B

58.3   A 32-year-old G1 P0 woman undergoes an IVF pregnancy cycle and
        becomes pregnant with triplets. She has been followed in a high-risk
        obstetrics clinic with an uncomplicated pregnancy course. She arrives
        to the hospital labor and delivery unit at 30 weeks' gestation with a
        blood pressure of 150/100 mm Hg, and 2+ proteinuria. Additionally
        she complains of dyspnea. Her oxygen saturation is 82% on room air.
        She is contracting every 4 minutes. The patient is diagnosed with
        preeclampsia. Which of the following statements is most accurate?
        A. The patient should be treated with IV heparin.
        B. The patient should be treated with IV furosemide.
        C. The patient should be treated with corticosteroids and a tocolytic
           agent.
        D. The patient likely has a concealed abruption.

ANSWERS

58.1   **C.** The ultrasound findings are consistent with monochorionic,
        diamniotic twins, since there is only a thin membrane between the two
        gestations. Since a dizygotic gestation always gives rise to a dichorionic
        diamniotic gestation, this patient must have a monozygotic pregnancy
        which split at 4 to 8 days after fertilization. A monozygotic pregnancy
        is at greater risk for IUGR, stillbirth, and TTT syndrome.

58.2   **C.** The large discrepancy of fetal weight and amniotic fluid volume
        between the two gestations is consistent with TTT syndrome. The
        best treatment is laser ablation of the shared vessels, but this proce-
        dure is only available at select centers. Another option is serial amni-
        otic fluid reduction. In TTT syndrome, one twin acts as the donor
        (smaller) and the other as the recipient (larger). A high stillbirth risk
        exists with this condition.

58.3   **B.** This patient likely has pulmonary edema due to the preeclampsia
        as well as the increased plasma volume due to the multiple gestations.

The higher the number of pregnancies, the more the plasma volume, and greater the risk of pulmonary edema. This patient should have intravenous furosemide to decrease intravascular volume, placed on magnesium sulfate, and plans made for delivery. Although DVT and pulmonary embolism is always a consideration in a pregnant patient, pulmonary edema would be more likely. The chest radiograph would be helpful to differentiate the two conditions (infiltrates with pulmonary edema, clear in pulmonary embolism). Tocolysis and corticosteroids would be useful in isolated preterm labor, although many experts avoid their use in multiple gestations because of the risk of pulmonary edema.

Clinical Pearls

> ➤ The two types of twin gestations are mono- and dizygotic. Monozygotic twins are associated with a higher rate of anomalies and maternal complications.
> ➤ Maternal effects of pregnancy are enhanced in twin gestation—increased nausea and vomiting, greater "physiologic" anemia, greater increase in blood pressure after 20 weeks, and greater increase in size and weight of the uterus.
> ➤ TTT syndrome should be suspected with a substantial discordance of the twins and discrepancy of the distribution of the amniotic fluid volume.
> ➤ Twin gestation without a dividing membrane is associated with a high stillbirth rate due to cord entanglement.
> ➤ Vasa previa is a serious condition that can cause rapid fetal demise after rupture of membranes.
> ➤ Prenatal diagnosis is best made by ultrasound with color Doppler, and management is planned cesarean delivery before rupture of membranes.

REFERENCES

Cunningham FG, Leveno KJ, Bloom SL, Hauth JC, Gilstrap LC III, Wenstrom KD. Abnormalities of the placenta, umbilical cord, and membranes. In: *Williams Obstetrics.* 22nd ed. New York, NY: McGraw-Hill; 2005:627-628.

Cunningham FG, Leveno KJ, Bloom SL, Hauth JC, Gilstrap LC III, Wenstrom KD. Multifetal gestation. In: *Williams Obstetrics.* 22nd ed. New York, NY: McGraw-Hill; 2005:911-935.

Oyelese Y, Sulian JC. Placent previa, placenta accreta, and vasa previa. ACOG *Clinical Expert Series.* April 2006;107:4.

Strehlow S, Uzelac P. Complications of labor & delivery. In: Decherny AH, Nathan L, Goodwin TM, Laufer N, eds. *Current Diagnosis & Treatment of Obstetrics & Gynecology.* 10th ed. New York, McGraw-Hill; 2007.

Case 59

A 35-year-old G2 P1001 woman is seen for her first prenatal visit. Based on her last menstrual period, she is at 15 weeks' gestation. She has no complaints, and has no significant medical history. She denies dysuria or urinary urgency. Her surgical history is remarkable only for "ear tubes" as a child. Her last delivery was a vaginal delivery and was uncompli-cated. She has had Pap smears each year which to her memory "have been normal." On examination, she is a well-appearing white female in no distress. Her blood pressure (BP) is 100/65 mm Hg, heart rate (HR) 90 beats per minute (bpm), respiratory rate (RR) 12 breaths per minute, temperature 98°F (36.6°C), weight 130 lb. Her general physical exami-nation is normal. The breasts are nontender and without masses or skin changes. The heart reveals II/VI systolic ejection murmur. The lungs are clear. Her abdomen is nontender and her fundal height is at the level of the umbilicus. Fetal heart tones are 140 bpm. The pelvic examination reveals a normal external genitalia, normal-appearing vagina and cervix. The bimanual examination shows adequate pelvimetry, and nontender uterus without adnexal or other masses. The cervix is normal in consistency and without masses. Her extremities are without edema. Prenatal laborato-ries are obtained and reveal the following:

CBC: Hgb 10.0 g/dL   MCV 82 fL   Plt 150,000   WBC 8,000
Rubella: nonimmune   **Hepatitis B surface antigen**: positive

Blood type: O, Rh negative   **Indirect Coombs (antibody screen)**: negative

HIV ELISA: negative   **UC&S**: 10,000 cfu/mL of group B streptococcus

RPR: negative   **Pap smear**: ASC-US
Gonorrhea assay: negative   **Chlamydia assay:** negative

➤ What items should be listed on the problems list?

➤ What is your next step for the problems listed?

➤ What other testing should be recommended to the patient?

ANSWERS TO CASE 59:
Prenatal Care

Summary: A 35-year-old G2 P1001 white female at 15 weeks' gestation whose prior delivery was normal. Her fundal height is at the umbilicus. Fetal heart tones are 140 bpm. Prenatal laboratory results indicate a hemoglobin level of 10.0 g/dL with MCV 82 fL; hepatitis surface antigen positive; Rh-negative blood type, negative indirect Coombs; urine culture revealing 10,000 cfu/mL of group B streptococcus; and a Pap smear showing ASC-US.

Problem List:
1. Advanced maternal age (AMA)–age 35 or greater at estimated time of delivery
2. Size greater than dates (fundal height at umbilicus corresponds to 20 weeks)
3. Mild microcytic anemia (Hgb < 10.5)
4. Hepatitis B surface antigen (HBsAg) positive
5. Rh-negative blood type with negative indirect Coombs
6. Urine culture with GBS 10,000 cfu/mL, asymptomatic
7. Pap smear showing atypical squamous cells of undetermined significance (ASC-US)
8. Rubella nonimmune

Next Steps:
1. AMA—genetic counseling and offer genetic amniocentesis
2. Size/dates—fetal ultrasound to assess gestational age, multiple gestation
3. Anemia—therapeutic trial of iron
4. HBsAg positive—check liver function tests, and hepatitis B serology to assess for active hepatitis versus chronic carrier status
5. Rh negative with indirect Coombs negative—Rhogam at 28 weeks and at delivery if the baby proves to be Rh positive
6. Urine culture with GBS—treat with ampicillin and re-culture urine, penicillin IV prophylaxis in labor
7. Pap smear ASC-US—observe and repeat Pap smear postpartum
8. Rubella status—vaccinate postpartum

Other Testing: Cystic fibrosis screening; consider early diabetic screen

ANALYSIS

Objectives

1. Describe the routine prenatal care and the key screening strategies.
2. Be able to understand the principle of developing a problem list and its importance.
3. Be able to describe the "next steps" with any abnormal finding and know its significance.

Considerations

This is a 35-year-old woman who is seen for her first prenatal visit. Since pregnancy and delivery is a normal physiological process, the purpose of the prenatal care is to educate and build rapport with the patient and family, establish gestational age, screen for possible conditions that may impact on maternal or fetal health, and monitor the progress of the pregnancy. During the first visit, a fairly extensive process is used to screen for at-risk conditions using a detailed history, general physical examination, and laboratory panel. This patient has a variety of conditions that need addressing. The best way to ensure that each issue is dealt with in a systematic manner and until resolution is to use a "problem list." Thus, numerous issues are written into the problem list, and investigation is performed until resolution of the problem. An understanding of the strategy and approach to addressing each issue is fundamental to the care of patients. Likewise, an understanding of the physiologic changes of pregnancy allows for interpretation of physical examination findings and impact of various diseases. (See Table 59–1).

For instance, this 35-year-old patient has an early systolic ejection murmur, very common in pregnancy due to the increased cardiac output. A diastolic murmur however would be abnormal. Although the American College of Obstetricians and Gynecologists recommends counseling every pregnant patient about cystic fibrosis screening, Caucasian patients are at particular risk with gene frequency being about 1 in 40. Also for women over the age of 30, some practitioners will perform a glucose screen for gestational diabetes early (for instance 18 weeks), and if negative then again at the time of universal screening, 26- to 28 weeks' gestation.

Table 59–1 PHYSIOLOGICAL CHANGES IN PREGNANCY

	PARAMETER		COMMENT
Cardiovascular	Cardiac output and plasma volume increased 50%	Systemic vascular resistance decreased	Mean arterial pressure unchanged/slightly lower	Pregnancy increases intravascular volume
Respiratory	Respiratory rate unchanged	Tidal volume increased	Minute ventilation increased	Ventilation exceeds needs
Arterial blood gas	pH 7.45 (increased)	P_{CO_2} 28 (decreased)	HCO_3 18 (decreased)	Primary respiratory alkylosis and partial metabolic compensation
Renal	GFR—increased 50%	Serum Cr decreased	Ureteral caliper dilated	GFR increased and creatinine clearance also increased
Hematologic	Hemoglobin decreased slightly	Platelet decreased slightly	Leukocyte count slightly increased	Physiologic anemia due to plasma volume increased more than red blood cell mass
Gastrointestinal	Delayed stomach emptying	Decreased lower esophageal sphincter tone	Decreased gut motility	

APPROACH TO
Prenatal Care

DEFINITIONS

ADVANCED MATERNAL AGE: Pregnant woman who will be 35 years or beyond at the estimated date of delivery.

ISOIMMUNIZATION: The development of specific antibodies as a result of antigenic stimulation by material from the red blood cells of another individual. For example, Rh isoimmunization means an Rh-negative woman who develops anti-D (Rh factor) antibodies in response to exposure to Rh (D) antigen.

ASYMPTOMATIC BACTERIURIA: Urine culture of 100,000 cfu/mL or more of a pure pathogen of a mid stream-voided specimen.

GENETIC COUNSELING: An educational process provided by a health-care professional for individuals and families who have a genetic disease or who are at risk for such a disease. It is designed to provide patients and their families with information about their condition or potential condition and help them make informed decisions.

VERTICAL TRANSMISSION: The passage of infection from mother to fetus, whether in utero, during labor and delivery, or postpartum.

ANTENATAL TESTING: A procedure that attempts to identify whether the fetus is at risk for uteroplacental insufficiency and perinatal death. Some of these tests include nonstress test and biophysical profile.

BASIC OBSTETRICAL ULTRASOUND: Sonographic examination focused on fetal biometry (dating and fetal weight), number of fetuses, fetal presentation, placental location, amniotic fluid volume, and limited fetal anatomical survey.

COMPREHENSIVE (OR TARGETED) ULTRASOUND: Detailed anatomical evaluation to assess a suspected structural anomaly.

CLINICAL APPROACH

Physiological Changes. Pregnancy is associated with numerous physiological changes. An understanding of these changes is critical in the interpretation of laboratory tests, or a rational awareness of how disease processes may impact the pregnant patient. Some "seemingly abnormal" findings will be normal in pregnancy such as glycosuria due to the increased glomerular filtration rate delivering more glucose to the kidneys. Other findings in pregnancy will appear to be normal, but are "worrisome" in pregnancy; for instance, when the P_{CO_2} level is 40 mm Hg (normal for nonpregnant), it indicates significant CO_2 retention and possibly impending respiratory failure.

Dating. The priorities of prenatal care includes establishment of gestational age since all of the monitoring, assessments, and milestones are based on gestational age. History of the LMP, regularity of menses, medication use that may affect ovulation, physical examination, and early ultrasound help this determination. On examination, the fundal height in centimeters corresponds to the gestational age from 20 to 34 weeks. An ultrasound will be obtained when there is a discrepancy of 3 cm or more.

Prevention. Much of prenatal care involves educating the patient, and measures to prevent hazardous conditions. Use of immunizations (influenza and Rhogam), prenatal vitamin with folate, iron supplementation, and a balanced diet are recommended.

Screening for Conditions of Risk. Much of the time spent in caring for the pregnant patient is involved in trying to identify high-risk conditions and taking the proper steps to reduce the risk, or minimize complications (see Table 59–2).

Because maternal and fetal health are both being considered, any high-risk condition must be balanced from both perspectives. Many of the cases involve antepartum, intrapartum, or postpartum complications (see Table 59–3).

Table 59–2 SUMMARY OF PRENATAL LABORATORIES, RAMIFICATIONS, AND EVALUATION

LAB TEST	FINDING	RAMIFICATIONS	NEXT STEP	COMMENTS
Hemoglobin	< 10.5 g/dL	Preterm delivery Low fetal iron stores Identify thalassemia	Mild–therapeutic trial of iron Moderate–ferritin and Hb electrophoresis	
Rubella	Negative	Nonimmune to rubella	Stay away from sick individuals, vaccinate postpartum	Live attenuated vaccine
Blood type	Any type	May help pediatricians identify ABO incompatibility		
Rh factor	Negative	May be susceptible to Rh disease	If antibody screen negative, give Rhogam at 28 weeks, and if baby is Rh positive, then also after delivery	
Antibody screen	Positive	May indicate isoimmunization	Need to identify the antibody, and then titer	Lewis lives, Kell kills, Duffy dies
HIV ELISA	Positive	May indicate infection with HIV	Western blot or PCR, if positive then place patient on anti-HIV medicines, offer elective cesarean, or IV ZDV in labor	Intervention reduces Vertical transmission from 25% to 2%
RPR	Positive	May indicate syphilis	Specific antibody such as MHA-TP, and if positive then stage disease	Less than 1 year, penicillin × 1; > 1 year or unknown, penicillin IM each week × 3

(Continued)

Table 59-2 SUMMARY OF PRENATAL LABORATORIES, RAMIFICATIONS, AND EVALUATION (CONTINUED)

LAB TEST	FINDING	RAMIFICATIONS	NEXT STEP	COMMENTS
Gonorrhea	Positive	May cause preterm labor, blindness	Ceftriaxone IM	
Chlamydia	Positive	May cause neonatal blindness, pneumonia	Azithromycin or amoxicillin orally – no doxy !	
Hepatitis B surface antigen	Positive	Patient is infectious	Check LFTs and hepatitis serology to determine if chronic carrier vs active hepatitis	Baby needs HBIG and hepatitis B vaccine
Urine culture	Positive	Asymptomatic bacteriuria may lead to pyelonephritis 25%	Treat with antibiotic and recheck urine culture	If GBS is organism, then give penicillin in labor
Pap smear	Positive	Only invasive cancer would alter management	ASC-US = re-Pap postpartum; LGSIL, HSIL=colposcopy	Reflexive HPV not recommended with ASC-US
Nuchal translucency (11-13 weeks)	Positive	May indicate trisomy	Offer karyotype and follow-up ultrasounds	Increased NT means increased risk, not definitive diagnosis

Test (timing)	Result	Indication	Action	Note
Trisomy screen (16-20 weeks)	Positive	At risk for trisomy or NTD	Basic ultrasound for dates; if dates confirmed, offer genetic amniocentesis	Most common reason for abnormal serum screening—wrong dates
1 h diabetic screen (26-28 weeks)	Positive (elevated)	May indicate gestational diabetes	Go to 3 h GTT	About 15% of those screened will be positive
3 h glucose tolerance test	2 abnormal values	Gestational diabetes	Try ADA diet, monitor blood sugars, if elevated may need meds or insulin	About 15% of abnormal 1 h GCT will have gestational diabetes
GBS culture (35-37 weeks)	Positive	GBS colonizing genital tract	Penicillin during labor	Helps to prevent early GBS sepsis of newborn

Table 59–3 ANTENATAL, INTRAPARTUM, AND POSTPARTUM

PREGNANCY PHASE	CONDITION	DIAGNOSIS	CASE NUMBER
PRENATAL			
	Normal	Routine prenatal care	59
	Vaginal bleeding < 20 weeks gestation	Threatened abortion Completed abortion Ectopic pregnancy Septic abortion	7 10 29 43
	Vaginal bleeding > 20-weeks gestation	Placenta previa Placenta abruption	14 15
	Serum screening	Congenital anomalies	55
	Multiple gestations	Twin gestation	58
	Anemia in pregnancy	Thalassemia	30
	Abdominal pain in pregnancy	Torsion of ovary Ruptured corpus luteum	28 39
	Hypertensive disease	Preeclampsia	25
	Pruritus	Cholestasis of pregnancy	20
	Thrombo-embolism	DVT in pregnancy Pulmonary embolism	35 22
	Thyroid disease	Hyperthyroidism in pregnancy	47
	Infectious	Chlamydia and HIV in pregnancy Pyelonephritis Parvovirus	48 34 49

(Continued)

Table 59–3 ANTENATAL, INTRAPARTUM, AND POSTPARTUM (CONTINUED)

PREGNANCY PHASE	CONDITION	DIAGNOSIS	CASE NUMBER
INTRAPARTUM			
	Labor	Normal and abnormal	6
	Fetal heart rate	Fetal bradycardia	18
	Preterm birth	Preterm labor	31
	Infection	Intraamniotic infection HSV in labor	52 23
DELIVERY			
	Complications of delivery	Shoulder dystocia	11
	Hemorrhage	Placenta accreta Postpartum hemorrhage (also under "Postpartum")	8 44
POSTPARTUM			
	Infection	Breast abscess Endometritis	46 50
	Hemorrhage	Postpartum hemorrhage (also under Delivery)	44

Comprehension Questions

59.1 A 24-year-old woman G2 P0010 had a pregnancy complicated by abruption placentae leading to fetal death at 38 weeks' gestation. There was no etiology found after a diligent search. Which of the following statements is most accurate regarding this pregnancy?

A. With no etiology found, the risk of abruption in this current pregnancy is the same as any other pregnant patient.

B. Antenatal testing with biophysical profile should be considered starting at 34- to 35 weeks' gestation.

C. Induction of labor should be considered at 37- to 38 weeks' gestation.

D. Weekly ultrasound examinations screening for retroplacental hemorrhage should be considered starting at 32 weeks' gestation.

59.2 A 27-year-old G0 P0 woman is contemplating becoming pregnant. In preparation, her obstetrician conducts a preconception counseling session and assesses rubella status, and prescribes supplemental folate. Which of the following is the best explanation of the purpose of the supplemental folate?

A. Avoidance of megaloblastic anemia

B. Decreasing fetal anomalies

C. Enhancing absorption of iron

D. Increasing maternal immune function

59.3 A 32-year-old G1 P0 woman at 15 weeks' gestation is a physiologist, and is questioning the physician about the adaptations that occur in pregnancy. Which of the following statements is most accurate regarding the changes in pregnancy?

A. Cardiac output is largely the same as the nonpregnant woman.

B. The plasma volume is increased by about 50%.

C. The systemic vascular resistance of a pregnant woman is slightly increased as compared to the nonpregnant woman.

D. The pregnant woman typically has a short diastolic murmur which is physiologic.

59.4 A 29-year-old G1 P0 woman at 18 weeks' gestation is noted to have a blood type of O, Rh positive. Her antibody screen (indirect Coombs) is positive. Identification of the antibody is anti-Lewis. Which of the following is the most accurate statement regarding this patient?

A. This fetus is at significant risk for fetal erythroblastosis if s/he is Lewis positive.

B. The father of the baby's Lewis antigen status should be evaluated.

C. Ultrasound for fetal hydrops should be performed.

D. Further testing is not indicated in this patient.

59.5   A 31-year-old G1 P0 woman at 15 weeks' gestation is noted to have a positive hepatitis B surface antigen. Which of the following would most significantly increase the risk of vertical transmission?
    A. Presence of positive hepatitis E antigen
    B. Presence of positive anti-hepatitis B surface antibody
    C. Presence of positive anti-hepatitis B core antibody
    D. Presence of elevated liver function tests

ANSWERS

59.1   **C.** A history of abruption that is unexplained confers an increased risk of abruption with subsequent pregnancies. Antenatal testing does not predict acute events such as abruption. Rather, fetal testing such as biophysical profile is designed to identify chronic uteroplacental insufficiency such as caused by chronic hypertension, renal insufficiency, or maternal lupus. Ultrasound has poor ability to identify retroplacental clots or abruption. Induction at or slightly before the time of abruption with the fetal loss if at term is a reasonable approach to avoid repeat abruption.

59.2   **B.** The main purpose of the supplemental folate prior to pregnancy is to help reduce fetal neural tube defects (NTD). These conditions include anencephaly, a fatal anomaly where there are no cerebral hemispheres or fetal skull, or spina bifida which often leads to debilitation and inability to control bowel or bladder. Because the neural tube closes at 21 to 28 days embryonic age (5-6 weeks gestational age), by the time the patient realizes she is pregnant, the "die is cast" regarding the neural tube. Folate supplementation reduces the risk of neural tube defects by 50%; thus, every woman in the reproductive age should take sufficient folate to reduce the risk of fetal NTDs.

59.3   **B.** In pregnancy, the plasma volume is increased by about 50%. The cardiac output likewise increases by 50%, as does the glomerular filtration rate. The stroke volume and heart rate both increase to account for this elevated CO. The mean arterial pressure is unchanged to slightly decreased, meaning that the systemic vascular resistance is markedly decreased as compared to the nonpregnant patient. An early systolic ejection murmur is physiologic, whereas a diastolic murmur usually indicates a pathological etiology.

59.4   **D.** No further testing is indicated in this patient, because anti-Lewis antibodies do not cause hemolytic disease of the newborn. This is because Lewis antibodies are IgM and do not cross the placenta, whereas anti-D (Rh) are IgG. Other worrisome antibodies include anti-Kell and anti-Duffy. "Lewis lives, Kell kills, Duffy dies." This highlights the need to identify the antibody when the indirect Coombs (antibody screen) is positive. When a worrisome antibody is identified, the titer should be evaluated to assess the potential severity of the isoimmunization potential. In general, fetal risk is not great unless the titer is 1:8 or higher.

59.5   **A.** This patient has a positive hepatitis B surface antigen, meaning that the patient has been infected with hepatitis B virus and currently still infectious (virus actively replicating). Liver function tests would indicate whether this is a chronic carrier status (normal LFT) versus active hepatitis (elevated LFT). The hepatitis antibodies also will give a clue regarding acute versus chronic hepatitis. The presence of hepatitis E antigen markedly increases the transmission. Regardless of whether E antigen is present, this baby when born should receive hepatitis B immune globulin (HBIG) to protect against immediate exposure, and then the active hepatitis B vaccine for life-long immunity. Hepatitis B infections to the neonate often lead to cirrhosis and hepatocellular carcinoma.

Clinical Pearls

➤ Pregnancy and delivery is a normal physiological process. The objective of prenatal care is to educate the patient, prevent complications, and screen for significant conditions that can affect maternal or fetal health.

➤ Assessment of a pregnant woman depends on knowledge of the physiologic changes in pregnancy.

➤ HIV, hepatitis B, and syphilis are three infectious diseases in which intervention can dramatically impact neonatal well being.

➤ Identification and treatment of asymptomatic bacteriuria markedly decreases the risk of pyelonephritis in pregnancy.

➤ The main objective in assessing for cervical dysplasia/neoplasia is to identify invasive cervical cancer, since that finding would change the management in pregnancy and treatment of other lesser findings would be deferred until after pregnancy.

➤ Advanced maternal age is defined as age of 35 or greater at the estimated date of delivery. These women are at increased risk for autosomal trisomies, and genetic counseling and genetic amniocentesis is usually offered.

➤ Screening for hypertension and proteinuria by semiquantitative urine dipstick at each prenatal visit is performed to screen for gestational hypertension or preeclampsia.

➤ Antepartum fetal testing is defined as a procedure that attempts to identify whether the fetus is at risk for uteroplacental insufficiency and perinatal death. Some of these tests include nonstress test and biophysical profile.

➤ Live attenuated vaccines should be avoided in pregnancy, but killed vaccines are acceptable, and some, such as influenza vaccine, are indicated in pregnancy.

REFERENCES

Cunningham FG, Leveno KJ, Bloom SL, Hauth JC, Gilstrap LC III, Wenstrom KD. Prenatal care. In: *Williams Obstetrics*. 22nd ed. New York, NY: McGraw-Hill; 2005:201-230.

Lu MC, Williams III, J, Hobel CJ. Antepartum care: preconception and prenatal care, genetic evaluation and teratology, and antenatal fetal assessment. In: Hacker NF, Gambone JC, Hobel CJ, eds. *Essentials of Obstetrics and Gynecology*, 5th ed. Philadelphia, PA: Saunders; 2009:71-90.

Case 60

A 51-year-old parous woman complains of a 4-year history of itching of her vagina. She scratches the area daily and reports that the itching is worse at nighttime. She has diabetes, well controlled, is postmenopausal of 3 years, denies any sexually transmitted disease or abnormal Pap smear history, and has four children delivered vaginally. On inspection and examination of the external female genitalia the following is revealed: atrophic-appearing external female genitalia, tissue over the labia minora is white and thin, the clitoris is hard to appreciate, excoriations are noted on bilateral labia majora, and some small bruising noted at the introitus. She is very tender on examination and it is difficult to insert a speculum as the introitus seems constricted. The cervix is visualized and no discharge is noted. Bimanual examination reveals a small uterus and no adnexal masses are appreciated.

➤ What is the most likely diagnosis?

➤ What is the next step in making the diagnosis?

➤ What is the most likely therapy?

ANSWERS TO CASE 60:
Lichen Sclerosis of Vulva

Summary: A 51-year-old woman is noted to have itching of the vagina for 4 years. Inspection of the external female genitalia reveals atrophic, white, thin excoriated tissue and retraction of the clitoris and constriction of the introitus with some bruising.

➤ **Most likely diagnosis:** Lichen sclerosis.

➤ **Next step:** Biopsy of the affected areas.

➤ **Most likely therapy:** Corticosteroid ointment.

ANALYSIS

Objectives

1. Describe the characteristics of patients that present with lichen sclerosis, and the natural history of the disease.
2. Recognize the anatomical boundaries of the vulva and aspects of good vulvar hygiene.
3. Identify current treatment regimes for lichen sclerosis (LS) and the follow-up that is requisite.

Considerations

This woman is suffering from lichen sclerosis given the history and physical findings that she presented with. The diagnosis is confirmed with biopsy of the affected vulvar tissue, which reveals a thinned epidermis, hyperkeratosis, and elongation of the rete pegs. Lichen planus can also present similarly, but usually involves the vagina which LS does not. An experienced dermatopathologist should be able to differentiate the two on biopsy specimen. Long-standing candidal infection of the vulva may lead to similar symptoms. Since our patient is postmenopausal, therefore lacking estrogen, the pH of the area is raised and not amenable to candidal infection unless she has poorly controlled diabetes or is immunosuppressed. Sometimes vaginal atrophy in the postmenopausal patient can lead to pruritus, but not to this extent. Psoriasis may present with pruritus but not usually, and the lesions are classically described as silver scales, and are also present on the extensor surfaces of the extremities. Cancer of the vulva or vulvar intraepithelial neoplasia commonly presents with pruritus and is often associated with LS which is why biopsy of the affected area and frequent surveillance of the vulva is crucial.

APPROACH TO
Vulvar Disorders

DEFINITIONS

LICHEN SCLEROSIS: Chronic, inflammatory dermatologic disease characterized by pruritus and pain, which mainly affects the anogenital region.

VULVA: The external genitalia of the female comprised of the mons pubis, the labia majora and minora, the clitoris, the vestibule of the vagina and its glands, and the opening of the urethra and of the vagina.

CLINICAL APPROACH

The anatomic boundaries of the vulva extend from the mons pubis superiorly to the anus inferiorly and the genitocrural folds laterally. It is made up from the labia majora and minora, mons pubis, clitoris, vestibule of the vagina, urethral meatus, Skene glands, vaginal orifice, hymen, and Bartholin glands.

Lichen Sclerosis

Lichen sclerosis is a chronic progressive inflammatory medical condition of which there is no definitive cure. LS is more common in women than men, and the onset is usually in the postmenopausal period, although it can occur at any age. LS usually presents in the anogenital region, with extragenital disease only 15% to 20% of the time. Women with the disease usually present with the complaint of itching which can be worse at night, and is described by the patient as vaginal itching. Appreciate that the itching is localized to the tissue of the vulva. **Differential diagnosis** of LS is **lichen planus, psoriasis, vulvar intraepithelial neoplasia, and vitiligo**. On examination of the external genitalia, a figure-eight pattern is seen around the vulva and anus. The skin is classically described as **"cigarette paper" as it appears crinkled and is fragile, thinned, and atrophic**. Tears may develop from scratching or attempted intercourse and ultimately scarring may cause narrowing or a complete closure of the vaginal introitus, even in the parous woman. The labia minora may fuse burying the clitoris behind the fused clitoral hood. The scratching of the areas worsens the disease and can also lead to dyschezia, from constriction of the anus.

Discussing components of vulvar hygiene including avoiding irritants to the skin such as soaps and bubble baths, cessation of scratching the lesions, and wearing all cotton, white underwear may help to alleviate symptoms. Ensure that the patient is aware of the chronicity of the disease and the need for yearly surveillance. Treatment of the disease is aimed at preventing relapses of intense pruritus and the mainstay is corticosteroids. Initially a potent steroid ointment, Clobetasol, may be necessary to provide relief, and should be used daily until relief and then tapered.

Bartholin Gland Abscess

The Bartholin or greater vestibular glands are located at the 5- and 7-o'clock locations of the labia majora. Usually they are too small to palpate but with inflammation, they can be enlarged and painful. The treatment options include incision and placement of a small balloon catheter into the gland, or marsupialization which is surgical fixation of the cyst wall everted against the mucosa of the vulva. The purpose of both of these techniques is to allow drainage of the infection for several weeks. A simple incision and drainage is prone to recurrence. Bartholin gland infections are usually polymicrobial and not usually sexually transmitted. Involvement in women over the age of 40 years can be associated with cancer and should have a biopsy.

Vulvar Cancer

Because vulvar cancer can present with no symptoms or with itching, any suspicious lesion of the vulva especially in a postmenopausal woman should undergo biopsy. If vulvar cancer is diagnosed, then the patient should have surgical staging, with the primary lesion removed and the adjacent inguinal lymph nodes. Most vulvar cancers are squamous cell, but melanoma, basal cell carcinoma, and other subtypes can occur.

Comprehension Questions

Match the vulvar lesion (A-E) to the clinical presentation (60.1-60.4).
    A. Lichen sclerosis
    B. Psoriasis
    C. Vulvar cancer
    D. Vulvar candidiasis
    E. Postmenopausal vulvar atrophy

60.1   A 55-year-old postmenopausal woman is recently remarried and has pain with intercourse.

60.2   A 52-year-old postmenopausal woman complains of intense itching around her vagina and anus which makes intercourse and defecating painful.

60.3   A 45-year-old woman with poorly controlled diabetes reports that she has tears on her vagina "lips" and burning on the outside skin with urination.

60.4   A 59-year-old postmenopausal woman presents with a 10-year history of vaginal itching, which she scratches frequently, and a bump near her clitoris.

60.5   A 54-year-old postmenopausal woman complains of itching in her vagina and the physician notices scaly lesions on both of her elbows.

ANSWERS

60.1   **E.** Complaints of dyspareunia, or painful intercourse, are not uncommon in the postmenopausal state. Without estrogen, the vaginal and vulvar tissue can atrophy leading to bruising, tearing, and even bleeding of the vulva vagina with intercourse. Topical estrogen can alleviate these symptoms.

60.2   **A.** Pruritus of the vulva is not unique to lichen sclerosis, although the predilection for the vulva and anus is. Examination of the vulva and anus with indicated biopsies and topical steroid ointment is the treatment of choice.

60.3   **D.** Diabetes can lead to candidal infection of the vulva which can cause fissures in the labial folds, and the scratching of the disease can sometimes spread the infection. Women who present with vulvar candidiasis should be checked for risk factors for diabetes.

60.4   **C.** Lichen sclerosis left unchecked and with repeated scratching can lead to carcinoma of the vulva. The "bump" that she has noticed is likely to be cancer of the vulva and excision of this is necessary, with indicated biopsies of other affected areas undertaken.

60.5   **B.** Psoriasis can affect the genital area and the silver plaques on the elbow are a dead giveaway to the disease. Treatment of this disease may prove difficult and consultation with an experienced dermatologist is requisite.

Clinical Pearls

➤ Itching of the vulva, especially in a postmenopausal woman, should prompt a thorough history and examination with indicated biopsies of the affected areas.

➤ Lichen sclerosis is a chronic condition characterized by thin, cigarette paper like, crinkly epithelium. Frequent surveillance of the vulva is necessary as to prevent squamous cell carcinoma of the vulva.

➤ Vulva cancer is staged surgically including dissecting the ipsilateral inguinal lymph nodes.

➤ Bartholin gland abscesses are treated by Word catheter or marsupialization so that drainage for several weeks can occur.

REFERENCES

American College of Obstetricians and Gynecologists. Diagnosis and management of vulvar skin disorders. ACOG *Practice Bulletin 93*. Washington, DC: 2008.

Brown D. Non-neoplastic epithelial disorders of the skin and mucosa (vulvar dystrophies). In: Kaufman R, Faro S, Brown D, eds. *Benign Diseases of the Vulva and Vagina*. 5th ed. Philadelphia, PA: Elsevier; 2005:274-290.

Frumovitz M, Bodurka DC. Neoplastic diseases of the vulva. In: Katz VL, Lentz GM, Lobo RA, Gersenson DM, eds. *Comprehensive Gynecology*. 5th ed. St. Louis, MO: Mosby-Year Book; 2007:781-800.

Listing of Cases

Listing by Case Number

Listing by Disorder (Alphabetical)

Page numbers followed by *f* or *t* indicate figures or tables, respectively.